W9-DDA-914

Clinical Hypertension and Vascular Diseases

Series Editor
William B. White

More information about this series at http://www.springer.com/series/7673

Venkatesh Aiyagari • Philip B. Gorelick
Editors

Hypertension and Stroke

Pathophysiology and Management

Second Edition

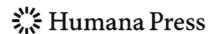 Humana Press

Editors
Venkatesh Aiyagari, MBBS, DM
Department of Neurological Surgery and
  Neurology and Neurotherapeutics
University of Texas Southwestern
  Medical Center
Dallas, TX, USA

Philip B. Gorelick, MD, MPH, FACP
Department of Translational Science and
  Molecular Medicine
College of Human Medicine
Michigan State University
Grand Rapids, MI, USA

Medical Director
Mercy Health Hauenstein Neurosciences
Grand Rapids, MI, USA

Clinical Hypertension and Vascular Diseases
ISBN 978-3-319-29150-5   ISBN 978-3-319-29152-9   (eBook)
DOI 10.1007/978-3-319-29152-9

Library of Congress Control Number: 2016947964

Printed on acid-free paper

This Humana Press imprint is published by Springer Nature
The registered company is Springer International Publishing AG Switzerland

Clinical Hypertension and Vascular Diseases

Blood Pressure Monitoring in Cardiovascular Medicine and Therapeutics, Second Edition
White, William B (Ed.)
2007

Lower Extremity Arterial Disease
Caralis, Dennis G, Bakris, George L. (Eds.)
2005

Hypertension in the Elderly
Prisant, L. Michael (Ed.)
2005

Pediatric Hypertension
Portman, Ronald J, Sorof, Jonathan M, Ingelfinger, Julie R. (Eds.)
2004

Secondary Hypertension
Mansoor, George A (Ed.)
2004

Blood Pressure Monitoring in Cardiovascular Medicine and Therapeutics
White, William B. (Ed.)
2000

William B. White, MD

Dedicated to my mother Shakuntala Aiyagari for her love and affection and to my wife Veena for her unwavering support and friendship.

Venkatesh Aiyagari, MBBS, DM

In honor of my family: Ruth and Harold, Bonnie, Jessica, David and Leah, Alissa, Kevin, Lilah Rose, and Emerson.

Philip B. Gorelick, MD, MPH, FACP

Foreword

Hypertension experts have long recognized the direct relationship between uncontrolled hypertension and both hemorrhagic and ischemic types of stroke. In just 5 years since the first edition of *Hypertension and Stroke* was published, the field related to hypertension and cerebrovascular disease has advanced in the understanding of pathophysiology and blood pressure goals as well as in improvements in imaging and intervention. Hence, the second edition of *Hypertension and Stroke* remains an important and clinically relevant textbook in the subject of stroke neurology—once again, this book brings together the basic pathophysiologic, epidemiologic, diagnostic, and therapeutic advances in the evaluation of hypertension in patients with stroke or who are at great risk of stroke.

Drs. Aiyagari and Gorelick, both of whom are experts in vascular neurology, have organized this volume into sections that cover the importance of blood pressure in patients with cerebrovascular disease including overviews of the epidemiology of stroke and its relationship to hypertension; clinical evaluation that covers a variety of topics such as brain imaging, diagnostic evaluation, and cognitive assessment; and pharmacologic approaches to the management of high blood pressure in primary and secondary stroke prevention. The treatment of stroke in acute settings is nicely detailed in this book and an area of great importance in hospital medicine. As the editors note, since the prior edition, there are new sections on blood pressure regulation, the evaluation and management of hypertensive encephalopathy including eclampsia, the importance of short- and long-term blood pressure variability, and recommendations for choice of antihypertensive therapies and goals of that therapy.

The chapters in *Hypertension and Stroke* have been written by many of the most well-known authors in the field of clinical hypertension, clinical trials, and stroke neurology who have provided comprehensive, scientifically sound, and clinically appropriate information. As series editor of *Clinical Hypertension and Vascular Diseases*, I am once again delighted by the publication of this second edition of

Hypertension and Stroke—I believe it is the foremost textbook in the field for specialists in neurology and cardiovascular medicine as well as any physician who takes care of older adults at risk for cerebrovascular disorders.

William B. White, MD
Hypertension and Clinical Pharmacology
Calhoun Cardiology Center
University of Connecticut School of Medicine
Farmington, CT, USA

Preface

Hypertension is one of the most prevalent public health problems of our time. It is estimated that in the year 2000, nearly a quarter of the world's population—nearly one billion individuals—had hypertension. This proportion is expected to increase to nearly 30 %—more than 1.5 billion individuals—by the year 2025. Hypertension is the most significant modifiable risk factor for cerebrovascular diseases and is linked to a variety of neurological conditions including ischemic and hemorrhagic stroke and cognitive impairment. It is estimated that nearly 50 % of strokes could be prevented by blood pressure control. Although improvements have been made in detection and treatment of hypertension in some developed countries, on a global scale, rates of control remain inadequate.

On a more practical level, the practitioner taking care of patients with hypertension and cerebrovascular disease is often faced with several questions. For example, when is it safe to initiate antihypertensive therapy after acute ischemic stroke? What should be the target blood pressure in patients presenting with acute cerebral hemorrhage? Which blood pressure lowering agent is most safe and efficacious for primary or secondary prevention of stroke? In this book we explore answers to these and several other important aspects of hypertension and stroke.

Since the publication of the first edition of *Hypertension and Stroke: Pathophysiology and Management*, there have been several advances in this area. Several large clinical trials addressing the management of hypertension in patients with ischemic and hemorrhagic stroke have been published, and several national guidelines on the management of hypertension and stroke have been revised or updated. In the second edition of *Hypertension and Stroke*, we have attempted to collate and synthesize this rapidly expanding knowledge base into an up-to-date handy reference for clinicians. The chapters in this multiauthor monograph have been written by leading experts in the fields of vascular neurology, neuroepidemiology, critical care neurology, cardiology, nephrology, pharmacology, neuropsychology, and cognitive function and brain imaging. Several international experts bring a unique perspective from different geographic regions and healthcare systems.

The book consists of four sections, and the corresponding chapters address the following subjects:

1. The epidemiology of hypertension and stroke in relation to the definition, diagnosis, and workup of hypertension and epidemiological and clinical studies exploring the link between hypertension and stroke
2. The role of the central nervous system in regulating blood pressure and the pathophysiologic effects of hypertension on the brain and the cerebral vasculature
3. The management of hypertension in the settings of different stroke subtypes, a guide to recurrent stroke prevention, and the choice of antihypertensive agents
4. The importance of blood pressure in cognitive function, a review of newer brain imaging modalities to assess the effect of hypertension on the brain, and the role of cerebral amyloid angiopathy and cerebral microhemorrhages on cognitive function

New to the second edition are sections on the central regulation of blood pressure, effects of hypertension on the cerebral vasculature, eclampsia, subarachnoid hemorrhage, blood pressure variability, and a practical guide to choosing the right antihypertensive agent for the right patient.

It is our firm belief that this text will provide current, relevant, and expert information to guide primary care physicians, internists, neurologists, emergency physicians, intensivists, and cardiologists, as well as epidemiologists and cardiovascular researchers. We anticipate that medical students, residents, and advance practice providers will also benefit from this treatise. As the global health challenges posed by hypertension and stroke rise, *Hypertension and Stroke* will be a handy ally in meeting these challenges.

Dallas, TX, USA   Venkatesh Aiyagari, MBBS, DM
Grand Rapids, MI, USA   Philip B. Gorelick, MD, MPH, FACP

Contents

Contributors

Venkatesh Aiyagari, MBBS, DM Departments of Neurological Surgery and Neurology and Neurotherapeutics, University of Texas Southwestern Medical Center, Dallas, TX, USA

Noha Aljehani, MBBS Department of Neurology and Rehabilitation, University of Illinois, College of Medicine at Chicago, Chicago, IL, USA

Hee-Joon Bae, MD, PhD Department of Neurology, Seoul National University Bundang Hospital, Gyeonggi-do, South Korea

George L. Bakris, MD ASH Comprehensive Hypertension Center, University of Chicago Medical Center, Chicago, IL, USA

Scott H. Carlson, PhD Department of Biology, Luther College, Decorah, IA, USA

Hugues Chabriat, MD, PhD Department of Neurology, CHU Lariboisière, Assistance Publique des Hôpitaux de Paris, Paris, France

Geoffrey A. Donnan, MD, FRCP, FRACP The Florey Institute of Neuroscience and Mental Health, Melbourne, VIC, Australia

Anne M. Dorrance, PhD Department of Pharmacology and Toxicology, Michigan State University, East Lansing, MI, USA

William J. Elliott, MD, PhD Department of Biomedical Sciences, The Pacific Northwest University of Health Sciences, Yakima, WA, USA

Muhammad U. Farooq, MD, FACP, FAHA Division of Stroke and Vascular Neurology, Mercy Health Hauenstein Neurosciences, Grand Rapids, MI, USA

Philip B. Gorelick, MD, MPH, FACP Translational Science and Molecular Medicine, Michigan State College of Human Medicine, Grand Rapids, MI, USA

Mercy Health Hauenstein Neurosciences, Grand Rapids, MI, USA

Steven M. Greenberg, MD, PhD Stroke Service, Department of Neurology, Massachusetts General Hospital Stroke Research Center, Harvard Medical School, Boston, MA, USA

J. Dedrick Jordan, MD, PhD Departments of Neurology and Neurosurgery, University of North Carolina School of Medicine, Chapel Hill, NC, USA

Beom Joon Kim, MD, PhD Department of Neurology, Seoul National University Bundang Hospital, Gyeonggi-do, South Korea

Luke J. Laffin, MD ASH Comprehensive Hypertension Center, University of Chicago Medical Center, Chicago, IL, USA

Thomas K.A. Linden, MD, PhD Institute of Neuroscience and Physiology, Gothenburg University, Gothenburg, Sweden

The Florey Institute of Neuroscience and Mental Health, Melbourne, VIC, Australia

Department of Neurology, Sahlgrenska University Hospital, Gothenburg, Sweden

Alejandro Magadán, MD Department of Neurology and Neurotherapeutics, University of Texas Southwestern Medical Center, Dallas, TX, USA

Zakraus K. Mahdavi, MD Department of Neurological Surgery, Neurology and Neurotherapeutics, The University of Texas Southwestern Medical Center, Dallas, TX, USA

Jiangyong Min, MD, PhD Division of Stroke and Vascular Neurology, Mercy Health Hauenstein Neurosciences, Grand Rapids, MI, USA

David L. Nyenhuis, PhD Hauenstein Neuroscience Center, Mercy Health Saint Mary's Health Care, Grand Rapids, MI, USA

Karen Orjuela, MD Department of Neurology, Loyola University Medical Center, Maywood, IL, USA

Dilip K. Pandey, MD, PhD Department of Neurology and Rehabilitation, University of Illinois, College of Medicine at Chicago, Chicago, IL, USA

Claudia A. Perez, MD, MS Department of Neurological Surgery, The University of Texas Southwestern Medical Center, Dallas, TX, USA

Department of Neurology and Neurotherapeutics, The University of Texas Southwestern Medical Center, Dallas, TX, USA

William J. Powers, MD Department of Neurology, University of North Carolina School of Medicine, Chapel Hill, NC, USA

Michael A. Rubin, MD, MA Department of Neurological Surgery, The University of Texas Southwestern Medical Center, Dallas, TX, USA

Department of Neurology and Neurotherapeutics, The University of Texas Southwestern Medical Center, Dallas, TX, USA

Sean D. Ruland, DO Department of Neurology, Stritch School of Medicine, Loyola University Chicago, Maywood, IL, USA

Domenic A. Sica, MD Division of Nephrology, Clinical Pharmacology and Hypertension, Virginia Commonwealth University Health System, Richmond, VA, USA

Youji Soga, MD, PhD Department of Neurology and Rehabilitation, University of Illinois, College of Medicine at Chicago, Chicago, IL, USA

Susan P. Steigerwalt, MD, FASH, FACP Division of Cardiovascular Medicine, University of Michigan, Ann Arbor, MI, USA

Sean Stocker, PhD Departments of Cellular and Molecular Physiology and Neural and Behavioral Sciences, Penn State College of Medicine, Hershey, PA, USA

Fernando D. Testai, MD, PhD Department of Neurology and Rehabilitation, College of Medicine at Chicago, University of Illinois, Chicago, IL, USA

Raymond R. Townsend, MD Renal Electrolyte and Hypertension Division, University of Pennsylvania, Philadelphia, PA, USA

Anand Viswanathan, MD, PhD Stroke Service and Memory Disorders Unit, Department of Neurology, Massachusetts General Hospital Stroke Research Center, Harvard Medical School, Boston, MA, USA

Lawrence K.S. Wong, MD. Department of Medicine and Therapeutics, Faculty of Medicine, Prince of Wales Hospital, Chinese University of Hong Kong, Hong Kong, China

J. Michael Wyss, PhD Departments of Cell Developmental and Integrative Biology and Medicine, University of Alabama at Birmingham, Birmingham, AL, USA

Part I
Blood Pressure and Hypertension as Antecedents of Stroke

Chapter 1
Blood Pressure: Definition, Diagnosis, and Management

Raymond R. Townsend and Susan P. Steigerwalt

The Definition of Hypertension

The many years of follow-up in the Framingham Heart Study have shown that the relationship between blood pressure and target organ damage is a smooth, and reasonably linear one so that the choice of where to place a marker that differentiates "above this point is hypertension and below this point is normal" will always be somewhat arbitrary [1]. The first attempts to define a point above which excess harm including loss of life would occur was undertaken by Life Insurance Companies who, by the first quarter of the twentieth century had made reasonable estimates that 140/90 mmHg represented a realistic value to define excessive lifetime risk from blood pressure elevation [2]. The classic paper of Perrera published in the first volume of the Journal of Chronic Diseases in 1955 verified that the presence of a sustained elevation in systolic blood pressure of > 140 mmHg or diastolic blood pressure of >90 mmHg resulted uniformly in death within 20 years of onset [3]. Soberingly, in 1950, an era prior to antihypertensive therapy, suggested that a 40-year-old man with a systolic blood pressure of 145 mmHg was estimated to have about 15 years of life left before succumbing to target organ damage from hypertension.

Despite the recognition of excess risk associated with blood pressure elevation, many thought that the increase in blood pressure associated with aging represented a natural adaptation to arterial stiffening and argued against treating elevated blood pressure until

R.R. Townsend, M.D.
Renal Electrolyte and Hypertension Division, University of Pennsylvania, Philadelphia, PA, USA

S.P. Steigerwalt, M.D., F.A.S.H., F.A.C.P. (✉)
Devision of Cardiovascular Medicine, University of Michigan, Ann Arbor, MI, USA
e-mail: spspnhp@med.umich.edu

© Springer International Publishing Switzerland 2016
V. Aiyagari, P.B. Gorelick (eds.), *Hypertension and Stroke*, Clinical Hypertension and Vascular Diseases, DOI 10.1007/978-3-319-29152-9_1

it entered a malignant phase [4]. Once it entered a malignant phase, in which the diastolic blood pressure generally exceeded 140 mmHg and the patient had signs of heart disease, stroke, or uremia, life expectancy was less than 25% at 1 year [5].

Compelling as actuarial data may be, and natural history studies such as those of Perrera, many remained skeptical about the value of treating high blood pressure. It was not until the VA Cooperative Study Group reported on the benefit of treating moderate to severe hypertension (diastolic blood pressure values of 115–129 mmHg) [6] and then less elevated diastolic values of 90–115 mmHg [7] that practitioners began to administer antihypertensive therapy and recommend lifestyle therapies with the intent of preserving target organ function. With the ability to lower blood pressure with an increasing number of classes of antihypertensive drugs, and multiple agents within some classes of antihypertensive drugs, attention turned to the need to educate physicians on how to diagnose and then manage hypertensive patients. This effort was espoused by the National Heart Lung and Blood Institute in the early 1970s and was known as the High Blood Pressure Education Program. An outgrowth of this Program was the first Joint National Committee Report, chaired by Dr. Marvin Moser, and published in 1977 in JAMA, in which a formal definition for hypertension was proposed. Since the purpose of this chapter is not to review the history and nuances of the definition of hypertension, we refer the reader for the next 37 years from 1977 to 2014 to Table 1.1, which represents a summary from both JNC 8 and the recent AHA/ACCF/ASH guidelines for hypertension [8, 9].

As reviewed in JNC 8 and the AHA scientific statements, the levels of evidence supporting the threshold to diagnose hypertension in each of the instances above varies from "E" (Expert Opinion) to "A" (Strong support from existing evidence). Level B evidence suggests that the benefit at that level of BP > risk, but supporting evidence is modest. A full review of the evidence supporting the thresholds for the diagnosis of hypertension is reviewed in the two primary sources cited [8, 10]. It should be pointed out that there is disagreement world-wide, and within the USA, on the some of the threshold values shown above [11, 12]. The JNC 8 statement reviews the recommendations for hypertension diagnosis in an extensively referenced table in the JAMA publication [8].

Table 1.1 Thresholds for diagnosis and treatment of hypertension

	mmHg	Level of evidence
General population 18–60 years old	140/90	For systolic blood pressure: E
		For diastolic blood pressure: A
General population ≥60 years old	150/90	For systolic blood pressure: A
		For diastolic blood pressure: A
Patients with CKD <70 years old	140/90	E
Patients with diabetes	140/90	E
Patients with coronary artery disease	140/90	A
Patients with heart failure	140/90	B
Patients with stroke	130/80	E

Diagnosis of Hypertension

Evaluation Goals

The first goal in the diagnosis of hypertension is to assure that the blood pressure elevation is real. There are many short-term influences on blood pressure and the general impression is that hypertension should be diagnosed after at least two, and preferably three, different encounters where blood pressure is measured and the average >140/90 mmHg.

Traditionally these measures have been conducted in an office setting. The reason for three visits, and the need to measure blood pressure at least twice and preferably three times during an office encounter is based on work from the UK supporting this type of measurement schedule [13].

Several countries have recommended that confirmation of an office BP elevation be undertaken using ambulatory blood pressure monitoring (ABPM) [14] or by the use of home blood pressure monitoring (HBPM) [15]. If HBPM or ABPM are used to validate the diagnosis of hypertension, somewhat different values are recommended for the threshold of what constitutes "hypertension." These are outlined in Table 1.2.

The diagnostic work-up of the patient with a sustained elevation of blood pressure is undertaken to address three questions:

- Is the BP elevation primary or is it secondary to an underlying cause?
- Is the BP elevation attended by additional cardiovascular (CV) risk factors?
- Is the BP elevation attended by target organ damage of the brain, heart, or kidneys?

Answers to these questions will influence therapeutic decisions and provide insight into the need for management of blood pressure to encompass associated risk factors. Common errors in blood pressure measurement technique tend to falsely increase the readings leading to an overestimate of blood pressure level.

How to Measure Blood Pressure

In the office setting blood pressure should be measured 2–3 times in the sitting position, and averaged for that visit. The sitting position has been the principal position used for randomized clinical trials demonstrating benefit of blood pressure

Table 1.2 Out of office thresholds relative to office values for hypertension diagnosis

Office threshold	24 h ABPM	Daytime ABPM	Home BPM series[a]
140 mmHg systolic	≥130 mmHg	≥135 mmHg	≥135 mmHg
90 mmHg diastolic	≥80 mmHg	≥85 mmHg	≥85 mmHg

[a]Series=two morning+two evening HBPM for 7 consecutive days; drop the first day and then average the remaining 6 days for the systolic and diastolic blood pressure values

reduction [16]. The dominant arm is best used as it tends to be the higher one; but at least once blood pressure should be measured in both arms. A difference of 5 mmHg in systolic blood pressure between arms is not uncommon; however, a difference of systolic blood pressure of 10 mmHg or higher should raise concern for generalized vascular disease and subsequent heightened vascular disease risk [17]. It is useful to assess the response of the blood pressure to standing for at least 1 min. Recent guidelines form the AHA/ACCF recommend checking for orthostatic hypotension on all elderly hypertensive patients [18].

Blood pressure assessment requires adherence to AHA-recommended steps in preparing a patient for such a determination. A correct-sized cuff, defined as encircling at least 80 % of the mid upper-arm circumference, is applied and calibrated equipment is used with good inflation and deflation technique in a patient seated comfortably with the back supported, feet on the floor, and arm at heart level. The urinary bladder should be empty. The AHA recommends 5 min of rest prior to measurement and abstention from caffeine and cigarettes for 30 min prior to measurement [19]. This yields the most reproducible blood pressure determination. Despite good technique, the average blood pressure varies day to day, thus, a running average of at least three different measurement sessions affords the best office estimate of blood pressure.

A sizable number of patients use home blood pressure cuffs. The AHA Call to Action provides a description of how to use such home-based results in hypertension diagnosis and management and stresses the need for attention to proper technique [20]. In the USA hypertension is still based on office blood pressure readings, but in many other venues, particularly Canada, out-of-office blood pressures are used to establish a diagnosis of hypertension [15]. In this regard ABPM has resurfaced as a valuable tool to secure the diagnosis of hypertension. Both the National Institute for Health and Clinical Excellence (NICE) guidelines from the UK and the recent United States Preventive Services Task Force (USPTFS) guidance statement recommend 24 h ABPM to confirm the diagnosis of hypertension prior to initiation of treatment [14, 21]. The use of ABPM allows an accurate diagnosis of white coat hypertension, and more importantly, masked hypertension. In the case of white coat hypertension blood pressures are better outside the office compared to office values [22]. Masked hypertension means that blood pressure recordings outside the office are higher than those recorded in the office setting [23].

Evaluation of the Hypertension: Addressing Three Key Questions

As previously mentioned there are three key questions to address in relation to the diagnosis of hypertension. These are asked to determine:

1. Does the patient have a secondary form of hypertension?
2. Are there associated cardiovascular risks or predisposition to such risks?
3. Is there any target organ damage?

Recognizing the presence of a secondary form of hypertension may direct curative therapy (e.g., removal of an aldosterone-producing adenoma) or provide insight into mechanisms which may help guide therapy (e.g., renal artery stenosis and the use of medications with block the renin–angiotensin system activity or endovascular intervention to correct renal artery stenosis).

Identification of the presence and severity of other cardiovascular risk factors is important for two reasons. First, we may wish to avoid using medications which can cause or worsen a risk factor (e.g., the use of beta-blocking drugs in patients with a low HDL cholesterol level which could lower HDL further or thiazide diuretics in a patient with impaired fasting glucose which could precipitate diabetes mellitus) [24]. Second, the presence of other risk factors (e.g., components of the metabolic syndrome) may heighten the risk of hypertension and warrant consideration of additional and more intensive therapy.

Finally, the presence of target organ damage is important to detect because it moves the treatment goal from *primary* prevention to *secondary* prevention. For example, a patient with a history of stroke has a risk of another stroke within the next 5 years which may be 30 % or higher, a value which far exceeds the average hypertensive patient's risk without such a history. Guidelines suggest the use of a diuretic and angiotensin-converting enzyme inhibitor for recurrent stroke prevention. This is discussed in further detail in subsequent chapters of this book.

General Principles of Diagnosis of Hypertension: Medical History

Patients with elevated blood pressure should have a thorough general history and physical examination and selected investigations (*see* Tables 1.3 and 1.4). The evaluation of a patient with elevated blood pressure begins with a complete medical history. The history should query the duration (when known) and severity of high blood pressure. Clues such as the sudden onset of severe blood pressure elevation when blood pressure was previously known to be normal raise suspicion for a secondary cause of hypertension. Knowledge of concomitant medical conditions and associated cardiovascular comorbidities and responses to various treatments should also be obtained. Information about dietary habits, alcohol consumption, tobacco use, level of physical activity, and sleep duration (which predicts both hypertension and CV events [25]) should be determined since there may be allied areas of lifestyle or other intervention. A family history of hypertension, renal disease, cardiovascular disease, and diabetes mellitus should be noted. Sleep-disordered breathing which is common in hypertension may be uncovered by queries about daytime sleepiness, snoring/gasping, fitful sleep, and nocturnal arousals with breathless symptoms. A screening tool such as the Epworth Sleepiness Scale™ [26] may be helpful.

In addition, it is important to obtain details of past medication use with particular attention to side effects and effectiveness in controlling blood pressure. Current medications, including over-the-counter preparations, should be reviewed. For example, nonsteroidal anti-inflammatory drugs (NSAIDs) can decrease the efficacy

Table 1.3 Medical history in the patient with elevated blood pressure

Item	Evaluation
Age at onset and duration of elevated blood pressure	Onset in younger patients (e.g., <30 years) may indicate a secondary cause; when blood pressure at onset is severe (e.g., stage 2 hypertension), this may also be a clue to a secondary cause
Lifestyle factors	High salt intake, physical inactivity, psychosocial stress, and sleep-disordered breathing (e.g., sleep apnea) may contribute to elevated blood pressure
Concurrent medications	Consider nonsteroidal anti-inflammatory drugs (NSAIDs), oral contraceptives, corticosteroids, licorice, cough/cold/weight-loss pills, and sympathomimetics
Risk factors for cardiovascular disease	Family history of premature cardiovascular disease especially in a first-degree relative (parent or sibling), diabetes, smoking, and elevated cholesterol
Symptoms or history which suggest possible secondary cause	Episodic sweating, heart racing/palpitations, and headache (e.g., pheochromocytoma); muscle weakness and increased urine volume (e.g., hyperaldosteronemia); family history of kidney disease (hereditary forms such as polycystic kidney disease); protein or blood in urine and/or ankle swelling (various types of renal disease); daytime somnolence, snoring/gasping during sleep (e.g., sleep-disordered breathing); prior stroke, heart attack, or peripheral arterial disease (e.g., renal artery stenosis); leg discomfort and claudication in young patient (e.g., coarctation of aorta); and heat intolerance and weight loss (e.g., hyperthyroidism)
Target organ damage	Chest pain or chest discomfort or known prior myocardial infarction (coronary artery disease); neurologic symptoms consistent with stroke or transient ischemic attack (cerebrovascular disease); dyspnea and easy fatigue (possible heart failure); claudication (peripheral arterial disease)

of antihypertensive drugs, presumably through mechanisms that inhibit the vasodilatory and natriuretic prostaglandin effects and the potentiation of angiotensin-II effects [27] (*see* Tables 1.3 and 1.5 for medications affecting blood pressure). It is important to assess the use of alternative medications and supplements, as individuals often do not consider or report these as "medications," and they may contain potent pressor substances such as sympathomimetics or European black licorice. A useful website for further information on complementary and alternative medicine is http://www.tangcenter.uchicago.edu.

General Principles of Diagnosis of Hypertension: Physical Examination

The physical examination of the patient begins with measurement of height and weight, waist circumference, and blood pressure in *both* arms. The blood pressure is recorded according to the arm with the higher blood pressure measurement. It is sometimes necessary to measure blood pressure in the leg in instances when

Table 1.4 Physical examination in the patient with elevated blood pressure

Item	Routine evaluation
General appearance, skin lesions, distribution of body fat	Waist circumference (may fit criteria for metabolic syndrome; adds to diabetic and CV risk); signs of prior stroke from gait/station, motor, and cognition exams; uncommonly secondary forms are evident as striae (Cushing's syndrome) or mucosal fibromas (multiple endocrine neoplasia type 2)
Fundus	Retinal arteriole caliber changes and presence of other retinal pathology reflects severity of hypertension
Neck (thyroid) and carotid arteries	Multinodular diffuse goiter (Graves' disease); presence of carotid bruits may be a clue to elevated stroke risk
Heart and lungs	Presence of rales and/or gallops (target organ damage), interscapular murmur (coarctation of the aorta); displacement of apex beat (point of maximal impulse suggestive of heart enlargement)
Abdomen	Palpable kidneys (polycystic kidney disease); midepigastric bruits (renal arterial disease); striae (Cushing's syndrome)
Neurologic examination	Reduced grip strength or other muscle weakness, hyperreflexia, spasticity, Babinski sign, gait disturbance, or cognitive impairment (previous stroke)
Pulse examination	Delayed/absent femoral pulses (coarctation of the aorta or atherosclerosis); loss of pedal pulses (atherosclerosis, particularly in smokers)

coarctation of the aorta is suspected. Although blood pressure measurements with the patient supine, sitting, and standing are usually undertaken in a hypertension specialty clinic, in a primary care setting where time constraints are germane, a seated blood pressure is carried out three times and averaged. In patients older than 60 years it is important to determine a standing blood pressure level as well. This helps identify orthostatic hypotension, a predictor of falls in the elderly, and possible intolerance to blood pressure lowering [28].

Key features of the general physical examination of the patient with elevated blood pressure are listed in Table 1.3 and below:

- Retina (to assess vascular impact of blood pressure)
- Pulses and vessels (searching for carotid bruits for known or subclinical stenosis; abdomen/midepigastric bruits for renovascular disease; femoral bruits for atherosclerosis; poor or delayed femoral pulses suspicious for aortic coarctation; and pedal pulses for peripheral arterial disease, particularly in smokers)
- Heart for gallop sounds and enlargement
- Lungs (rales; unusual in the early phase of hypertension)
- Legs for edema
- Abbreviated neurologic exam for strength, gait, and cognition

Cardiac examination may show a displaced apical impulse, reflecting left ventricular enlargement. When sustained, the apical impulse may indicate left ventricular hypertrophy (LVH). Auscultation of an S_4 gallop may document early physical findings of hypertension.

Table 1.5 Drugs associated with development of or worsening of elevated blood pressure

Drug class or drug	Proposed mechanism of action
Nonsteroidal anti-inflammatory agents [39]	Prostaglandin inhibition causing renal sodium retention and decrease in GFR
High-dose corticosteroids [40]	Mineralocorticoid receptor (MR) stimulation (sodium retention) and sodium–potassium ATPase inhibition (vasoconstriction)
Oral contraceptives [41]	Unknown, usually trivial elevations of blood pressure
Prescribed sympathomimetics (Meridia™, Ritalin, Provigil™, etc.) [42, 43]	Vasoconstriction and sodium retention
Selective serotonin reuptake inhibitors (SSRIs), selective norepinephrine reuptake inhibitors (SSNIs) [44, 45]	Increase of serotonin or norepinephrine via reuptake inhibition
Erythrocyte-stimulating agents [46]	Vasoconstriction
Tacrolimus, cyclosporine [47]	Vasoconstriction, sodium retention, decrease in GFR
Highly active anti-retroviral therapy (HAART) [48]	Unknown
European black licorice (often contained in alternative medications and chewing tobacco) [49]	Indirectly causes activation of MR, sodium retention, and enhanced vascular reactivity
Cocaine, ecstasy, methamphetamines, and other recreational drugs [50, 51]	Sympathetic activation/vasoconstriction
VEGF inhibitors [52, 53]	FLT-1

VEGF vascular endothelial growth factor, *GFR* glomerular filtration rate

Frequency of Blood Pressure Monitoring After the Initial Examination

After the initial examination, blood pressure monitoring is recommended at specified intervals. We recommend subsequent blood pressure monitoring according to the Joint National Committee 7 guidelines as shown in Table 1.6 [3].

Laboratory Studies in the Evaluation of the Patient with Hypertension or Elevated Blood Pressure

A number of select laboratory tests are recommended for routine evaluation of the patient with elevated blood pressure. At a minimum these should include the following diagnostic studies: hemoglobin or hematocrit, urinalysis with microscopic examination, serum creatinine and electrolytes, serum glucose, a fasting lipid profile, and a 12-lead electrocardiogram (ECG). Other studies such as thyroid hormone concentrations are guided by a history suggesting thyroid excess or the discovery of

Table 1.6 Follow-up recommendations for subsequent blood pressure monitoring

Initial BP		
SBP	DBP	Follow-up recommendation
<120	<80	Recheck in 2 years
120–139	80–89	Recheck in 1 year
140–159	90–99	Confirm within 2 months
≥160	≥100	Evaluate within 1 month; for those with higher blood pressures (e.g., ≥180/110 mmHg), evaluate and treat immediately or within 1 week depending on clinical situation and complications

From Chobanian AV, Bakris GL, Black HR, et al. Seventh report of the joint national committee on prevention, detection, evaluation, and treatment of high blood pressure. Hypertension. 2003;42:1206–52, with permission

SBP systolic blood pressure, *DBP* diastolic blood pressure, *BP* blood pressure

a thyroid nodule on examination of the neck. The urine studies and the electrolytes/creatinine determinations (and calculated MDRD eGFR) may reflect target organ damage to the kidney. The glucose and the lipid profile may reveal the presence of other cardiovascular risk factors. The 12-lead ECG may show LVH or the presence of a prior myocardial infarction, both of which represent valuable information in planning treatment.

The use of spot urine albumin/creatinine (ACR) in diabetic patients is well established [29]. In nondiabetic patients, early morning spot urine ACR may be a marker for increased cardiovascular risk, systemic inflammation, and renal failure [30]. Both population-based studies such as PREVEND [31] and clinical trials such as HOPE [32] show increased cardiovascular event rates associated with presence of increased ACR. We recommend screening for ACR in patients with hypertension, repeating it twice to confirm the abnormality. Elevated ACR requires special attention to control of blood pressure, lipids, and evidence of systemic inflammation.

Evaluation for Secondary Causes of Hypertension or Elevated Blood Pressure

In some instances medical history, physical examination, or the initial diagnostic testing leads one to suspect a secondary cause of hypertension. Table 1.4 includes physical findings that may lead one to suspect a secondary cause of hypertension. The reader is referred to several authoritative reviews of secondary causes of hypertension which cover this topic in detail [33, 34].

Obstructive sleep apnea (OSA) is probably the most common cause of secondary hypertension. It occurs more frequently in men (9 % of men and 4 % of women in the US population) and is often associated with obesity [20, 35]. In patients with hypertension, 30–80% have at least moderate grades of sleep apnea [35]. In population studies, OSA is associated with congestive heart failure, stroke, coronary artery disease, and sudden cardiac death. Post stroke, 43–91 % of patients may have OSA [21, 36]. In uncontrolled hypertensives, treatment of OSA has been shown to decrease blood pressure on average by 5/3 mmHg [22, 37]. Bradley and Floras have said: "OSA appears to increase the risk of cardiovascular disease, and its treatment has the potential to decrease risk. Prospective clinical trials are needed." The reader is referred to an informative recent review for more details [38].

Summary: Evaluation of Elevated Blood Pressure

For proper diagnosis of hypertension or elevated blood pressure, multiple blood pressure readings should be taken at various times to confirm the diagnosis. The accurate measurement of blood pressure is made with the correct cuff size, patient position, and technique. ABPM is increasingly being used to verify a diagnosis of hypertension. The medical history, physical exam, and initial diagnostic test strategy should address three key questions: (1) Is increased blood pressure primary or secondary? (2) Are other cardiovascular risk factors present? and (3) Is there any evidence of target organ damage?

References

1. Muldoon MF, Rutan GH. Defining hypertension: never as simple as it seems. J Hypertens. 2003;21(3):473–4.
2. Fisher JW. The diagnostic value of the sphygmomanometer in examinations for life insurance. JAMA. 1914;63:1752–4.
3. Perera GA. Hypertensive vascular disease; description and natural history. J Chronic Dis. 1955;1:33–42.
4. Goldring W, Chasis H. Antihypertensive drug therapy: an appraisal. In: Ingelfinger FJ, Relman AS, editors. Controversies in international medicine. Philadelphia: Saunders; 1966. p. 83.
5. Keith NM, Wagener HP, Barker NW. Some different types of essential hypertension: their course and prognosis. Am J Med Sci. 1939;197:332–43.
6. Effects of treatment on morbidity in hypertension. Results in patients with diastolic blood pressures averaging 115 through 129 mm Hg. JAMA 1967; 202(11):1028–34.
7. Effects of treatment on morbidity in hypertension. II. Results in patients with diastolic blood pressure averaging 90 through 114 mm Hg. JAMA 1970;213(7):1143–152.
8. James PA, Oparil S, Carter BL, Cushman WC, Dennison-Himmelfarb C, Handler J, Lackland DT, Lefevre ML, Mackenzie TD, Ogedegbe O, Smith Jr SC, Svetkey LP, Taler SJ, Townsend RR, Wright Jr JT, Narva AS, Ortiz E. 2014 Evidence-based guideline for the management of high blood pressure in adults: report from the Panel Members Appointed to the Eighth Joint National Committee (JNC 8). JAMA. 2014;311(5):507–20.
9. Chirinos JA, Segers P, Duprez DA, Brumback L, Bluemke DA, Zamani P, Kronmal R, Vaidya D, Ouyang P, Townsend RR, Jacobs DR. Late systolic central hypertension as a predictor of incident heart failure: the multi-ethnic study of atherosclerosis. J Am Heart Assoc. 2015;4(3), e001335.

10. Rosendorff C, Lackland DT, Allison M, Aronow WS, Black HR, Blumenthal RS, Cannon CP, de Lemos JA, Elliott WJ, Findeiss L, Gersh BJ, Gore JM, Levy D, Long JB, O'Connor CM, O'Gara PT, Ogedegbe O, Oparil S, White WB. Treatment of hypertension in patients with coronary artery disease: a scientific statement from the American Heart Association, American College of Cardiology, and American Society of Hypertension. Circulation. 2015;131(19): e435–e470.

11. Wright Jr JT, Fine LJ, Lackland DT, Ogedegbe G, Dennison Himmelfarb CR. Evidence supporting a systolic blood pressure goal of less than 150 mm Hg in patients aged 60 years or older: the minority view. Ann Intern Med. 2014;160(7):499–503.

12. Flack JM, Sica DA, Bakris G, Brown AL, Ferdinand KC, Grimm Jr RH, Hall WD, Jones WE, Kountz DS, Lea JP, Nasser S, Nesbitt SD, Saunders E, Scisney-Matlock M, Jamerson KA. Management of high blood pressure in Blacks: an update of the International Society on Hypertension in Blacks consensus statement. Hypertension. 2010;56(5):780–800.

13. Hartley RM, Velez R, Morris RW, D'Souza MF, Heller RF. Confirming the diagnosis of mild hypertension. Br Med J (Clin Res Ed). 1983;286(6361):287–9.

14. http://www.nice.org.uk/guidance/cg127. http://www.nice.org.uk/guidance/cg127. 2014.

15. Cloutier L, Daskalopoulou SS, Padwal RS, Lamarre-Cliche M, Bolli P, McLean D, Milot A, Tobe SW, Tremblay G, McKay DW, Townsend R, Campbell N, Gelfer M. A new algorithm for the diagnosis of hypertension in Canada. Can J Cardiol. 2015;31:620–30.

16. Mosenkis A, Townsend RR. Sitting on the evidence: what is the proper patient position for the office measurement of blood pressure? J Clin Hypertens (Greenwich). 2005;7(6):365–6.

17. Clark CE, Taylor RS, Shore AC, Ukoumunne OC, Campbell JL. Association of a difference in systolic blood pressure between arms with vascular disease and mortality: a systematic review and meta-analysis. Lancet. 2012;379(9819):905–14.

18. Aronow WS, Fleg JL, Pepine CJ, Artinian NT, Bakris G, Brown AS, Ferdinand KC, Ann FM, Frishman WH, Jaigobin C, Kostis JB, Mancia G, Oparil S, Ortiz E, Reisin E, Rich MW, Schocken DD, Weber MA, Wesley DJ. ACCF/AHA 2011 expert consensus document on hypertension in the elderly: a report of the American College of Cardiology Foundation Task Force on Clinical Expert Consensus documents developed in collaboration with the American Academy of Neurology, American Geriatrics Society, American Society for Preventive Cardiology, American Society of Hypertension, American Society of Nephrology, Association of Black Cardiologists, and European Society of Hypertension. J Am Coll Cardiol. 2011;57(20):2037–114.

19. Pickering TG, Hall JE, Appel LJ, Falkner BE, Graves J, Hill MN, Jones DW, Kurtz T, Sheps SG, Roccella EJ. Recommendations for blood pressure measurement in humans and experimental animals: part 1: blood pressure measurement in humans: a statement for professionals from the Subcommittee of Professional and Public Education of the American Heart Association Council on High Blood Pressure Research. Circulation. 2005;111(5):697–716.

20. Pickering TG, Miller NH, Ogedegbe G, Krakoff LR, Artinian NT, Goff D. Call to action on use and reimbursement for home blood pressure monitoring: executive summary: a joint scientific statement from the American Heart Association, American Society of Hypertension, and Preventive Cardiovascular Nurses Association. Hypertension. 2008;52(1):1–9.

21. Piper MA, Evans CV, Burda BU, Margolis KL, O'Connor E, Whitlock EP. Diagnostic and predictive accuracy of blood pressure screening methods with consideration of rescreening intervals: a systematic review for the U.S. Preventive Services Task Force. Ann Intern Med. 2015;162(3):192–204.

22. Pickering TG, James GD, Boddie C, Harshfield GA, Blank S, Laragh JH. How common is white coat hypertension? JAMA. 1988;259:225–8.

23. Pickering TG, Davidson K, Gerin W, Schwartz JE. Masked hypertension. Hypertension. 2002;40(6):795–6.

24. Papadakis JA, Mikhailidis DP, Vrentzos GE, Kalikaki A, Kazakou I, Ganotakis ES. Effect of antihypertensive treatment on plasma fibrinogen and serum HDL levels in patients with essential hypertension. Clin Appl Thromb Hemost. 2005;11:139–46.

25. Eguchi K, Pickering TG, Schwartz JE, et al. Short sleep duration as an independent predictor of cardiovascular events in Japanese patients with hypertension. Arch Intern Med. 2008;168:2225–31.
26. Manni R, Politini L, Ratti MT, Tartara A. Sleepiness in obstructive sleep apnea syndrome and simple snoring evaluated by the Epworth Sleepiness Scale. J Sleep Res. 1999;8:319–20.
27. Fierro-Carrion GA, Ram CV. Nonsteroidal anti-inflammatory drugs (NSAIDs) and blood pressure. Am J Cardiol. 1997;80:775–6.
28. The Consensus Committee of the American Autonomic Society and the American Academy of Neurology. Consensus statement on the definition of orthostatic hypotension, pure autonomic failure, and multiple system atrophy. Neurology. 1996;46:1470.
29. Singh P, Aronow WS, Mellana WM, Gutwein AH. Prevalence of appropriate management of diabetes mellitus in an academic general medicine clinic. Am J Ther. 2009;17(1):42–5.
30. van der Velde M, Halbesma N, DeCharro FT, et al. Screening for albuminuria identifies individuals at increased renal risk. J Am Soc Nephrol. 2009;20:852–62.
31. Hillege HL, Fidler V, Diercks GF, et al. Urinary albumin excretion predicts cardiovascular and noncardiovascular mortality in general population. Circulation. 2002;106:1777–82.
32. Gerstein HC, Mann JF, Yi Q, et al. Albuminuria and risk of cardiovascular events, death, and heart failure in diabetic and nondiabetic individuals. JAMA. 2001;286:421–6.
33. Onusko E. Diagnosing secondary hypertension. Am Fam Physician. 2003;67:67–74.
34. Aurell M. Screening for secondary hypertension. Curr Hypertens Rep. 1999;1:461.
35. Fletcher EC, DeBehnke RD, Lovoi MS, Gorin AB. Undiagnosed sleep apnea in patients with essential hypertension. Ann Intern Med. 1985;103:190–5.
36. Bassetti CL, Milanova M, Gugger M. Sleep-disordered breathing and acute ischemic stroke: diagnosis, risk factors, treatment, evolution, and long-term clinical outcome. Stroke. 2006;37:967–72.
37. Pepperell JC, Ramdassingh-Dow S, Crosthwaite N, et al. Ambulatory blood pressure after therapeutic and subtherapeutic nasal continuous positive airway pressure for obstructive sleep apnoea: a randomised parallel trial. Lancet. 2002;359:204–10.
38. Qaseem A, Dallas P, Owens DK, Starkey M, Holty JC, Shekelle P, et al. Diagnosis of obstructive sleep apnea in adults: a clinical practice guideline from the American College of Physicians. Ann Intern Med. 2014;161:210–20. doi:10.7326/M12-3187.
39. Farkouh ME, Verheugt FW, Ruland S, et al. A comparison of the blood pressure changes of lumiracoxib with those of ibuprofen and naproxen. J Clin Hypertens (Greenwich). 2008;10:592–602.
40. Panoulas VF, Douglas KM, Stavropoulos-Kalinoglou A, et al. Long-term exposure to medium-dose glucocorticoid therapy associates with hypertension in patients with rheumatoid arthritis. Rheumatology (Oxford). 2008;47:72–5.
41. Shufelt CL, Bairey Merz CN. Contraceptive hormone use and cardiovascular disease. J Am Coll Cardiol. 2009;53:221–31.
42. Taneja I, Diedrich A, Black BK, Byrne DW, Paranjape SY, Robertson D. Modafinil elicits sympathomedullary activation. Hypertension. 2005;45:612–8.
43. Idelevich E, Kirch W, Schindler C. Current pharmacotherapeutic concepts for the treatment of obesity in adults. Ther Adv Cardiovasc Dis. 2009;3:75–90.
44. Kisely S, Cox M, Campbell LA, Cooke C, Gardner D. An epidemiologic study of psychotropic medication and obesity-related chronic illnesses in older psychiatric patients. Can J Psychiatry. 2009;54:269–74.
45. Johnson EM, Whyte E, Mulsant BH, et al. Cardiovascular changes associated with venlafaxine in the treatment of late-life depression. Am J Geriatr Psychiatry. 2006;14:796–802.
46. Krapf R, Hulter HN. Arterial hypertension induced by erythropoietin and erythropoiesis-stimulating agents (ESA). Clin J Am Soc Nephrol 2009;4(2):470–480.
47. Kramer BK, Boger C, Kruger B, et al. Cardiovascular risk estimates and risk factors in renal transplant recipients. Transplant Proc. 2005;37:1868–70.
48. Baekken M, Os I, Sandvik L, Oektedalen O. Hypertension in an urban HIV-positive population compared with the general population: influence of combination antiretroviral therapy. J Hypertens. 2008;26:2126–33.

49. Templin C, Westhoff-Bleck M, Ghadri JR. Hypokalemic paralysis with rhabdomyolysis and arterial hypertension caused by liquorice ingestion. Clin Res Cardiol. 2009;98:130–2.
50. Urbina A, Jones K. Crystal methamphetamine, its analogues, and HIV infection: medical and psychiatric aspects of a new epidemic. Clin Infect Dis. 2004;38:890–4.
51. Gahlinger PM. Club drugs: MDMA, gamma-hydroxybutyrate (GHB), Rohypnol, and ketamine. Am Fam Physician. 2004;69:2619–26.
52. Veronese ML, Mosenkis A, Flaherty KT, et al. Mechanisms of hypertension associated with BAY 43-9006. J Clin Oncol. 2006;24:1363–9.
53. Bono P, Elfving H, Utriainen T, et al. Hypertension and clinical benefit of bevacizumab in the treatment of advanced renal cell carcinoma. Ann Oncol. 2009;20:393–4.

Chapter 2
The Link Between Hypertension and Stroke: Summary of Observational Epidemiological Studies

Dilip K. Pandey, Noha Aljehani, and Youji Soga

Stroke is the leading cause of disability in the USA. It ranked seventh among 30 leading diseases and injuries contributing to the years of life lost due to premature mortality (YLLs) in the USA in 2010, and third for contributing to the reduced disability-adjusted life years (DALYs) [1]. Among modifiable risk factors for ischemic and hemorrhagic stroke, hypertension is the most robust one across age, gender, and race [2, 3]. Hypertension has made its way from being the fourth-leading risk factor in 1990, as quantified by DALYs, to being the leading risk factor in 2010 [4]. Hypertension is also a highly prevalent health condition. As many as 80 million adult Americans (one in three US adults) have hypertension defined as elevated blood pressure (systolic blood pressure ≥ 140 mmHg or diastolic blood pressure ≥ 90 mmHg) or taking antihypertensive medicine or being told at least twice by a physician or other health professional that one has high blood pressure [5–7]. The prevalence of hypertension increases rapidly above the age of 65 years. The age-adjusted prevalence of hypertension in 2009–2012 was 80 % for women and 76 % for men over 75 years of age [8, 9]. The prevalence of hypertension also varies by race and is highest amongst non-Hispanic Blacks (Fig. 2.1). The lifetime risk for developing hypertension is 90 % among individuals who are normotensive at 55 years of age [10]. A recent prediction model showed that every 10 % increases in hypertension treatment could prevent an additional 14,000 deaths per year in the adult population ages 25–79 [11]. Projections show that by 2030, about 41.4 % of US adults will have hypertension, an increase of 8.4 % from 2012 estimates (unpublished AHA computation, based on methodology described by Hiedenreich et al.) [11].

D.K. Pandey, M.D., Ph.D. (✉) • N. Aljehani, M.B.B.S. • Y. Soga, M.D., Ph.D.
Department of Neurology and Rehabilitation, University of Illinois College of
Medicine at Chicago, Chicago, IL, USA
e-mail: dpandey@uic.edu

© Springer International Publishing Switzerland 2016
V. Aiyagari, P.B. Gorelick (eds.), *Hypertension and Stroke*, Clinical
Hypertension and Vascular Diseases, DOI 10.1007/978-3-319-29152-9_2

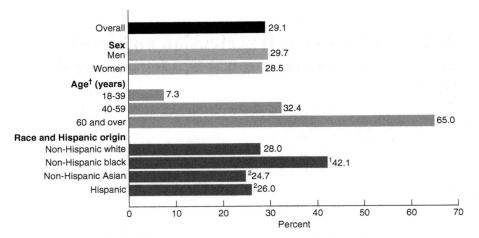

Fig. 2.1 Age-specific and age-adjusted prevalence of hypertension among adult aged 18 and over, United States 2011–2012 (*Source*: CDC/NCHS, National Health and Nutrition Examination Survey, 2011–2012. Accessed on 15 April 2015 at http://www.cdc.gov/nchs/data/databriefs/db133. pdf)

Hypertension as a Risk Factor for Stroke

There is compelling evidence from observational and interventional studies, suggesting that hypertension is a significant and strong risk factor for stroke. It has been estimated that about 54 % of strokes worldwide are attributable to high blood pressure (BP) [12]. The Framingham Heart Study in 1970 observed a significant relationship between risk of stroke and blood pressure ≥160/95 mmHg in both sexes and at all ages [13]. Persons with a normal BP (<120/80 mmHg) had been reported approximately half the lifetime risk of stroke compared to those with high BP (≥140/90 mmHg) [14]. A meta-analysis of 12 prospective cohort studies with 518,520 participants found that prehypertension is associated with incident stroke. The risk is particularly noted in nonelderly people and for those with BP values in the higher prehypertension range [15].

Detailed analyses of large cohort studies have shown that the relationship between BP and risk of stroke is continuous, consistent, and independent of other risk factors. Earlier epidemiological studies used diastolic pressure as a measurement rather than systolic pressure and consistently showed its association with the risk of stroke [16, 17]. In a meta-analysis of nine prospective observational studies published between 1958 and 1990, MacMahon et al. concluded that as BP decreased so did the risk of stroke. A decrease in diastolic BP by 5, 7.5, and 10 mmHg was associated with a decreased risk of stroke at least by 34, 46, and 56 %, respectively [16]. The Eastern Stroke and Coronary Heart Disease Collaborative Research Group, a subset of Asia Pacific Cohort Studies Collaboration (APCSC), also showed a positive relationship between diastolic BP and the risk of stroke. Overall, individuals in the group with the highest diastolic BP (DBP≥ 110) had a risk of stroke about 13 times greater than those in the group with the lowest diastolic BP (DBP≤ 79). For each 5 mm decrease in diastolic BP, the risk was almost halved for both ischemic strokes (odds ratio (OR) 0.61, 95 % confidence interval (CI): 0.57–0.66) and hemorrhagic strokes (OR 0.54, 95 % CI: 0.50–0.58) [18]. Systolic BP gained attention around the 1990s after several epidemiological studies suggested that systolic BP might represent a stronger risk factor for stroke than diastolic BP. Moreover, systolic BP increases with advancing age, whereas diastolic BP levels off at approximately age 50 years and decreases after the age of 60 years. Systolic BP has been shown to be a better predictor of coronary heart disease after the age of 50 years [19].

Systolic BP was more strongly correlated with 12-year risk of stroke mortality than diastolic BP in the Framingham Heart Study [20]. Also, the prospective population-based Copenhagen City Heart study reported that systolic BP is a better predictor of stroke than diastolic BP [21]. The APCSC, which analyzed 37 cohort studies conducted in the Asia Pacific region, reported a continuous, log-linear association between systolic BP and risk of stroke down to at least 115 mmHg. After standardizing for age, a 10 mmHg decrease in systolic BP was associated with a 41 % (95 % CI: 40–42 %) lower risk of stroke in Asia and a 30 % (95 % CI: 22–37 %) lower risk of stroke in Australasia [22]. In an analysis of 61 prospective cohort studies by the Prospective Study Collaboration (PSC), there was greater than a twofold reduction in stroke mortality with each 20 mmHg decrease in systolic BP for those aged 40–69 years (*see* Table 2.1) [23, 24].

An important finding from the above studies is that the association between BP and risk of stroke is continuous and log linear at all ages, and there is no evidence of a threshold below which levels of BP are no longer associated with lower risk of stroke, down to approximately 115 mmHg for systolic BP or 75 mmHg for diastolic BP [25]. This finding suggests that whether blood pressure meets the usual definition of hypertension (systolic BP ≥140 mmHg or diastolic BP ≥90 mmHg) or falls within the range of what is typically considered normal, in epidemiological observational studies a lower level of blood pressure has a lower risk of stroke. This steady increase in risk of stroke with increasing systolic BP is also reflected in the stroke risk appraisal score developed by the Framingham Heart study [26, 27].

Age is an important cofactor of the stroke and hypertension relationship. The positive relationship between elevated BP and risk of stroke is weaker in older aged persons compared to middle-aged individuals. The APCSC reported that in the age groups <60, 60–69, and ≥70 years, a 10 mmHg decrease in systolic BP was associated with a 54, 36, and 25 % lower risk of stroke, respectively (Table 2.1) [22]. A similar trend was observed in the PSC and in the nested case–control study from the Rochester Epidemiology Project (Fig. 2.2, Table 2.1) [23, 28]. Data from NHANES 2005 to 2010 found that 76.5 % of US adults ≥80 years of age had hypertension. Of this population, 43.9 % had isolated systolic hypertension (ISH) and 2.0 % had systolic and diastolic hypertension [29]. Although there is a decreased association between risk of stroke and hypertension among older populations, lowering BP is still beneficial due to the high incidence of stroke and high morbidity/mortality rates seen in this group [25].

Table 2.1 Overview of risk of stroke associated with hypertension

	MacMahon et al. [11]		APCSC [17]		PSC [18]		Rochester Epidemiology Project [22]	
Study type	Meta-analysis of 9 prospective cohort studies published between 1963 and 1989		Meta-analysis of 37 prospective cohort studies conducted between 1961 and 1992		Meta-analysis of 61 prospective cohort studies conducted between 1958 and 1990		Nested case–control study	
Number of participants	418,343		425,325		958,074		1862 (931 cases)	
Cases of stroke	843 strokes of all type		5178 strokes of all type		11,960 strokes of all type		931 ischemic strokes	
Age at baseline	25–84		20–107		NR		Age matched controls	
Follow-up period (mean)	6–25 years (10 years)		2–27 years (7 years)		4–25 years (12 years)		15 years[a]	
Sex	Male 96%		Male 57%		NR		Sex matched controls	
Study population	USA, Europe, Puerto Rico		China, Japan, Hong Kong, Taiwan, Singapore, South Korea, New Zealand, Australia		Europe, USA, Japan, China, Australia		USA	
Results	5 mmHg ↓ DBP	34% ↓ risk	*Age*	*10 mmHg ↓ SBP*	*Age*	*20 mmHg ↓ SBP*	*Age*	*OR (cases vs. controls)*
	7.5 mmHg ↓ DBP	46% ↓ risk	<60	54% ↓ stroke risk	40–49	64% ↓ risk	50	4.8
	10 mmHg ↓ DBP	56% ↓ risk	60–69	36% ↓ stroke risk	50–59	62% ↓ risk	60	3.2
			≥70	25% ↓ stroke risk	60–69	57% ↓ risk	70	2.2
					70–79	50% ↓ risk	80	1.5
					80–89	33% ↓ risk	90	1.0
					Age	*10 mmHg ↓ DBP*		
					40–49	65% ↓ risk		
					50–59	66% ↓ risk		
					60–69	60% ↓ risk		
					70–79	52% ↓ risk		
					80–89	37% ↓ risk		

APCSC Asia Pacific Cohort Studies Collaboration, *PSC* Prospective Studies Collaboration, *SBP* systolic blood pressure, *DBP* diastolic blood pressure, *OR* odds ratio, *NR* not reported

[a] Ischemic strokes identified from 15 years follow-up of Rochester Epidemiology Project

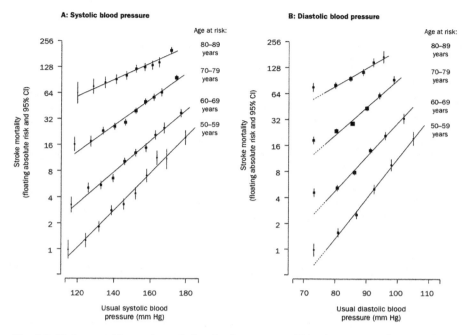

Fig. 2.2 Stoke mortality rate in each decade of age vs. usual blood pressure at the start of that decade. Rates are plotted on a floating absolute scale, and each *square* has area inversely proportional to the effective variance of the log mortality rate (From Lewington S, Clarke R, Qizilbash N, Peto R, Collins R, Prospective Studies C. Age-specific relevance of usual blood pressure to vascular mortality: a meta-analysis of individual data for one million adults in 61 prospective studies. *Lancet.* Dec 14 2002; 360(9349):1903–1913, with permission)

Racial differences in hypertension and risk of stroke have been reported from several observational studies in the United States. The Northern Manhattan Stroke Study showed that hypertension was an independent risk factor for ischemic stroke in whites (OR 1.8), blacks (OR 2.0), and Caribbean Hispanics (OR 1.2) [30]. The Baltimore-Washington Cooperative Young Stroke Study, population-based case–control study (patients aged 18–44 years), showed a positive association between hypertension and risk of ischemic stroke in whites and blacks for both men and women. Age-adjusted ORs (95 % CI) for ischemic stroke for a history of hypertension for white men, white women, black men, and black women were 1.6 (0.7–3.2), 2.5 (1.1–5.9), 3.8 (1.8–7.9), and 4.2 (2.4–7.5), respectively [31]. The same increment in SBP is associated with a higher stroke risk in Blacks than for Whites [32]. For example, for 10 mmHg increase in levels of SBP, the increased stroke risk in whites is ≈8 %; however, a similar 10 mmHg increase in SBP in African Americans is associated with a 24 % increase in stroke risk, an impact three times greater than in whites [33].

Treating hypertension is an important therapeutic target in the prevention of stroke that has been supported by several studies [34–38]. Since stroke is more dependent on blood pressure than coronary heart disease, the relationship between absolute risk of events and number of events prevented is stronger for stroke than coronary heart disease [39–41]. A long-term decrease of 5–6 mmHg in diastolic BP after 2–3 years of continuous treatment was associated with about 35–40% less stroke [40]. In the Hypertension Detection and Follow-up Program study, patients with hypertension receiving standardized antihypertensive therapy had a 5-year incidence of stroke of 1.9 per 100 persons compared to 2.9 per 100 persons among those receiving routine community cares [42]. In the Systolic Hypertension in the Elderly Program, the 5-year incidence of all strokes was 5.2 per 100 with antihypertensive treatment vs. 8.2 per 100 with placebo treatment [43]. A report from the Hypertension in the Very Elderly Trial suggests that patients with hypertension who are 80 years of age or older also benefit from antihypertensive treatment to prevent stroke [44, 45]. The BP-reduction component of the SPS3 trial showed that targeting a SBP <130 mmHg reduce recurrent stroke overall by ≈20% ($P=0.08$) but statistically significantly reduced ICH by two-thirds.

Hypertension as a Risk of Stroke by Stroke Subtype

Stroke is usually classified into two major categories: ischemic stroke and hemorrhagic stroke. Hemorrhagic stroke can be further divided into strokes caused by an intracerebral hemorrhage (ICH) or a subarachnoid hemorrhage (SAH). Approximately 80% of strokes are ischemic, 15% are ICH, and 5% are SAH [46].

Hypertension and Ischemic Stroke

Various schemes have been developed to classify ischemic strokes into further subtypes according to its etiology [47, 48]. Among these stroke subtypes, differences in incidence, recurrence rate, long-term survival, and race have been reported [49, 50]. Several epidemiological studies have also addressed the relationship between risk factors and different stroke subtypes [51–54]. BP is a powerful determinant of risk for both ischemic stroke and intracranial hemorrhage [55]. Differences in the strength of association between hypertension and risk of stroke among stroke subtypes, especially lacunar vs. non-lacunar infarction (or small-vessel disease vs. large-vessel disease), have drawn attention. By using the Stroke Data Bank of the National Institute of Neurological and Communicative Disorders and Stroke, Mast et al. determined that lacunar infarcts, especially multiple ones, were strongly related to hypertension (OR 2.5, 95% CI: 1.1–6.0) [56]. Hsu et al. compared the risk factors of lacunar infarct with those of other stroke subtypes among 240 patients admitted to a stroke unit and noted that lacunar patients were more likely to have hypertension [57]. Among the 5017 patients enrolled in the German Stroke Data Bank, hypertension was significantly more common in microangiopathy (79.4%) than in macroangiopathy (70.0%) cases [58].

However, several studies and a systematic review appear to contradict these results. Schulz et al. observed no differences between stroke subtypes in regards to the association of hypertension and risk of stroke among hospitalized and non-hospitalized ischemic stroke patients [54]. Ohira et al. reported that the impact of baseline hypertension on the incidence of ischemic stroke did not vary according to ischemic stroke subtype in the Atherosclerosis Risk in Communities (ARIC) study data [59]. Similarly, study by Lai et al. showed that while hypertension was the most common risk factor in first-time or recurrent stroke patients, and the history of hypertension was not statistically different by stroke subtypes [60]. A systematic review of 28 studies comparing risk factors in patients with lacunar vs. non-lacunar infarction showed that the association between hypertension and lacunar infarction is only marginally greater than that of non-lacunar infarction when subtypes were defined independently of risk factors [48].

Hemorrhagic Stroke

Intracerebral Hemorrhage

Evidence from several epidemiological studies demonstrates a strong relationship between ICH and hypertension [61–69]. A case–control study of 331 consecutive primary ICH cases enrolled in the Melbourne Risk Factor Study (MERFS) reported a twofold-increased risk of ICH with elevated BP [70]. Another case–control study by Feldmann et al. observed that hypertension is an independent risk factor that confers a sixfold higher risk (OR 5.71, 95 % CI: 3.61–9.05) of ICH among men and women aged 18–49 years (Table 2.2) [71]. A systematic review of 11 case–control and 3 cohort studies on risk factors for ICH in the general population showed a positive association between hypertension and ICH with an overall OR of 3.68 in case–control studies. Among cohort studies, all studies showed a positive association between hypertension and ICH, and two studies showed an increasing risk of ICH with an increasing degree of hypertension (Table 2.2) [72]. This increase in risk of ICH with increase in degree of hypertension has been seen in other epidemiological studies as well. A pooled analysis of the ARIC and the Cardiovascular Health Study (CHS) data also reported this trend. Compared to normal-high normal BP, relative risk (RR) (95 % CI) of ICH was 1.43 (0.90–2.26) for BP 140–159/90–99 mmHg, 2.71 (1.58–4.67) for BP 160–179/100–109 mmHg, and 5.55 (3.07–10.03) for BP ≥ 160/110 mmHg (Table 2.2) [73].

A prospective cohort study carried out within the Alpha-Tocopherol, Beta-Carotene Cancer Prevention (ATBC) Study also found a similar trend. The RR (95 % CI) of ICH was 2.20 (2.28–6.25) for systolic BP 140–159 mmHg and 3.78 (2.28–6.25) for systolic BP ≥ 160 mmHg, compared to systolic BP ≤ 139 mmHg. RR was 2.10 (1.34–3.31) for diastolic BP 90–99 mmHg and 4.17 (2.58–6.74) for diastolic BP ≥ 100 mmHg, compared to diastolic BP ≤ 89 mmHg (Table 2.2) [52]. Sue et al. and others found a similar association in Asians (Table 2.2) [74–76].

Table 2.2 Overview of risk of intracerebral hemorrhage associated with hypertension

	Ariesen et al. [59]	Sturgeon et al. [60]	Suh et al. [61]	Leppälä et al. [40]	Feldmann et al. [58]
Study type	Systematic Review of 11 case–control and 3 cohort studies from 1966 to 2001	Pooled analysis of ARIC and CHS	Prospective cohort study	Prospective cohort study	Case–control study
Number of participants	*Case–control studies* 72–662 *Cohort studies* 28,519–114,793	21,680 (15,792 ARIC, 5888 CHS)	114,793	28,519	636[a]
Cases of ICH	*Case–control studies* 24–331 *Cohort studies* 112–386	135 (61 ARIC, 74 CHS)	372	112	217
Study population		USA	South Korea	Finland	USA
Age	Age matched on most of case–control studies	Mean age 54 (ARIC) Mean age 73 (CHS)	35–59	50–69	18–49

Sex	Sex matched on most of case–control studies	44.8 % male (ARIC) 42.4 % male (CHS)		Male only		Male only		56 % male
Results		*BP*	*RR*	*BP*	*RR*	*SBP*	*RR*	Adjusted OR 5.71
	Case–control studies							
	Overall crude OR 3.68	SBP <140/DBP<90	1.0	SBP<130/DBP<85	1.0	≤139	1.0	
	Cohort studies	SBP140–159/DBP90–99	1.43	SBP130–139/DBP85–89	2.16	140–159	2.20	
	Adjusted RR 1.14–33 by different levels of blood pressure	SBP160–179/DBP100–109	2.71	SBP140–159/DBP90–99	5.32	≥160	3.78	
		SBP≥160/DBP≥110	5.55	SBP160–179/DBP100–109	10.44	*DBP*	*RR*	
		BP as continuous measure		SBP≥180/DBP≥110	33.32	≤89	1.0	
		10 mmHg ↑ SBP: 25 % ↑ risk				90–99	2.10	
		10 mmHg ↑ DBP: 47 % ↑ risk				≥100	4.17	

ICH intracerebral hemorrhage, *SBP* systolic blood pressure, *DBP* diastolic blood pressure, *BP* blood pressure, *OR* odds ratio, *RR* relative risk, *ARIC* Atherosclerosis Risk in Communities Study, *CHS* Cardiovascular Health Study

aCases and controls matched on race, age, and gender

The increased risk associated with blood pressure does not seem to be restricted to clinical hypertension. Studies have shown that blood pressure increases within the normal range are also associated with a linear increase in the risk of ICH [52]. Additionally, the risk of ICH increases with hypertension, in persons who are not compliant with antihypertensive medication, are 55 years of age or younger, or are smokers [77]. Improved control of hypertension appears to reduce the incidence of ICH [78]. Given the strength of association, the high prevalence of hypertension, and the readily available treatment options, blood pressure control is considered the main option for prevention of ICH [79].

Patients receiving long-term oral anticoagulation medication are also at increased risk for ICH [80]. Several risk factors of anticoagulation-associated bleeding have been investigated: advanced age, history of myocardial infarction or ischemic heart disease, diabetes, cerebrovascular disease, concomitant use of antiplatelet agents, intensity of anticoagulation, and hypertension [81, 82]. A retrospective study by Wintzen et al. found that hypertension was present in 80 % of the anticoagulant-associated ICH patients and was the most important predisposing condition [83]. Given that warfarin use has rapidly increased in the last decades, studies have also shown a drastic increase in ICH related to warfarin use, though this notion is contested by other studies [80, 84]. Launbjerg et al. found that hypertension was an independent risk factor for anticoagulant-related bleeding in a multivariate analysis of 551 anticoagulated patients in 1010 treatment years of follow-up [85]. Analysis of pooled data from five randomized trials indicates that the patients who had an ICH while taking warfarin had higher systolic and diastolic BPs at study entry than those warfarin-treated patients who did not have ICH [86]. On the other hand, a case–control study, comparing 170 patients who developed ICH during warfarin therapy and 1020 matched anticoagulated patients who did not have ICH, found no statistical difference in the prevalence of diagnosed hypertension [87].

The effect of hypertension on mortality in anticoagulation-associated ICH has also been investigated. A retrospective study by Fric-Shamji et al. reported that higher initial mean arterial pressure was correlated with the propensity of hematoma to expand after initial imaging and might partially explain the effect on mortality [87].

Subarachnoid Hemorrhage

Smoking, hypertension, and excessive alcohol use are the most important modifiable risk factors for SAH [88]. An overview of all observational studies of risk factors for SAH published in English from 1966 through March 2005 reported a positive relationship between hypertension and SAH in both cohort (RR 2.5, 95 % CI: 2.0–3.1) and case–control studies (OR 2.6, 95 % CI: 2.0–3.1) (Table 2.3) [88]. In 1996, a review of 9 longitudinal and 11 case–control studies identified preexisting hypertension as a significant risk factor for the development of SAH, with a relative risk of 2.8 (for longitudinal studies; 95 % confidence interval [CI], 2.1–3.6) and an OR of 2.9 (for case control studies; 95 % CI 2.4–3.7). Associations between diurnal variations in blood pressure and risk of aSAH have also been reported [89, 90]. A reanalysis of patient data in the APCSC demonstrated that hypertension was an independent risk factor for SAH (hazard ratio (HR) 2.0, 95 % CI: 1.5–2.7) (refer Table 2.3). The risk of SAH increases sharply with the increase in systolic BP [91]. This trend was also seen in a large cohort study among Asian populations for both men and women (Table 2.3) [75].

Since the rupture of a cerebral aneurysm causes most SAHs, several studies have attempted to identify risk factors for the rupture/growth of an aneurysm. Chronically elevated systolic blood pressure (SBP) has been shown to be a strong predictor of intracranial aneurysm rupture. In a recent publication from the Nord-Trøndelag Health (HUNT) study, a large population-based study in Norway, both mild (SBP 130–139 mmHg) and severe (SBP > 170 mmHg) chronic elevations of SBP were associated with an increased risk of aSAH in the 22-year follow-up period compared with those with SBP of less than 130 mmHg (hazard ratios of 2.3 and 3.3, respectively) [92]. Family history, age and modifiable risk factors, including cigarette smoking, and hypertension have been thought to increase the risk of rupture [93–95]. Among patients with small aneurysms (≤7 mm), hypertension, relatively young age, and posterior circulation location have been reported as significant risk factors for rupture [96]. However, a few studies, using magnetic resonance angiography or computed tomography angiography to assess aneurysm growth, did not find any relation between aneurysmal growth and hypertension [97–99].

Hypertension and Stroke Recurrence

Ischemic Stroke Recurrence

Despite extensive translational and clinical research, concerted patient education with regard to vascular risk factors and lifestyle modifications, and a serious effort on the part of health care professionals over the last few decades, only one-third of hypertensive patients have blood pressure (BP) controlled to recommended levels of <140/90 mmHg for uncomplicated hypertension and <130/80 mmHg for patients with diabetes mellitus or renal disease. For those with uncontrolled hypertension, the risk of stroke is dramatically increased. In a US population-based study, the estimation of population attributable risks has revealed that 9–16 % of all ischemic stroke cases can be avoided by eliminating hypertension alone [100].

Since lowering BP might worsen cerebral perfusion if autoregulation is impaired or if a severe carotid artery stenosis is present, lowering BP during the acute phase of ischemic stroke has been debated. However, several trials have confirmed that long-term BP control can reduce stroke recurrence [25, 35]. A meta-analysis by Gueyffier et al. reported a 28 % reduction in the risk of stroke recurrence without any significant adverse effect with antihypertensive drug treatment in hypertensive stroke patients [101]. The United Kingdom Transient Ischemic Attack Collaborative

Table 2.3 Overview of risk of subarachnoid hemorrhage associated with hypertension

	KMIC Study [62]	Feigin et al. [77]	Asia Pacific Cohort Studies Collaboration [78]
Study type	Prospective cohort study	Systematic review of 14 cohort and 23 case–control studies published between 1966 and 2005	Meta analysis of 26 cohort studies
Cases of SAH	308	3936 (cohort 892 case–control 3044)	236
Study population	South Korea	Cohort studies: USA, Japan, UK, South Korea, Finland. Case–control studies: Finland, UK, USA, NZ, Portugal, Norway, Japan, Australia, Germany, WHO (Africa/Asia/Europe/Latin America)	Japan, China, Taiwan, South Korea, Singapore, Australia, NZ

Results

KMIC Study [62]

BP	RR
Male	
SBP<120/DBP<80	1.0
SBP 120–129/DBP 80–84	1.46
SBP 130–139/DBP 85–89	2.41
SBP 140–159/DBP 90–99	2.92
SBP 160–179/DBP 100–109	3.66
SBP≥160/DBP≥110	5.12
Female	
SBP<120/DBP<80	1.0
SBP 120–129/DBP 80–84	1.77
SBP 130–139/DBP 85–89	2.60
SBP 140–159/DBP 90–99	3.82
SBP 160–179/DBP 100–109	9.06
SBP≥160/DBP≥110	20.49

Feigin et al. [77]

Cohort studies		
Sex	RR	
Female	3.3	
Male	2.3	
Total	2.5	
Case–control studies		
Sex	OR	
Female	3.3	
Male	2.1	
Total	2.6	

Asia Pacific Cohort Studies Collaboration [78]

BP	HR
SBP<140	1.0
SBP≥140	2.0
10-mmHg ↑ SBP: 31 % ↑ risk	

KMIC Korea Medical Insurance Corporation, *SAH* subarachnoid hemorrhage, *SBP* systolic blood pressure, *DBP* diastolic blood pressure, *BP* blood pressure, *RR* relative risk, *OR* odds ratio, *HR* hazard ratio

Group, which followed patients with a recent history of transient ischemic attack, amaurosis fugax, or minor stroke for average of 4 years, reported a direct and continuous relationship of both diastolic and systolic pressure with recurrence of stroke. Each 5 mmHg reduction in diastolic pressure and each 10 mmHg reduction in systolic pressure were associated with 34 and 28 % fewer strokes, respectively [101]. A systematic review of seven randomized control trials reported a 24 % (95 % CI: 8–37) reduction in recurrent strokes in patients with prior ischemic or hemorrhagic stroke or transient ischemic attack with lowering blood pressure or treating hypertension with a variety of antihypertensive agents [102]. In the Perindopril Protection Against Recurrent Stroke Study (PROGRESS), antihypertensive treatment resulted in a 43 % (95 % CI: 30–54) reduction in stroke recurrence in hypertensive and non-hypertensive patients with history of stroke or transient ischemic attack [103].

Hemorrhagic Stroke Recurrence

Both European and Asian studies have suggested that hypertension is a risk factor for recurrence of ICH [104–108]. Yen et al. reported a high prevalence of hypertension among recurrent ICH patients in the Taiwanese population (88.2 %) [109]. Poor control of arterial hypertension was detected in 7 % of hypertensive patients without rebleeding and in 47 % of hypertensive patients with rebleeding in a cohort of 112 survivors of a first primary ICH in an average 84.1 months of follow-up [110]. After a review of 43 recurrent ICH patients admitted to their hospital, Bae et al. reported an increased risk of recurrent hemorrhage among patients who had antihypertensive therapy of less than 3 months after the initial ICH compared to those with long-term therapy [111]. This finding suggests that long-term control of hypertension is necessary to prevent a recurrence of hemorrhage.

In this section, we have discussed hypertension as a risk of stroke recurrence on ischemic and hemorrhagic stroke separately. However, hypertension has also been reported as an independent risk factor of ICH among ischemic stroke patients (SBP $\geq$ 140 HR 2.07, 95 % CI: 1.23–3.83) [112].

Importance of Systolic Blood Pressure in Elderly

Aging is associated with an increase in systolic BP and, consequently, ISH (systolic BP $\geq$ 140 mmHg and diastolic BP < 90 mmHg) is the most common subtype of hypertension in elderly populations. As the elderly population of most developed countries is projected to increase [113], ISH will continue to gain attention. The rise in systolic BP in ISH is mainly due to a decreased elasticity of the large arteries and is not necessarily accompanied by a rise in mean arterial blood pressure or in peripheral resistance [114].

Epidemiological studies have indicated that ISH is an independent risk factor for stroke and a potent modifiable target for reducing the risk for stroke. In the Framingham Heart study, individuals with ISH had an increased incidence of stroke independent of age and arterial rigidity [20]. In the Honolulu Heart program, the RR of stroke from ISH in Japanese-American men aged 45–54 years and men aged 55–68 years was 4.8 and 1.2, respectively [115]. In the NHANES long-term follow-up study, stroke risk was significantly higher in individuals with ISH (RR 2.7, 95 % CI: 2.0–3.4) [116]. Meta-analysis of eight clinical trials including 15,693 patients with ISH showed that the HR for stroke associated with a 10 mmHg higher initial systolic BP was 1.22 and active treatment of hypertension reduced stroke by 30 % [117].

Conclusion

In this chapter, current data pertinent to hypertension and its risk of stroke are reviewed. The prevention and management of hypertension are major public health challenges [118]. Despite the availability of therapies, it has been reported that even in developed countries, many patients with hypertension remain undetected or untreated [119] The 2009–2012 data from NHANES/NCHS in comparison to 2005–2006 data showed an increase of 4 % (from 78.7 to 82.7 %) of adult Americans with hypertension had awareness of their condition, 76.5 % were under current treatment, and almost 9 % (45.4–54.1 %) had it under control (NCHS and National Heart, Lung, and Blood Institute (NHLBI)) [120]. Data from the Framingham Heart study show that control rates of BP in men <60, 60–79, and ≥80 years of age were 38 %, 36 %, and 38 %, respectively. For women in the same age groups, they were 38 %, 28 %, and 23 %, respectively [120].

It is not surprising that nontreatment or nonoptimal treatment of hypertension is associated with an excess risk of stroke. Compared with treated and controlled hypertensives, the RR of stroke for treated and uncontrolled hypertensives and for untreated hypertensives who needed treatment was 1.30 (95 % CI: 0.70–2.44) and 1.76 (95 % CI: 1.05–2.94), respectively [121]. It has been reported that there is a lack of blood pressure control, particularly in the early morning hours in patients receiving seemingly effective antihypertensive therapy [122, 123]. This so-called "morning blood pressure surge" is reported to coincide with a higher prevalence of multiple silent infarcts on magnetic resonance imaging and an increased risk for stroke [124]. Elliott et al. performed a meta-analysis of 31 publications and reported a 79 % (95 % CI: 72–87 %) increase in stroke of all types between 6:00 a.m. and noon compared to the other 18 h of the day [125]. Current evidence suggests that ambulatory blood pressure monitoring may provide a more sensitive means of detecting patients at risk and monitoring therapeutic effect [126]. More studies on how to effectively control hypertension are needed to prevent stroke.

References

1. US Burden of Disease Collaborators. The State of US Health, 1990-2010. Burden of disease, injuries, and risk factors. JAMA. 2013;310(6):519–608.
2. Dahlof B. Prevention of stroke in patients with hypertension. Am J Cardiol. 2007;100:17J–24.
3. Sacco RL. Identifying patient populations at high risk for stroke. Neurology. 1998;51:S27–30.
4. Murray CJ, et al. Disability-adjusted life years (DALYs) for 291 diseases and injuries in 21 regions, 1990-2010: a systematic analysis for the Global Burden of Disease Study 2010. Lancet. 2012;380:2197–223.
5. Mozaffarian D, Benjamin EJ, Go AS, Arnett DK, Blaha MJ, Cushman M, de Ferranti S, Despres JP, Fullerton HJ, Howard VJ, Huffman MD, Judd SE, Kissela BM, Lackland DT, Lichtman JH, Lisabeth LD, Liu S, Mackey RH, Matchar DB, McGuire DK, Mohler III ER, Moy CS, Muntner P, Mussolino ME, Nasir K, Neumar RW, Nichol G, Palaniappan L, Pandey DK, Reeves MJ, Rodriguez CJ, Sorlie PD, Stein J, Towfighi A, Turan TN, Virani SS, Willey JZ, Woo D, Yeh RW, Turner MB, American Heart Association Statistics Committee, Stroke Statistics Subcommittee. Heart disease and stroke statistics—2015 update: a report from the American Heart Association. Circulation. 2015;131:e29–322.
6. Lloyd-Jones D, Adams R, Carnethon M, De Simone G, Ferguson TB, Flegal K, Ford E, Furie K, Go A, Greenlund K, Haase N, Hailpern S, Ho M, Howard V, Kissela B, Kittner S, Lackland D, Lisabeth L, Marelli A, McDermott M, Meigs J, Mozaffarian D, Nichol G, O'Donnell C, Roger V, Rosamond W, Sacco R, Sorlie P, Stafford R, Steinberger J, Thom T, Wasserthiel-Smoller S, Wong N, Wylie-Rosett J, Hong Y, American Heart Association Statistics Committee, Stroke Statistics Subcommittee. Heart disease and stroke statistics—2009 update: a report from the American Heart Association Statistics Committee and Stroke Statistics Subcommittee. Circulation. 2009;119:e21–181.
7. Fields LE, Burt VL, Cutler JA, Hughes J, Roccella EJ, Sorlie P. The burden of adult hypertension in the United States 1999 to 2000: a rising tide. Hypertension. 2004;44:398–404.
8. Ervin RB. Prevalence of metabolic syndrome among adults 20 years of age and over, by sex, age, race and ethnicity, and body mass index: United States, 2003-2006. Natl Health Stat Rep. 2009;13:1–7.
9. Kuczmarski RJ, Ogden CL, Grummer-Strawn LM, Flegal KM, Guo SS, Wei R, Mei Z, Curtin LR, Roche AF, Johnson CL. CDC growth charts: United States. Adv Data. 2000;314:1–27.
10. Vasan RS, Beiser A, Seshadri S, Larson MG, Kannel WB, D'Agostino RB, Levy D. Residual lifetime risk for developing hypertension in middle-aged women and men: The Framingham Heart Study. JAMA. 2002;287:1003–10.
11. Cook S, Auinger P, Li C, Ford ES. Metabolic syndrome rates in United States adolescents, from the National Health and Nutrition Examination Survey, 1999-2002. J Pediatr. 2008;152:165–70.
12. Krishnamoorthy S, Lip GY. Hypertension, stroke and the impact of atrial fibrillation. Expert Rev Cardiovasc Ther. 2008;6:1287–9.
13. Kannel WB, Wolf PA, Verter J, McNamara PM. Epidemiologic assessment of the role of blood pressure in stroke. The Framingham study. JAMA. 1970;214:301–10.
14. Seshadri S, Beiser A, Kelly-Hayes M, Kase CS, Au R, Kannel WB, Wolf PA. The lifetime risk of stroke: estimates from the Framingham Study. Stroke. 2006;37:345–50.
15. Lee M, Saver JL, Chang B, Chang KH, Hao Q, Ovbiagele B. Presence of baseline prehypertension and risk of incident stroke: a meta-analysis. Neurology. 2011;77:1330–7.
16. MacMahon S, Peto R, Cutler J, Collins R, Sorlie P, Neaton J, Abbott R, Godwin J, Dyer A, Stamler J. Blood pressure, stroke, and coronary heart disease. Part 1, Prolonged differences in blood pressure: prospective observational studies corrected for the regression dilution bias. Lancet. 1990;335:765–74.
17. Anonymous. Cholesterol, diastolic blood pressure, and stroke: 13,000 strokes in 450,000 people in 45 prospective cohorts. Prospective studies collaboration. Lancet. 1995;346:1647–53.
18. Anonymous. Blood pressure, cholesterol, and stroke in eastern Asia. Eastern Stroke and Coronary Heart Disease Collaborative Research Group. Lancet. 1998;352:1801–7.

19. Franklin SS, Larson MG, Khan SA, Wong ND, Leip EP, Kannel WB, Levy D. Does the relation of blood pressure to coronary heart disease risk change with aging? The Framingham Heart Study. Circulation. 2001;103:1245–9.
20. Kannel WB, Wolf PA, McGee DL, Dawber TR, McNamara P, Castelli WP. Systolic blood pressure, arterial rigidity, and risk of stroke. The Framingham study. JAMA. 1981;245:1225–9.
21. Nielsen WB, Lindenstrom E, Vestbo J, Jensen GB. Is diastolic hypertension an independent risk factor for stroke in the presence of normal systolic blood pressure in the middle-aged and elderly? Am J Hypertens. 1997;10:634–9.
22. Lawes CM, Rodgers A, Bennett DA, Parag V, Suh I, Ueshima H, MacMahon S, Asia Pacific Cohort Studies Collaboration. Blood pressure and cardiovascular disease in the Asia Pacific region. J Hypertens. 2003;21:707–16.
23. Lewington S, Clarke R, Qizilbash N, Peto R, Collins R, Prospective Studies Collaboration. Age-specific relevance of usual blood pressure to vascular mortality: a meta-analysis of individual data for one million adults in 61 prospective studies. Lancet. 2002;360:1903–13.
24. SPS3 Study Group, Benavente OR, Coffey CS, Conwit R, Hart RG, McClure LA, Pearce LA, Pergola PE, Szychowski JM. Blood-pressure targets in patients with recent lacunar stroke: the SPS3 randomised trial. Lancet. 2013;382:507–15.
25. Lawes CM, Bennett DA, Feigin VL, Rodgers A. Blood pressure and stroke: an overview of published reviews. Stroke. 2004;35:776–85.
26. D'Agostino RB, Wolf PA, Belanger AJ, Kannel WB. Stroke risk profile: adjustment for antihypertensive medication. The Framingham Study. Stroke. 1994;25:40–3.
27. Wolf PA, D'Agostino RB, Belanger AJ, Kannel WB. Probability of stroke: a risk profile from the Framingham Study. Stroke. 1991;22:312–8.
28. Whisnant JP, Wiebers DO, O'Fallon WM, Sicks JD, Frye RL. A population-based model of risk factors for ischemic stroke: Rochester, Minnesota. Neurology. 1996;47:1420–8.
29. Chen W, Srinivasan SR, Li S, Xu J, Berenson GS. Clustering of long-term trends in metabolic syndrome variables from childhood to adulthood in Blacks and Whites: the Bogalusa Heart Study. Am J Epidemiol. 2007;166:527–33.
30. Sacco RL, Boden-Albala B, Abel G, Lin IF, Elkind M, Hauser WA, Paik MC, Shea S. Race-ethnic disparities in the impact of stroke risk factors: the northern Manhattan stroke study. Stroke. 2001;32:1725–31.
31. Rohr J, Kittner S, Feeser B, Hebel JR, Whyte MG, Weinstein A, Kanarak N, Buchholz D, Earley C, Johnson C, Macko R, Price T, Sloan M, Stern B, Wityk R, Wozniak M, Sherwin R. Traditional risk factors and ischemic stroke in young adults: the Baltimore-Washington Cooperative Young Stroke Study. Arch Neurol. 1996;53:603–7.
32. Go AS, Mozaffarian D, Roger VL, Benjamin EJ, Berry JD, Blaha MJ, Dai S, Ford ES, Fox CS, Franco S, Fullerton HJ, Gillespie C, Hailpern SM, Heit JA, Howard VJ, Huffman MD, Judd SE, Kissela BM, Kittner SJ, Lackland DT, Lichtman JH, Lisabeth LD, Mackey RH, Magid DJ, Marcus GM, Marelli A, Matchar DB, McGuire DK, Mohler III ER, Moy CS, Mussolino ME, Neumar RW, Nichol G, Pandey DK, Paynter NP, Reeves MJ, Sorlie PD, Stein J, Towfighi A, Turan TN, Virani SS, Wong ND, Woo D, Turner MB, American Heart Association Statistics Committee, Stroke Statistics Subcommittee. Heart disease and stroke statistics—2014 update: a report from the American Heart Association. Circulation. 2014;129:e28–292.
33. Howard G, Lackland DT, Kleindorfer DO, Kissela BM, Moy CS, Judd SE, Safford MM, Cushman M, Glasser SP, Howard VJ. Racial differences in the impact of elevated systolic blood pressure on stroke risk. JAMA Intern Med. 2013;173:46–51.
34. Howard G, Cushman M, Kissela BM, Kleindorfer DO, McClure LA, Safford MM, Rhodes JD, Soliman EZ, Moy CS, Judd SE, Howard VJ, REasons for Geographic And Racial Differences in Stroke (REGARDS) Investigators. Traditional risk factors as the underlying cause of racial disparities in stroke: lessons from the half-full (empty?) glass. Stroke. 2011;42:3369–75.
35. Zhang H, Thijs L, Staessen JA. Blood pressure lowering for primary and secondary prevention of stroke. Hypertension. 2006;48:187–95.
36. Grassi G, Arenare F, Trevano FQ, Dell'Oro R, Mancia AG. Primary and secondary prevention of stroke by antihypertensive treatment in clinical trials. Curr Hypertens Rep. 2007;9:299–304.

37. Kubo M, Hata J, Doi Y, Tanizaki Y, Iida M, Kiyohara Y. Secular trends in the incidence of and risk factors for ischemic stroke and its subtypes in Japanese population. Circulation. 2008;118:2672–8.
38. Campbell NR, Brant R, Johansen H, Walker RL, Wielgosz A, Onysko J, Gao RN, Sambell C, Phillips S, McAlister FA, Canadian Hypertension Education Program Outcomes Research Task Force. Increases in antihypertensive prescriptions and reductions in cardiovascular events in Canada. Hypertension. 2009;53:128–34.
39. Messerli FH, Williams B, Ritz E. Essential hypertension. Lancet. 2007;370:591–603.
40. Collins R, Peto R, MacMahon S, Hebert P, Fiebach NH, Eberlein KA, Godwin J, Qizilbash N, Taylor JO, Hennekens CH. Blood pressure, stroke, and coronary heart disease. Part 2, Short-term reductions in blood pressure: overview of randomised drug trials in their epidemiological context. Lancet. 1990;335:827–38.
41. James PA, Oparil S, Carter BL, Cushman WC, Dennison-Himmelfarb C, Handler J, Lackland DT, LeFevre ML, MacKenzie TD, Ogedegbe O, Smith Jr SC, Svetkey LP, Taler SJ, Townsend RR, Wright Jr JT, Narva AS, Ortiz E. 2014 evidence-based guideline for the management of high blood pressure in adults: report from the panel members appointed to the Eighth Joint National Committee (JNC 8). JAMA. 2014;311:507–20.
42. Anonymous. Five-year findings of the hypertension detection and follow-up program. III. Reduction in stroke incidence among persons with high blood pressure. Hypertension Detection and Follow-up Program Cooperative Group. JAMA. 1982;247:633–8.
43. Anonymous. Prevention of stroke by antihypertensive drug treatment in older persons with isolated systolic hypertension. Final results of the Systolic Hypertension in the Elderly Program (SHEP). SHEP Cooperative Research Group. JAMA. 1991;265:3255–64.
44. Bromfield SG, Bowling CB, Tanner RM, Peralta CA, Odden MC, Oparil S, Muntner P. Trends in hypertension prevalence, awareness, treatment, and control among US adults 80 years and older, 1988-2010. J Clin Hypertens (Greenwich). 2014;16:270–6.
45. Beckett NS, Peters R, Fletcher AE, Staessen JA, Liu L, Dumitrascu D, Stoyanovsky V, Antikainen RL, Nikitin Y, Anderson C, Belhani A, Forette F, Rajkumar C, Thijs L, Banya W, Bulpitt CJ, HYVET Study Group. Treatment of hypertension in patients 80 years of age or older. N Engl J Med. 2008;358:1887–98.
46. Warlow C, Sudlow C, Dennis M, Wardlaw J, Sandercock P. Stroke. Lancet. 2003;362:1211–24.
47. Adams Jr HP, Bendixen BH, Kappelle LJ, Biller J, Love BB, Gordon DL, Marsh III EE. Classification of subtype of acute ischemic stroke. Definitions for use in a multicenter clinical trial. TOAST. Trial of Org 10172 in Acute Stroke Treatment. Stroke. 1993;24:35–41.
48. Jackson C, Sudlow C. Are lacunar strokes really different? A systematic review of differences in risk factor profiles between lacunar and nonlacunar infarcts. Stroke. 2005;36:891–901.
49. Kolominsky-Rabas PL, Weber M, Gefeller O, Neundoerfer B, Heuschmann PU. Epidemiology of ischemic stroke subtypes according to TOAST criteria: incidence, recurrence, and long-term survival in ischemic stroke subtypes: a population-based study. Stroke. 2001;32:2735–40.
50. Markus HS, Khan U, Birns J, Evans A, Kalra L, Rudd AG, Wolfe CD, Jerrard-Dunne P. Differences in stroke subtypes between black and white patients with stroke: the South London Ethnicity and Stroke Study. Circulation. 2007;116:2157–64.
51. Sacco RL. Risk factors, outcomes, and stroke subtypes for ischemic stroke. Neurology. 1997;49:S39–44.
52. Leppala JM, Virtamo J, Fogelholm R, Albanes D, Heinonen OP. Different risk factors for different stroke subtypes: association of blood pressure, cholesterol, and antioxidants. Stroke. 1999;30:2535–40.
53. Kirshner HS. Differentiating ischemic stroke subtypes: risk factors and secondary prevention. J Neurol Sci. 2009;279:1–8.
54. Schulz UG, Rothwell PM. Differences in vascular risk factors between etiological subtypes of ischemic stroke: importance of population-based studies. Stroke. 2003;34:2050–9.

55. White CL, Pergola PE, Szychowski JM, Talbert R, Cervantes-Arriaga A, Clark HD, Del Brutto OH, Godoy IE, Hill MD, Pelegri A, Sussman CR, Taylor AA, Valdivia J, Anderson DC, Conwit R, Benavente OR, SPS3 Investigators. Blood pressure after recent stroke: baseline findings from the secondary prevention of small subcortical strokes trial. Am J Hypertens. 2013;26:1114–22.

56. Mast H, Thompson JL, Lee SH, Mohr JP, Sacco RL. Hypertension and diabetes mellitus as determinants of multiple lacunar infarcts. Stroke. 1995;26:30–3.

57. Hsu LC, Hu HH, Chang CC, Sheng WY, Wang SJ, Wong WJ. Comparison of risk factors for lacunar infarcts and other stroke subtypes. Zhonghua Yi Xue Za Zhi (Taipei). 1997;59:225–31.

58. Grau AJ, Weimar C, Buggle F, Heinrich A, Goertler M, Neumaier S, Glahn J, Brandt T, Hacke W, Diener HC. Risk factors, outcome, and treatment in subtypes of ischemic stroke: the German stroke data bank. Stroke. 2001;32:2559–66.

59. Ohira T, Shahar E, Chambless LE, Rosamond WD, Mosley Jr TH, Folsom AR. Risk factors for ischemic stroke subtypes: the Atherosclerosis Risk in Communities study. Stroke. 2006;37:2493–8.

60. Lai SL, Weng HH, Lee M, Hsiao MC, Lin LJ, Huang WY. Risk factors and subtype analysis of acute ischemic stroke. Eur Neurol. 2008;60:230–6.

61. Abu-Zeid HA, Choi NW, Maini KK, Hsu PH, Nelson NA. Relative role of factors associated with cerebral infarction and cerebral hemorrhage. A matched pair case-control study. Stroke. 1977;8:106–12.

62. Brott T, Thalinger K, Hertzberg V. Hypertension as a risk factor for spontaneous intracerebral hemorrhage. Stroke. 1986;17:1078–83.

63. Calandre L, Arnal C, Ortega JF, Bermejo F, Felgeroso B, del Ser T, Vallejo A. Risk factors for spontaneous cerebral hematomas. Case-control study. Stroke. 1986;17:1126–8.

64. Zia E, Pessah-Rasmussen H, Khan FA, Norrving B, Janzon L, Berglund G, Engstrom G. Risk factors for primary intracerebral hemorrhage: a population-based nested case-control study. Cerebrovasc Dis. 2006;21:18–25.

65. Giroud M, Creisson E, Fayolle H, Andre N, Becker F, Martin D, Dumas R. Risk factors for primary cerebral hemorrhage: a population-based study—the Stroke Registry of Dijon. Neuroepidemiology. 1995;14:20–6.

66. Juvela S, Hillbom M, Palomaki H. Risk factors for spontaneous intracerebral hemorrhage. Stroke. 1995;26:1558–64.

67. Qureshi AI, Suri MA, Safdar K, Ottenlips JR, Janssen RS, Frankel MR. Intracerebral hemorrhage in blacks. Risk factors, subtypes, and outcome. Stroke. 1997;28:961–4.

68. Hanggi D, Steiger HJ. Spontaneous intracerebral haemorrhage in adults: a literature overview. Acta Neurochir (Wien). 2008;150:371–9, discussion 379.

69. Woo D, Sauerbeck LR, Kissela BM, Khoury JC, Szaflarski JP, Gebel J, Shukla R, Pancioli AM, Jauch EC, Menon AG, Deka R, Carrozzella JA, Moomaw CJ, Fontaine RN, Broderick JP. Genetic and environmental risk factors for intracerebral hemorrhage: preliminary results of a population-based study. Stroke. 2002;33:1190–5.

70. Thrift AG, McNeil JJ, Forbes A, Donnan GA. Risk factors for cerebral hemorrhage in the era of well-controlled hypertension. Melbourne Risk Factor Study (MERFS) Group. Stroke. 1996;27:2020–5.

71. Feldmann E, Broderick JP, Kernan WN, Viscoli CM, Brass LM, Brott T, Morgenstern LB, Wilterdink JL, Horwitz RI. Major risk factors for intracerebral hemorrhage in the young are modifiable. Stroke. 2005;36:1881–5.

72. Ariesen MJ, Claus SP, Rinkel GJ, Algra A. Risk factors for intracerebral hemorrhage in the general population: a systematic review. Stroke. 2003;34:2060–5.

73. Sturgeon JD, Folsom AR, Longstreth Jr WT, Shahar E, Rosamond WD, Cushman M. Risk factors for intracerebral hemorrhage in a pooled prospective study. Stroke. 2007;38:2718–25.

74. Suh I, Jee SH, Kim HC, Nam CM, Kim IS, Appel LJ. Low serum cholesterol and haemorrhagic stroke in men: Korea Medical Insurance Corporation Study. Lancet. 2001;357:922–5.

75. Kim HC, Nam CM, Jee SH, Suh I. Comparison of blood pressure-associated risk of intracerebral hemorrhage and Subarachnoid hemorrhage (SAH): Korea Medical Insurance Corporation study. Hypertension. 2005;46:393–7.
76. Woodward M, Huxley H, Lam TH, Barzi F, Lawes CM, Ueshima H, Asia Pacific Cohort Studies Collaboration. A comparison of the associations between risk factors and cardiovascular disease in Asia and Australasia. Eur J Cardiovasc Prev Rehabil. 2005;12:484–91.
77. Thrift AG, McNeil JJ, Forbes A, Donnan GA. Three important subgroups of hypertensive persons at greater risk of intracerebral hemorrhage. Melbourne Risk Factor Study Group. Hypertension. 1998;31:1223–9.
78. Furlan AJ, Whisnant JP, Elveback LR. The decreasing incidence of primary intracerebral hemorrhage: a population study. Ann Neurol. 1979;5:367–73.
79. Ikram MA, Wieberdink RG, Koudstaal PJ. International epidemiology of intracerebral hemorrhage. Curr Atheroscler Rep. 2012;14:300–6.
80. Flaherty ML, Kissela B, Woo D, Kleindorfer D, Alwell K, Sekar P, Moomaw CJ, Haverbusch M, Broderick JP. The increasing incidence of anticoagulant-associated intracerebral hemorrhage. Neurology. 2007;68:116–21.
81. Cavallini A, Fanucchi S, Persico A. Warfarin-associated intracerebral hemorrhage. Neurol Sci. 2008;29 Suppl 2:S266–8.
82. Hylek EM, Singer DE. Risk factors for intracranial hemorrhage in outpatients taking warfarin. Ann Intern Med. 1994;120:897–902.
83. Wintzen AR, de Jonge H, Loeliger EA, Bots GT. The risk of intracerebral hemorrhage during oral anticoagulant treatment: a population study. Ann Neurol. 1984;16:553–8.
84. Huhtakangas J, Tetri S, Juvela S, Saloheimo P, Bode MK, Hillbom M. Effect of increased warfarin use on warfarin-related cerebral hemorrhage: a longitudinal population-based study. Stroke. 2011;42:2431–5.
85. Launbjerg J, Egeblad H, Heaf J, Nielsen NH, Fugleholm AM, Ladefoged K. Bleeding complications to oral anticoagulant therapy: multivariate analysis of 1010 treatment years in 551 outpatients. J Intern Med. 1991;229:351–5.
86. Anonymous. Risk factors for stroke and efficacy of antithrombotic therapy in atrial fibrillation. Analysis of pooled data from five randomized controlled trials. Arch Intern Med. 1994;154:1449–57.
87. Fric-Shamji EC, Shamji MF, Cole J, Benoit BG. Modifiable risk factors for intracerebral hemorrhage: study of anticoagulated patients. Can Fam Physician. 2008;54:1138–9, 1139. e1–4.
88. Feigin VL, Rinkel GJ, Lawes CM, Algra A, Bennett DA, van Gijn J, Anderson CS. Risk factors for Subarachnoid hemorrhage (SAH): an updated systematic review of epidemiological studies. Stroke. 2005;36:2773–80.
89. Fogelholm RR, Turjanmaa VM, Nuutila MT, Murros KE, Sarna S. Diurnal blood pressure variations and onset of subarachnoid haemorrhage: a population-based study. J Hypertens. 1995;13:495–8.
90. Teunissen LL, Rinkel GJ, Algra A, van Gijn J. Risk factors for Subarachnoid hemorrhage (SAH): a systematic review. Stroke. 1996;27:544–9.
91. Feigin V, Parag V, Lawes CM, Rodgers A, Suh I, Woodward M, Jamrozik K, Ueshima H, Asia Pacific Cohort Studies Collaboration. Smoking and elevated blood pressure are the most important risk factors for subarachnoid hemorrhage in the Asia-Pacific region: an overview of 26 cohorts involving 306,620 participants. Stroke. 2005;36:1360–5.
92. Sandvei MS, Romundstad PR, Muller TB, Vatten L, Vik A. Risk factors for aneurysmal subarachnoid hemorrhage in a prospective population study: the HUNT study in Norway. Stroke. 2009;40:1958–62.
93. Clarke M. Systematic review of reviews of risk factors for intracranial aneurysms. Neuroradiology. 2008;50:653–64.
94. Juvela S, Porras M, Poussa K. Natural history of unruptured intracranial aneurysms: probability of and risk factors for aneurysm rupture. J Neurosurg. 2000;93:379–87.

95. Morita A, Fujiwara S, Hashi K, Ohtsu H, Kirino T. Risk of rupture associated with intact cerebral aneurysms in the Japanese population: a systematic review of the literature from Japan. J Neurosurg. 2005;102:601–6.
96. Nahed BV, DiLuna ML, Morgan T, Ocal E, Hawkins AA, Ozduman K, Kahle KT, Chamberlain A, Amar AP, Gunel M. Hypertension, age, and location predict rupture of small intracranial aneurysms. Neurosurgery. 2005;57:676–83, discussion 676–83.
97. Burns JD, Huston III J, Layton KF, Piepgras DG, Brown Jr RD. Intracranial aneurysm enlargement on serial magnetic resonance angiography: frequency and risk factors. Stroke. 2009;40:406–11.
98. Matsubara S, Hadeishi H, Suzuki A, Yasui N, Nishimura H. Incidence and risk factors for the growth of unruptured cerebral aneurysms: observation using serial computerized tomography angiography. J Neurosurg. 2004;101:908–14.
99. Juvela S, Poussa K, Porras M. Factors affecting formation and growth of intracranial aneurysms: a long-term follow-up study. Stroke. 2001;32:485–91.
100. Kissela BM, Khoury J, Kleindorfer D, Woo D, Schneider A, Alwell K, Miller R, Ewing I, Moomaw CJ, Szaflarski JP, Gebel J, Shukla R, Broderick JP. Epidemiology of ischemic stroke in patients with diabetes: the greater Cincinnati/Northern Kentucky Stroke Study. Diabetes Care. 2005;28:355–9.
101. Rodgers A, MacMahon S, Gamble G, Slattery J, Sandercock P, Warlow C. Blood pressure and risk of stroke in patients with cerebrovascular disease The United Kingdom Transient Ischaemic Attack Collaborative Group. BMJ. 1996;313:147.
102. Rashid P, Leonardi-Bee J, Bath P. Blood pressure reduction and secondary prevention of stroke and other vascular events: a systematic review. Stroke. 2003;34:2741–8.
103. PROGRESS Collaborative Group. Randomised trial of a perindopril-based blood-pressure-lowering regimen among 6,105 individuals with previous stroke or transient ischaemic attack. Lancet. 2001;358:1033–41.
104. Lee KS, Bae HG, Yun IG. Recurrent intracerebral hemorrhage due to hypertension. Neurosurgery. 1990;26:586–90.
105. Buhl R, Barth H, Mehdorn HM. Risk of recurrent intracerebral hemorrhages. Neurol Res. 2003;25:853–6.
106. Neau JP, Ingrand P, Couderq C, Rosier MP, Bailbe M, Dumas P, Vandermarcq P, Gil R. Recurrent intracerebral hemorrhage. Neurology. 1997;49:106–13.
107. Chen ST, Chiang CY, Hsu CY, Lee TH, Tang LM. Recurrent hypertensive intracerebral hemorrhage. Acta Neurol Scand. 1995;91:128–32.
108. Gonzalez-Duarte A, Cantu C, Ruiz-Sandoval JL, Barinagarrementeria F. Recurrent primary cerebral hemorrhage: frequency, mechanisms, and prognosis. Stroke. 1998;29:1802–5.
109. Yen CC, Lo YK, Li JY, Lin YT, Lin CH, Gau YY. Recurrent primary intracerebral hemorrhage: a hospital based study. Acta Neurol Taiwan. 2007;16:74–80.
110. Passero S, Burgalassi L, D'Andrea P, Battistini N. Recurrence of bleeding in patients with primary intracerebral hemorrhage. Stroke. 1995;26:1189–92.
111. Bae H, Jeong D, Doh J, Lee K, Yun I, Byun B. Recurrence of bleeding in patients with hypertensive intracerebral hemorrhage. Cerebrovasc Dis. 1999;9:102–8.
112. Ariesen MJ, Algra A, Warlow CP, Rothwell PM, Cerebrovascular Cohort Studies Collaboration (CCSC). Predictors of risk of intracerebral haemorrhage in patients with a history of TIA or minor ischaemic stroke. J Neurol Neurosurg Psychiatr. 2006;77:92–4.
113. Asmar R. Benefits of blood pressure reduction in elderly patients. J Hypertens Suppl. 2003;21:S25–30.
114. Staessen J, Amery A, Fagard R. Isolated systolic hypertension in the elderly. J Hypertens. 1990;8:393–405.
115. Petrovitch H, Curb JD, Bloom-Marcus E. Isolated systolic hypertension and risk of stroke in Japanese-American men. Stroke. 1995;26:25–9.

116. Qureshi AI, Suri MF, Mohammad Y, Guterman LR, Hopkins LN. Isolated and borderline isolated systolic hypertension relative to long-term risk and type of stroke: a 20-year follow-up of the national health and nutrition survey. Stroke. 2002;33:2781–8.

117. Staessen JA, Gasowski J, Wang JG, Thijs L, Den Hond E, Boissel JP, Coope J, Ekbom T, Gueyffier F, Liu L, Kerlikowske K, Pocock S, Fagard RH. Risks of untreated and treated isolated systolic hypertension in the elderly: meta-analysis of outcome trials. Lancet. 2000; 355:865–72.

118. Chobanian AV, Bakris GL, Black HR, Cushman WC, Green LA, Izzo Jr JL, Jones DW, Materson BJ, Oparil S, Wright Jr JT, Roccella EJ, Joint National Committee on Prevention, Detection, Evaluation, and Treatment of High Blood Pressure, National Heart, Lung, and Blood Institute, and National High Blood Pressure Education Program Coordinating Committee. Seventh report of the Joint National Committee on Prevention, Detection, Evaluation, and Treatment of High Blood Pressure. Hypertension. 2003;42:1206–52.

119. Mancia G, Ambrosioni E, Rosei EA, Leonetti G, Trimarco B, Volpe M, ForLife Study Group. Blood pressure control and risk of stroke in untreated and treated hypertensive patients screened from clinical practice: results of the ForLife study. J Hypertens. 2005;23:1575–81.

120. Lloyd-Jones D, Adams R, Carnethon M, De Simone G, Ferguson TB, Flegal K, Ford E, Furie K, Go A, Greenlund K, Haase N, Hailpern S, Ho M, Howard V, Kissela B, Kittner S, Lackland D, Lisabeth L, Marelli A, McDermott M, Meigs J, Mozaffarian D, Nichol G, O'Donnell C, Roger V, Rosamond W, Sacco R, Sorlie P, Stafford R, Steinberger J, Thom T, Wasserthiel-Smoller S, Wong N, Wylie-Rosett J, Hong Y, American Heart Association Statistics Committee, Stroke Statistics Subcommittee. Heart disease and stroke statistics—2009 update: a report from the American Heart Association Statistics Committee and Stroke Statistics Subcommittee. Circulation. 2009;119:480–6.

121. Klungel OH, Stricker BH, Paes AH, Seidell JC, Bakker A, Voko Z, Breteler MM, de Anthonius B. Excess stroke among hypertensive men and women attributable to undertreatment of hypertension. Stroke. 1999;30:1312–8.

122. Redon J, Roca-Cusachs A, Mora-Macia J. Uncontrolled early morning blood pressure in medicated patients: the ACAMPA study. Analysis of the control of blood pressure using abulatory blood pressure monitoring. Blood Press Monit. 2002;7:111–6.

123. Millar-Craig MW, Bishop CN, Raftery EB. Circadian variation of blood-pressure. Lancet. 1978;1:795–7.

124. Kario K, Pickering TG, Umeda Y, Hoshide S, Hoshide Y, Morinari M, Murata M, Kuroda T, Schwartz JE, Shimada K. Morning surge in blood pressure as a predictor of silent and clinical cerebrovascular disease in elderly hypertensives: a prospective study. Circulation. 2003;107:1401–6.

125. Elliott WJ. Circadian variation in the timing of stroke onset: a meta-analysis. Stroke. 1998;29:992–6.

126. Inoue R, Ohkubo T, Kikuya M, Metoki H, Asayama K, Obara T, Hirose T, Hara A, Hoshi H, Hashimoto J, Totsune K, Satoh H, Kondo Y, Imai Y. Stroke risk in systolic and combined systolic and diastolic hypertension determined using ambulatory blood pressure. The Ohasama study. Am J Hypertens. 2007;20:1125–31.

Chapter 3
Blood Pressure Control and Primary Prevention of Stroke: Summary of Clinical Trial Data

William J. Elliott

Hypertension, or high blood pressure (BP), is the most important modifiable risk factor for stroke [1–5], accounting for 54 % of the population-attributable risk worldwide in a recent global health model [6]. Stroke is the second leading cause of death worldwide (although recently fifth, after heart disease, cancer, chronic lower respiratory diseases, and unintentional injuries in the USA [7]) and ranks very highly as a cause of adult disability in all countries. As developing nations overcome problems related to sanitation and infant mortality, hypertension is expected to become the most important risk factor worldwide for premature mortality and morbidity among adults. The purpose of this chapter is to review the existing clinical trial evidence supporting the use of antihypertensive drug therapy to prevent a first stroke. Unfortunately, many such clinical trials enrolled individuals with a history of a prior stroke (who are typically at 3–4 times the risk of stroke as people without such a history), and reported only the aggregated results. Some investigators have attempted to retrieve the numbers of such subjects (and the numbers who suffered a recurrent stroke) from some of the earlier clinical trials [8]. Two trials (e.g., the Heart Outcomes Prevention Evaluation and the Study on Cognition and Prognosis in the Elderly) have reported sufficient data in different publications to be able to calculate these parameters [9–12]. Since the results of many recent and large trials have not disclosed results in this fashion, only the small set of clinical trials can be examined for which there are data about primary strokes (i.e., those studies that excluded subjects with a history of a prior stroke, or studies that reported the numbers of subjects with prior stroke who suffered a recurrent stroke). Fortunately, the results of these meta-analyses differ very little from the overall conclusions (which are based on *all* studies that reported aggregated primary and recurrent strokes).

W.J. Elliott, M.D., Ph.D. (✉)
Department of Biomedical Sciences, The Pacific Northwest University of Health Sciences, Yakima, WA, USA
e-mail: wj.elliott@yahoo.com

© Springer International Publishing Switzerland 2016
V. Aiyagari, P.B. Gorelick (eds.), *Hypertension and Stroke*, Clinical Hypertension and Vascular Diseases, DOI 10.1007/978-3-319-29152-9_3

Clinical Trials Involving Placebo or No Treatment

There have been 35 trials that observed strokes and involved comparisons of placebo or no treatment (hereinafter called "Placebo") with active antihypertensive agents (Table 3.1). The importance of the link between BP-lowering and stroke can be illustrated by the fact that many of these important clinical trials used "incident fatal or nonfatal stroke" as their pre-specified primary endpoint, and based their power calculation on an estimate of the efficacy of BP-lowering drugs in preventing stroke [20, 24, 25, 29, 30, 35, 40, 43]. Many of these trials were performed during the last millennium, when placebo or no treatment was still ethical in outcomes studies; most recent trials have compared outcomes in subjects whose established antihypertensive medication regimen was augmented by the addition of a placebo or one or more active antihypertensive agents, as an attempt to control BP was considered mandatory [9–12, 31–34, 36–42, 44, 45]. It is likely, therefore, that the early studies (in which placebo-treated patients typically were allowed to receive "rescue" active antihypertensive drug therapy only if the BP exceeded thresholds) showed a larger impact of antihypertensive drugs on primary stroke prevention than more recent studies, because efforts to control BP were made in both randomized groups. An exception to the generally beneficial effect of antihypertensive drug therapy on primary stroke prevention was seen in the Efficacy of Candesartan on Outcome in Saitama Trial (ECOST [39]), which showed significant secondary (but not primary) prevention of stroke in subjects given candesartan; some meta-analyses exclude this study, because it was single-blind, did not include placebo, and the comparator was ill-defined. The other major *caveat* about these results is that, in all trials, some subjects chose to discontinue their assigned treatment; in each arm this decision "biases the result of the trial toward the null." As a consequence, the estimates of the effectiveness of antihypertensive drug therapy are typically biased in a pessimistic direction, i.e., the results obtained in general medical practice with patients who follow their healthcare providers' recommendations are likely to be even *better* than those shown here.

A good example of these challenges is the earliest, multicenter, placebo-controlled long-term trial of antihypertensive drug treatment that recorded stroke outcomes, the Veterans Administration's Cooperative Study Group on Antihypertensive Agents [13]. In the 143 subjects with diastolic BPs between 115 and 129 mmHg (after 7 days of hospitalization, bed rest, and a low-sodium diet), there were 11 with a prior thrombotic stroke. It has not been revealed if the five strokes observed before the study's early termination (at 18 months) occurred in individuals with a prior history of stroke. Among those randomized to placebo, seven experienced "treatment failure" necessitating termination of participation (at an average of 17 months), and active antihypertensive drugs were given.

The results of these trials can be summarized in many different ways (Fig. 3.1), but the results are quite similar. If one restricts the meta-analysis to the nine studies that randomized subjects to *initial* therapy with either placebo

Table 3.1 Placebo-controlled trials of primary stroke prevention involving antihypertensive drugs

Trial acronym, year	Years of follow-up	Subjects with HTN (%)	ΔSBP (mmHg)	Active arm Agent	Active arm # of First strokes/# of subjects	Control arm Agent	Control arm # of First strokes/# of subjects	Comments (# with prior strokes)
VA I, 1967 [13]	1.5	100	30	Diuretic + others	1/73	Placebo + "rescue"	3/70	(6/5)
VA II, 1970 [14]	3.3	100	31.4	Diuretic + others	5/186	Placebo + "rescue"	20/194	(NR/NR)
USPHS, 1977 [15]	7	100	16	Diuretic + others	1/193	Placebo	6/196	(0/0)
Oslo, 1980 [16]	5.5	100	17	Diuretic	0/406	No treatment	5/379	(0/0)
ANBP-1, 1980 [17]	3	100	NR	Diuretic	13/1721	Placebo	22/1706	(0/0)
Kuramoto, 1981 [18]	4	100	20	Diuretic	3/44	Placebo	4/47	(0/0)
HDFP[a], 1982 [19]	5	100	10	Diuretic	87/5364	Placebo	142/5333	(N/A)
EWPHE[a], 1985 [20]	4.6	100	21	Diuretic	16/386	Placebo	22/405	(N/A)
MRC-1, 1985 [21]	5.5	100	~13 ~9.5	Diuretic or β-blocker	18/4297 42/4203	Placebo	109/8654	(32 or 31/61)
IPPPSH, 1985 [22]	4	100	3.8	β-Blocker	45/3185	Placebo	46/3172	(0/0)
Coope & Warrender[a], 1986 [23]	4.4	100	18.0	β-Blocker	18/410	No treatment	38/460	(N/A)
SHEP Pilot, 1989 [24]	2.8	100	15	Diuretic	11/443	Placebo + "rescue"	6/108	(8)
SHEP[a], 1991 [25]	4.5	100	11.1	Diuretic	95/2314	Placebo + "rescue"	152/2338	(N/A)
STOP-1, 1991 [26]	2.1	100	19.5	Diuretic or β-blocker	28/782	Placebo	49/784	(32/36)
MRC-E, 1992 [27]	5.7	100	15 15	Diuretic or β-blocker	45/1081 56/1102	Placebo	134/2213	(NR or NR/NR)
STONE, 1996 [28]	2.5	100	9.5	CCB	16/817	Placebo	36/815	(NR/NR); Not randomized
Syst-EUR, 1997 [29]	2.5	100	10.7	CCB + other	49/2398	Placebo + other	80/2297	(103)

(continued)

Table 3.1 (continued)

Trial acronym, year	Years of follow-up	Subjects with HTN (%)	ΔSBP (mmHg)	Active arm		Control arm		Comments (# with prior strokes)
				Agent	# of First strokes/# of subjects	Agent	# of First strokes/# of subjects	
Syst-China, 1998 [30]	2.8	100	8.0	CCB+other	45/1253	Placebo+other	59/1141	(45), Not randomized
HOPE[a], 2000 [9, 10]	4.5	46	3	Other+ACE-I	113/4188	Other+placebo	175/4190	Add-on (N/A)
PART2, 2000 [31]	4.7	?	6.0	Other+ACE-I	7/308	Other+placebo	4/309	Add-on (34/28)
IDNT, 2001 [32]	2.6	100	3 4	(ARB or CCB)+other	28/579 15/567	Placebo+other	26/569	(NR/NR)
RENAAL, 2001 [33]	3.4	100	2	ARB+other	47/751	Placebo+other	50/762	(0/1)
EUROPA, 2003 [34]	4.2	27? (BP>160/95)	5.0	Other+ACE-I	98/6110	Other+placebo	102/6108	Add-on (210/199)
HY-VET Pilot, 2003 [35]	1.1	100	23.0 23.0	ACE-I or diuretic	6/426 12/431	Placebo+Rescue	18/426	(18 or 18/22)
SCOPE[a], 2003 [11, 12]	3.5	100	3.2	ARB+other	83/2386	Placebo+other	100/2378	(N/A)
DIAB-HYCAR, 2004 [36]	3.3	55	1.3	Other+ACE-I	118/2443	Other+placebo	116/2469	Add-on (107/100)
PEACE, 2004 [37]	4.8	45	3.0	Other+ACE-I	71/4158	Other+placebo	92/4132	Add-on (291/248)
ACTION, 2005 [38]	4.9	100	6.6	Other+CCB	50/1975	Other+placebo	75/2002	Add-on (NR/NR)
E-COST, 2005 [39]	3.0	100	1.7	ARB+other	47/1053	No ARB+other	77/995	(23/69)
FEVER, 2005 [40]	3.3	100	3.5	Diuretic+CCB	177/4841	Diuretic+placebo	251/4870	Second-line (685/753)
ADVANCE, 2007 [41]	4.3	68	5.6	Other+diuretic+ACE-I	215/5569	Other+placebo	218/5571	Combination (502/520)

Trial acronym, year	Years of follow-up	Subjects with HTN (%)	ΔSBP (mmHg)	Active arm		Control arm		Comments (# with prior strokes)
				Agent	# of First strokes/# of subjects	Agent	# of First strokes/# of subjects	
Jikei, 2007 [42]	3.1	88	1.0	Other+ARB	25/1541	Other	43/1540	Add-on (NR/NR)
HYVET, 2008 [43]	1.8	100	15.0	Diuretic	51/1933	Placebo	69/1912	(130/131)
TRANSCEND, 2008 [44]	4.7	76	4.0	Other+ARB	112/2842	Other+placebo	136/2836	Add-on (648/654)
NAVIGATOR, 2010 [45]	5.0	78	2.8	Other+ARB	105/4631	Other+placebo	132/4675	Add-on (143/132)

HTN hypertension, *SBP* systolic blood pressure

[a]Denotes study for which the number of observed primary (as opposed to both primary and secondary) strokes can be calculated. (N/A) indicates that the number of subjects with prior stroke has been reported and subtracted from the total number of subjects in the trial. *VA I* First Veterans Administration Cooperative Study Group on Antihypertensive Agents, *VA II* Veterans Administration Cooperative Study Group on Antihypertensive Agents, *USPHS* United States Public Health Service trial, *ANBP-1* First Australian National Blood Pressure trial, *HDFP* Hypertension Detection and Follow-up Program, *EWPHE* European Working Party on Hypertension in the Elderly, *MRC-1* First Medical Research Council trial (in "mild" hypertensives), *IPPPSH* International Prospective Primary Prevention Study in Hypertension, *SHEP* Systolic Hypertension in the Elderly Program, *STOP-1* First Swedish Trial in Old Patients with Hypertension, *MRC-E* Medical Research Council trial (in elderly hypertensives), *STONE* Shanghai Trial of Nifedipine in the Elderly trial, *Syst-EUR* Systolic Hypertension in Europe trial, *Syst-China* Systolic Hypertension in China trial, *HOPE* Heart Outcomes Prevention Evaluation, *PART2* Prevention of Atherosclerosis with Ramipril study #2, *IDNT* Irbesartan Diabetic Nephropathy Trial, *RENAAL* Reduction of Endpoints in Non-insulin Dependent Diabetes Mellitus with the Angiotensin II Antagonist Losartan, *EUROPA* EUropean trial on Reduction of cardiac events with Perindopril in patients with stable coronary Artery disease, *HYVET* Hypertension in the Very Elderly Trial, *SCOPE* Study on Cognition and Prognosis in the Elderly trial, *DIAB-HYCAR* non-insulin–dependent DIABetes, HYpertension, microalbuminuria or proteinuria, Cardiovascular events And Rampril study, *PEACE* Prevention of Events with Angiotensin Converting Enzyme inhibition trial, *ACTION* a Coronary disease Trial Investigating Outcome with Nifedipine GITS trial. *E-COST* Efficacy of Candesartan on Outcome in Saitama Trial, *FEVER* Felodipine EVEnt Reduction study, *ADVANCE* Action in Diabetes and Vascular disease: preterAx and diamicroN-MR Controlled Evaluation, *TRANSCEND* Telmisartan Randomised AssessmeNt Study in ACE iNtolerant subjects with cardiovascular Disease trial, *NAVIGATOR* Nateglinide and Valsartan in Impaired Glucose Tolerance Outcomes Research, *CCB* calcium channel blocker, *ACE-I* angiotensin converting-enzyme inhibitor, *ARB* angiotensin receptor blocker, *BP* blood pressure, *NR* not reported

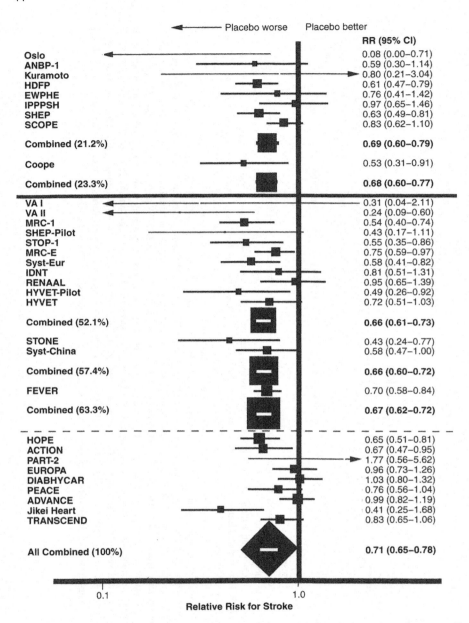

Fig. 3.1 Meta-analysis of placebo-controlled clinical trials of antihypertensive drugs that reported first (or first and recurrent) strokes. The trials above the *broad horizontal line* include only hypertensive subjects suffering a first stroke. The distinctions between groups of trials are discussed in the *text*. The "*boxes*" (representing the point estimates of relative risk, RR) are drawn in proportion to the number of strokes, and the *horizontal lines* represent the 95 % confidence intervals for each trial. The meta-analytic results (drawn in the figure as *squares*) above the *dashed horizontal line* (above "HOPE") showed no significant inhomogeneity in fixed-effects models. When trials that

or antihypertensive drug therapy, *and* included only subjects with no prior history of stroke [11, 12, 15–20, 22, 25], there is no significant inhomogeneity across studies [P (homogeneity) = 0.28], and the combined relative risk for a first stroke is 0.69 (95 % confidence interval: 0.60–0.79, $P<0.0001$). If one then adds the trial that used no treatment (rather than placebo) in the control group [23], there is little change (combined relative risk = 0.68, 95 % CI: 0.60–0.77). After adding data from a study that simply added an angiotensin converting-enzyme (ACE)-inhibitor or placebo to whatever other antihypertensive therapy was required [9, 10], the combined relative risk for *all* 11 studies that reported only *initial* strokes is therefore 0.67 (95 % CI: 0.60–0.75), with the P (homogeneity) = 0.37 (data not shown).

This conclusion is relatively robust to adding the results of clinical trials that included subjects with a history of prior strokes, but for which the numbers of subjects with recurrent strokes has not been revealed. Below the thick horizontal line in Fig. 3.1 are included, in sequence, the placebo-controlled studies that used initial therapy [13, 14, 21, 24, 26, 27, 29, 32, 33, 35, 39, 43], the two non-randomized studies [28, 29], the trial that randomized hypertensive subjects to placebo or a calcium antagonist as second-line therapy [40], and the trial that added either placebo or a calcium antagonist to whatever other antihypertensive drugs were already being taken [38]. The combined relative risk for stroke for these trials is 0.66 (95 % CI: 0.62–0.71), with a P (homogeneity) = 0.32. Lastly, one can add the results of trials in which "add-on" placebo or antihypertensive drug was given, but the subjects were not all hypertensive; [31, 34, 36, 37, 41–43, 45] many object to this, however, because the study populations become much less homogeneous. This may be the reason for the significant inhomogeneity ($P<0.002$) in the fixed-effects meta-analysis of these data. Nonetheless, using a random-effects model, the pooled relative risk for stroke across all 34 trials involving placebo or no treatment (whether primary or mixed primary/secondary stroke prevention) is 0.73 (95 % CI: 0.70–0.77, $P<0.0001$).

One of the most important conclusions from this dataset can be illustrated in Fig. 3.2. Across all trials, the number of strokes prevented (per 1000 subject-years) is directly proportional to the absolute risk of stroke (per 1000 subject-years, in the placebo-treated group). The corollaries to this are: "It is difficult, if not impossible, to prevent a stroke in a person who has a very low risk of a stroke," and conversely, "The higher the baseline risk of stroke, the greater the number of people who will benefit from treatment." The relationship is strengthened even further if placebo-controlled trials of secondary stroke prevention (e.g., the Perindopril pROtection aGainst REcurrent Stroke Study) are added.

---◄───

Fig. 3.1 (continued) included non-hypertensive subjects were added (below the *dashed horizontal line*; see text for details), the random-effects model showed a similar overall result (drawn as a *rhombus*) as the prior meta-analyses, despite significant inhomogeneity in the fixed-effects model. These data suggest that the point estimates and confidence limits for these meta-analyses are robust to many alterations in the dataset (and the rigor with which trials are included or excluded). For expansions of acronyms of trials, see Tables 3.1 and 3.2

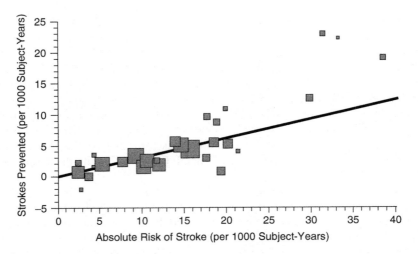

Fig. 3.2 Relationship of the absolute risk of stroke (calculated as strokes per 1000 subject-years in the placebo-treated group) and the number of strokes prevented by treatment (per 1000 subject-years). Data from individual trials are plotted as *squares*, with the area of each square proportional to the number of strokes reported for each trial. The correlation coefficients for this relationship were 0.86, $P < 0.001$ for unweighted data, and 0.89, $P < 0.001$ for weighted data

Clinical Trials Comparing Two or More Active Antihypertensive Drugs

Thirty-four clinical trials that reported strokes compared two or more active antihypertensive drugs in primarily hypertensive patients (Table 3.2). Note that three trials included a placebo-arm (and are therefore also listed in Table 3.1) [21, 27, 35], and that all except ONTARGET had hypertension as an inclusion criterion. Only five of these studies were planned as primary prevention trials [46, 47, 51, 52, 54]. The other 29 have enrolled at least one subject with a prior stroke, and none have reported the numbers of subjects that suffered a first vs. second stroke.

The lack of solid data about primary stroke prevention in hypertension trials can be illustrated by the results of a network meta-analysis of the data (nine placebo-controlled trials, six actively controlled trials). Unfortunately, the numbers of trials reporting observed first strokes is one with an angiotensin receptor blocker (ARB), and only two each for a calcium antagonist or an ACE-inhibitor. This leads to a high degree of "incoherence" ($\omega = 0.136$) in the model, and nonsignificant point estimates for regimens beginning with anything but a diuretic or β-blocker (data not shown).

These results stand in sharp contrast to those obtained from those derived from "the preponderance of the evidence," i.e., all trials comparing an *initial* placebo and/ or *initial* antihypertensive drugs in trials involving only hypertensive subjects (Fig. 3.3). For this more extensive network (involving 50 trials, 62 comparisons,

Table 3.2 Actively controlled trials of primary stroke prevention involving initial antihypertensive drugs

Trial acronym, year	Years of follow-up	Subjects with HTN (%)	ΔSBP (mmHg)	Arm 1 Agent	Arm 1 # of First strokes/# of subjects	Arm 2 (or Arm 3) Agent	Arm 2 (or Arm 3) # of First strokes/# of subjects	Comments (# with prior strokes)
MRC-1, 1985 [21]	5.5	100	4.5	Diuretic	18/4297	β-Blocker	42/4203	(32/31)
HAPPHY, 1987 [46]	3.8	100	0	Diuretic	41/3297	β-Blocker	32/3276	(0/0)
MAPHY, 1988 [47]	5.0	100	0.3	Diuretic	25/1625	β-Blocker	23/1609	(0/0)
MRC-E, 1992 [27]	5.7	100	0	Diuretic	45/1081	β-Blocker	56/1102	(NR/NR)
MIDAS, 1996 [48]	3.0	100	3.5	Diuretic	3/441	CCB	6/442	(NR/NR)
VHAS, 1997 [49]	2.0	100	1.0	Diuretic	4/707	CCB	5/707	(NR/NR)
ABCD, 1998 [50]	5.0	100	0	ACE-I	7/235	CCB	11/235	(2/3)
FACET, 1998 [51]	2.5	100	-4	ACE-I	4/189	CCB	10/191	(0/0)
UKPDS, 1998 [52]	8.4	100	-1	β-Blocker	17/358	ACE-I	21/400	(0/0)
CAPPP, 1999 [53]	6.1	100	2	β-Blocker/diuretic	148/5493	ACE-I	189/5492	(39/50)
NICH-ES, 1999 [54]	4.2	100	0	Diuretic	8/215	CCB	8/214	(0/0)
STOP-2, 1999 [55]	5.0	100	1	β-Blocker/diuretic	237/2213	ACE-I	215/2205	(86/86
			1			or CCB	207/2196	or 83)
INSIGHT, 2000 [56]	3.5	100	0	Diuretic	74/3164	CCB	67/3157	(NR/NR)
NORDIL, 2000 [57]	4.5	100	-3	β-Blocker/diuretic	196/5471	CCB	159/5410	(88/74)
AASK, 2001, 2002 [58, 59]	4.4 or 3.6	100	0	β-Blocker	23/441	ACE-I	23/436	(NR/NR)
			2			or CCB	9/217	
IDNT, 2001 [35]	2.6	100	1	CCB	28/579	ARB	15/567	(NR/NR)
LIFE, 2002 [60]	4.7	100	-1.1	β-Blocker	309/4588	ARB	232/4605	(359/369)
ELSA, 2002 [61]	3.8	100	-0.2	β-Blocker	14/1157	CCB	9/1177	(NR/NR)
ALLHAT, 2002 [62]	4.9	100	2	Diuretic	675/15255	ACE-I	457/9054	(NR/NR
			1			or CCB	377/9048	or NR)

(continued)

Table 3.2 (continued)

Trial acronym, year	Years of follow-up	Subjects with HTN (%)	ΔSBP (mmHg)	Arm 1 Agent	Arm 1 # of First strokes/# of subjects	Arm 2 (or Arm 3) Agent	Arm 2 (or Arm 3) # of First strokes/# of subjects	Comments (# with prior strokes)
ANBP-2, 2003 [63]	4.1	100	1	Diuretic	107/3039	ACE-I	112/3044	(~152/~122)
CONVINCE, 2003 [64]	3.0	100	0.1	Diuretic or β-blocker	58/3831 60/4466	CCB	79/3986 54/4393	(393/370)
SHELL, 2003 [65]	3.6	100	-1.6	Diuretic	38/940	CCB	37/942	(NR/NR)
INVEST, 2003 [66]	2.7	100	0.3	β-Blocker	201/11309	CCB	176/11267	(567/595)
HYVET-Pilot, 2003 [35]	1.1	100	0	Diuretic	6/426	ACE-I	12/431	(18/18)
JMIC-B, 2004 [67]	3.0	100	-2	ACE-I	16/822	CCB	16/828	(NR/NR)
VALUE, 2004 [68]	4.2	100	2.23	CCB	281/7596	ARB	322/7649	(1501/1513)
DETAIL, 2004 [69]	5.0	100	-4	ACE-I	6/130	ARB	6/120	(NR/NR)
ASCOT, 2005 [70]	5.5	100	1.6	β-Blocker	422/9618	CCB	327/9639	(1063/1050)
CASE-J, 2008 [71]	3.2	100	1.7	CCB	50/2349	ARB	61/2354	(225/248)
ONTARGET, 2008 [72]	4.7	69	0.9	ACE-I	405/8576	ARB	369/8642	(1805/1758)
ACCOMPLISH, 2008 [73]	3.0	100	0.9	ACE-I+diuretic	133/5762	ACE-I+CCB	112/5744	(736/762)
VART, 2010 [74]	3.4	100	0.0	ARB+other	10/510	CCB+other	10/511	(NR/NR)
COPE, 2011 [75]	3.2	100	-0.8 -0.7	CCB+ARB	17/1110	CCB+β-blocker CCB+diuretic	27/1089 12/1094	
Nagoya Heart Study, 2012 [76]	3.2	100	1.0	ARB	13/575	CCB	16/575	(24/30)

HTN hypertension, *SBP* systolic blood pressure

[a]Denotes study that has reported the number of observed primary (as opposed to both primary and secondary) strokes. *MRC-1* Medical Research Council trial (in "mild" hypertensives), *HAPPHY* Heart Attack Primary Prevention in Hypertensives study, *MAPHY* Metoprolol Atherosclerosis Prevention in Hypertensives trial, *NR* not reported, *MRC-E* Medical Research Council trial (in elderly hypertensives), *MIDAS* Multicenter Isradipine Diuretic Atherosclerosis Study, *VHAS* Verapamil Hypertension Atherosclerosis Study, *ABCD* Appropriate Blood pressure Control in Diabetes study, *FACET* Fosinopril Amlodipine Cardiac Events randomized Trial, *UKPDS* United

Kingdom Prospective Diabetes Study, *CAPPP* CAPtopril Primary Prevention Project, *NICH-ES* National Intervention Cooperative Study in Elderly Hypertensives, *STOP-2* Second Swedish Trial in Old Patients with hypertension, *INSIGHT* International Nifedipine GITS study: Intervention as a Goal in Hypertension Treatment, *NORDIL* NORdic DILtiazem study, *AASK* African American Study on Kidney disease and hypertension trial, *IDNT* Irbesartan Diabetic Nephropathy Trial, *LIFE* Losartan Intervention for Endpoint reduction trial, *ELSA* European Lacidipine Study on Atherosclerosis, *ALLHAT* Antihypertensive and Lipid-Lowering to prevent Heart Attack Trial, *ANBP-2* Second Australian National Blood Pressure trial, *CONVINCE* Controlled-ONset Verapamil INvestigation of Cardiovascular Endpoints trial, *SHELL* Systolic Hypertension in the Elderly: Lacidipine Long-term study, *INVEST* INternational Verapamil-trandolapril STudy, *HYVET* Hypertension in the Very Elderly trial, *JMIC-B* Japan Multicenter Investigation for Cardiovascular Diseases-B study, *VALUE* Valsartan Antihypertensive Long-term Use Evaluation, *DETAIL* Diabetics Exposed to Telmisartan and enalapriL study, *ASCOT* Anglo-Scandinavian Cardiac Outcomes Trial, *CASE-J* Candesartan Antihypertensive Survival Evaluation in Japan study, *ONTARGET* Ongoing Telmisartan Alone and in combination with Ramipril Global Endpoint Trial, *ACCOMPLISH* Avoiding Cardiovascular events with COMbination therapy in People LIving with Systolic Hypertension. *CCB* calcium channel blocker, *VART* Valsartan Amlodipine Randomized Trial, *COPE* Combination therapy of hypertension to Prevent cardiovascular Events, *ACE-I* angiotensin converting-enzyme inhibitor, *ARB* angiotensin receptor blocker, *NR* not reported

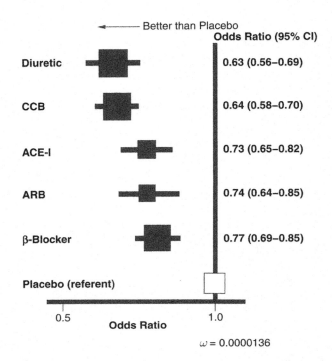

Fig. 3.3 Results of network meta-analysis of 50 clinical trials in 275,103 hypertensive subjects comparing placebo (or no treatment) and/or initial active antihypertensive drugs for prevention of stroke. When available, the numbers of subjects at risk for and suffering first strokes were used; otherwise the total numbers of subjects at risk for and suffering a first or recurrent stroke were used. The "*box*" corresponding to the point estimate of the effect size (relative to placebo) is drawn in proportion to the number of strokes observed with that class of antihypertensive drugs across all trials; the *horizontal lines* through the "boxes" correspond to the 95 % confidence intervals for each point estimate. Note that this model has a high degree of internal consistency (as the incoherence value, $\omega < 0.000004$). *CI* confidence interval, *CCB* calcium channel blocker, *ACE-I* angiotensin converting-enzyme inhibitor, *ARB* angiotensin receptor blocker

8877 strokes, and 275,103 subjects), the incoherence value was very small ($\omega < 0.000004$), suggesting a high degree of internal consistency. All five classes of antihypertensive drugs significantly (all $P < 0.00001$) prevented stroke, better than placebo (Fig. 3.3). If the referent agent was arbitrarily changed to "Diuretic," the incoherence does not change, and all pair-wise comparisons (except the calcium antagonist and ARB) remained significant, indicating that Placebo (odds ratio 1.64, 95 % confidence interval: 1.47–1.83, $P < 0.0001$), β-Blocker (odds ratio: 1.20, 95 % CI: 1.09–1.33, $P < 0.0004$), ACE-inhibitor (odds ratio: 1.16, 95 % CI: 1.05–1.28, $P < 0.005$) were significantly inferior to a Diuretic in preventing stroke. The differences between the Diuretic and Calcium Antagonist (odds ratio 0.99, 95 % CI: 0.90–1.08, $P = 0.75$), or between the Diuretic and ARB (odds ratio 1.06, 95 % CI: 0.92–1.23, $P = 0.43$), were not significant. These conclusions were robust to a wide range of changes in the dataset (e.g., omit ACCOMPLISH, as it studied initial combinations of agents; allocate the results of Scandinavian trials [26, 53, 55, 57] that used the physician's choice of either an initial β-blocker or an initial diuretic as "Conventional Therapy") to β-Blocker, Diuretic, or a 60:40 attribution of risk (similar to the reported distribution of initial treatments; data not shown).

If one broadens the criteria for entry into the network meta-analysis in a stepwise fashion, including trials that enrolled only hypertensive subjects, randomized anti-hypertensive agents as second- or third-line therapy, and reported first strokes, and next including other trials that included non-hypertensive subjects [9, 10, 31, 34, 36, 37, 41, 42, 44, 72], the incoherence value increases ($\omega = 0.049$, then 0.074), suggesting that the model progressively deteriorates, similarly to the inhomogeneity of fixed-effects meta-analysis of all placebo-controlled trials, discussed above. However, the overall conclusions regarding efficacy in stroke prevention remain stable (i.e., all classes of antihypertensive drugs are significantly superior to placebo, with very similar rank-ordering). Intuitively, this result makes sense (and is consistent with Fig. 3.2), because giving antihypertensive drugs to individuals who do not have elevated BPs, and/or are unlikely to lower their BPs very much with these drugs, should be less likely to prevent strokes than giving the same drugs to hypertensive individuals.

Blood Pressure Lowering: Relationship to Primary Stroke Prevention

The traditional way to try to interrelate BP-lowering and stroke prevention is a meta-regression analysis, plotting the difference in achieved (systolic) BP (as the independent variable) and the odds ratio for stroke (as the dependent variable; see Fig. 3.4 for an example). The reason for using systolic, rather than diastolic BP is that many of the studies in older patients enrolled subjects with near-normal diastolic BPs, and therefore the differences in diastolic BPs are not nearly as impressive as the differences in systolic BP. If one includes enough comparisons, there is a significant curvilinear relationship: trials having a larger difference in achieved (systolic) BP show lower odds ratios for stroke [77–79]. Although estimated central aortic pressure (rather than systolic BP) differences for each comparison correlated nearly linearly with stroke prevention [80], central aortic pressure was directly estimated in hypertensive subjects in a substudy of a single outcomes-based trial [81].

Some have claimed that calcium antagonists significantly prevent stroke, independent of their BP-lowering effects. Most, however, would agree with the overall conclusion of the Task Force for the Management of Arterial Hypertension of the European Society of Hypertension and the European Society of Cardiology, which was first made public in 2007 (and ratified twice since then): "Comparative randomized trials show that for similar blood pressure reductions, differences in the incidence of cardiovascular morbidity and mortality between different drug classes are small, thus strengthening the conclusion that their benefit depends largely on blood

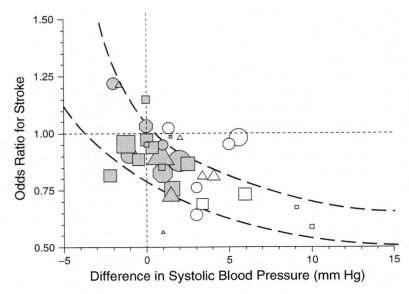

Fig. 3.4 Meta-regression plot of the relationship between the difference in achieved systolic blood pressure between randomized arms vs. the odds ratio for stroke for the larger trials in Tables 3.1 and 3.2. Note that trials with fewer than 58 strokes (5 % of those observed in the chlorthalidone-lisinopril comparison in the Antihypertensive and Lipid-Lowering to prevent Heart Attack Trial) are not shown, as their symbols are below the resolution of the figure. Trials involving an angiotensin receptor blocker are denoted by a *triangle*, calcium antagonists by *squares*, ACE-inhibitors by *circles*, and both of the latter by an *octagon*. *Open symbols* denote placebo-controlled trials. The area of each symbol is proportional to the number of strokes observed in each trial. The identity of each symbol can be ascertained by reference to Tables 3.1 and 3.2. Note that 91 % of the area for all symbols falls within the *dark, curved, dotted lines*, representing the upper and lower 95 % confidence limits for the significant ($P < 0.0001$) meta-regression analysis that was based on the results of placebo-controlled trials of diuretic and/or β-blocker reported before the year 2000. (Data from Staessen JA, Wang J-G, Thijs L. Cardiovascular prevention and blood pressure reduction: A quantitative overview updated until 01 March 2003. J Hypertens. 2003;21:1055-1076)

pressure lowering per se" [82]. This international panel of experts estimated the "BP-independent effect" of calcium antagonists on stroke or ACE-inhibitors on CHD as 5–10 % of the "dominant protective effect exerted by blood pressure lowering" [82]. Nonetheless, a meta-analysis and meta-regression analysis of 22 trials that measured changes in carotid intima-medial thickness indicated a significantly lower rate of carotid intima-media thickening in trials involving calcium antagonists, which was apparently independent of their BP-lowering effects [83]. While this information is consistent with (and may provide a pathophysiological explanation for) the idea that calcium antagonists have a "BP-independent effect" on preventing stroke, it does not prove that the phenomenon is true.

There has also been much discussion in the recent literature that ARBs might be particularly protective against stroke, especially a second stroke [39, 84, 85]. In primary stroke prevention, the Losartan Intervention For Endpoint reduction (LIFE) trial showed a significant lowering of stroke (with very little long-term BP difference) [60], and other studies involving ARBs showed (individually) a nonsignificant benefit for stroke prevention [11, 12, 44, 45]. More recent and much larger studies of ARBs for primary or secondary stroke prevention have failed to verify these earlier observations [44, 68, 72, 74, 75, 86]. Yet the data from each of these large trials fall quite within the expected ranges in the meta-regression plots of differences in observed systolic BP vs. odds ratio for stroke.

So far, only two trials have directly tested the hypothesis that greater BP-lowering (using very similar, if not identical, drug regimens) would result in a different risk of stroke [87, 88]. Some believe that there must be a BP below which further BP-lowering should be harmful, as few people survive long with systolic BPs < 60 mmHg. However, when 17,980 hypertensive subjects in the Hypertension Optimal Treatment Study were randomized to diastolic BP targets of ≤80, ≤85, or ≤90 mmHg, treated intensively with multiple-drug regimens (calcium antagonist initially, followed by an ACE-inhibitor), and then followed prospectively in an open-label fashion for 3.8 years, there were no significant differences in stroke across the three groups ($P = 0.74$) [87]. Although the *actual* differences in diastolic BPs across the groups were much less than originally planned (~2 vs. 5 mmHg), the clear conclusion was that lowering BP further than what is currently recommended would be neither helpful or harmful with respect to stroke for the general hypertensive population [87]. In contrast, the HOT study clearly showed the benefits of the lower-than-usual BP for diabetics, as those randomized to the lowest target (diastolic BP ≤ 80 mmHg) enjoyed a significant 51 % reduction in cardiovascular events, compared to those treated to the "conventional" target (diastolic BP ≤ 90 mmHg) [87]. Similar conclusions were derived from the more recent and larger Action to Control Cardiovascular Risk in Diabetics (ACCORD) trial [88]. A significant benefit for the lower systolic BP target (achieved: 119.3 mmHg) was seen for stroke (41 % reduction in any stroke, 37 % reduction in nonfatal stroke), compared to those treated to the conventional systolic BP target (achieve 133.5 mmHg), but the overall 12 % reduction in major cardiovascular events was not significant ($P = 0.20$). These data are but part of the rationale for why recent hypertension guidelines [1–4] have abandoned the lower-than-usual BP targets that had been recommended previously for high-risk groups (e.g., patients with diabetes, chronic kidney disease, and coronary heart disease).

Conclusions

Although *first* strokes have been reported in only 9 of the 35 placebo-controlled clinical trials (and constitute only 21 % of the number of strokes), the conclusion that antihypertensive drug therapy prevents about 32 % of strokes in these nine trials falls close to the 95 % confidence limits for the result of the meta-analysis across all 35 placebo-controlled trials (23–30 %), many of which included non-hypertensive subjects, or gave randomized drugs as second-line therapy. In network meta-analysis of 50 trials involving 275,103 subjects (all of whom had hypertension), 62 pair-wise comparisons, and 8877 strokes, all five major antihypertensive drug classes showed significant prevention of stroke, compared to placebo or no treatment, with an initial diuretic or calcium antagonist being more effective than other drug classes. Nearly all of the trials have shown better stroke prevention in the arm(s) that achieved a lower systolic BP, although calcium antagonists may have a small (but significant) BP-independent effect on stroke prevention. Since elevated BP is the most common population-based remediable risk factor for stroke, more attention to achieving and maintaining a BP < 140/90 mmHg should be a high-priority public health goal.

Disclosures

Sadly, the preparation of this manuscript was not supported by any entity, commercial or non-profit. The author's "Real or Potential Conflicts of Interest" are summarized on the enclosed "RUSH University Standard Financial Disclosure Form," and "Financial Disclosures" (involving only the last 12 months).

References

1. James PA, Oparil S, Carter BL, et al. 2014 Evidence-based guidelines for the management of high blood pressure in adults: report from the panel members appointed to the Eighth Joint National Committee (JNC 8). JAMA. 2014;311:507–20.
2. Weber MA, Schiffrin EL, White WB, et al. Clinical practice guidelines for the management of hypertension in the community: a statement by the American Society of Hypertension and the International Society of Hypertension. J Clin Hypertens (Greenwich). 2014;16:14–26.
3. Mancia G, Fagard R, Narkiewicz K, et al. 2013 Practice guidelines for the management of arterial hypertension of the European Society of Hypertension (ESH) and the European Society of Cardiology (ESC): ESH/ESC Task Force for the management of arterial hypertension. J Hypertens. 2013;31:1925–38.
4. Meschia JF, Bushnell C, Boden-Albala B, et al. Guidelines for the primary prevention of stroke: a guideline for healthcare professionals from the American Heart Association/American Stroke Association. Stroke. 2014;45:3754–832.
5. Mozaffarian D, Benjamin EJ, Go AS, et al. Heart Disease and Stroke Statistics—2015 update. A Report from the American Heart Association. Circulation. 2015;131:e1–295.
6. World Health Organisation. A global brief on hypertension: silent killer, global public health crisis. Geneva: WHO; 2013. p. 40. http://www.apps.who.int/iris/bitstream/10665/79059/1/WHO_DCO_WHD_2013.2_eng.pdf. Accessed 20 Feb 2015.
7. Kochanek KD, Murphy SL, Zu J, Arias E. Mortality in the United States, 2013. NCHS Data Brief. 2014;178:1–8. http://www.cdc.gov/nchs/data/databriefs/db178.pdf. Accessed 16 Feb 2015.
8. Gueyffier F, Boissel JP, Boutitie F, et al. Effect of antihypertensive treatment in patients having already suffered from stroke: gathering the evidence. The INDANA Project Collaborators. Stroke. 1997;28:2557–62.

9. Effects of an angiotensin-converting-enzyme inhibitor, ramipril, on death from cardiovascular causes, myocardial infarction, and stroke in high-risk patients. The Heart Outcomes Prevention Evaluation (HOPE) Study Investigators. N Engl J Med. 2000;342:145–53.
10. Bosch J, Yusuf S, Pogue J, et al. Use of ramipril in preventing stroke: double blind randomised trial. BMJ. 2002;324:699–702.
11. Lithell H, Hansson L, Skoog I, et al. The Study on Cognition and Prognosis in the Elderly (SCOPE): principal results of a randomized double-blind intervention trial. J Hypertens. 2003;21:875–86.
12. Trenkwalder P, Elmfeldt D, Hofman A, et al., for the Study on Cognition and Prognosis in the Elderly (SCOPE) Investigators. The Study on Cognition and Prognosis in the Elderly: major cardiovascular events and stroke in subgroups of patients. Blood Press. 2005;14:31–7.
13. Veterans Administration Cooperative Study Group on Antihypertensive Agents. Effects of treatment on morbidity in hypertension: results in patients with diastolic blood pressure averaging 115 through 129 mm Hg. JAMA. 1967;202:1028–34.
14. Veterans Administration Cooperative Study Group on Antihypertensive Agents. II. Effects of treatment results in patients with diastolic blood pressure averaging 90 through 114 mm Hg. JAMA. 1970;213:1143–52.
15. Smith WM. Treatment of mild hypertension: results of a ten-year intervention trial. Circ Res. 1977;40(5 Suppl 1):I98–105.
16. Helgeland A. Treatment of mild hypertension: a five-year controlled drug trial: the Oslo Study. Am J Med. 1980;69:725–32.
17. The Australian Therapeutic Trial in Mild Hypertension. Report by the Management Committee. Lancet. 1980;1:1261–7.
18. Kuramoto K, Matsushita S, Kuwajima I, Murakami M. Prospective study on the treatment of mild hypertension in the aged. Jpn Heart J. 1981;22:75–85.
19. Hypertension Detection and Follow-up Program Cooperative Group. Five-year findings of the Hypertension Detection and Follow-up Program: III. Reduction in stroke incidence among persons with high blood pressure. JAMA. 1982;247:633–8.
20. Amery A, Birkenhäger W, Brixko P, et al. Mortality and morbidity from the European Working Party on High Blood Pressure in the Elderly Trial. Lancet. 1985;1:1349–54.
21. MRC Trial of treatment of mild hypertension: principal results. Medical Research Council Working Party. Br Med J (Clin Res). 1985;291:97–104.
22. The IPPPSH Collaborative Group. Cardiovascular risk and risk factors in a randomised trial of treatment based on the beta-blocker oxprenolol: The International Prospective Primary Prevention Study in Hypertension (IPPPSH). J Hypertens. 1985;3:379–92.
23. Coope J, Warrender TS. Randomised trial of treatment of hypertension in elderly patients in primary care. BMJ. 1986;293:1145–51.
24. Perry Jr HM, Smith WM, McDonald RH, et al. Morbidity and mortality in the Systolic Hypertension in the Elderly Program (SHEP) pilot study. Stroke. 1989;20:4–13.
25. The SHEP Cooperative Study Group. Prevention of stroke by antihypertensive drug treatment in older persons with isolated systolic hypertension. JAMA. 1991;265:3255–64.
26. Dahlöf B, Lindholm LH, Hansson L, et al. Morbidity and mortality in the Swedish Trial in Old Patients with Hypertension (STOP-Hypertension). Lancet. 1991;338:1281–5.
27. Medical Research Council Trial of treatment of hypertension in older adults: principal results. MRC Working Party. BMJ. 1992;304:405–12.
28. Gong L, Zhang W, Zhu Y, et al. Shanghai trial of nifedipine in the elderly (STONE). J Hypertens. 1996;14:1237–45.
29. Staessen JA, Fagard R, Thijs L, et al., for the Systolic Hypertension in Europe (Syst-EUR) Trial Investigators. Morbidity and mortality in the placebo-controlled European Trial on Isolated Systolic Hypertension in the Elderly. Lancet. 1997;360:757–64.
30. Liu L, Wang J, Gong L, Liu G, Staessen JA, for the Systolic Hypertension in China (Syst-China) Collaborative Group. Comparison of active treatment and placebo in older Chinese patients with isolated systolic hypertension. J Hypertens. 1998;16:1823–9.

31. MacMahon S, Sharpe N, Gamble G, et al. Randomized, placebo-controlled trial of the angiotensin-converting enzyme inhibitor, ramipril, in patients with coronary or other occlusive arterial disease. J Am Coll Cardiol. 2000;36:438–43.
32. Lewis EJ, Hunsicker LG, Clarke WR, et al. Renoprotective effect of the angiotensin-receptor antagonist irbesartan in patients with nephropathy due to Type 2 diabetes. Collaborative Study Group. N Engl J Med. 2001;345:851–60.
33. Brenner BM, Cooper ME, de Zeeuw D, et al. Effects of losartan on renal and cardiovascular outcomes in patients with Type 2 diabetes and nephropathy. Reduction of Endpoints in Non-Insulin Dependent Diabetes Mellitus with the Angiotensin II Antagonist Losartan (RENAAL) Study Group. N Engl J Med. 2001;345:861–9.
34. Fox KM, and the EUROPA investigators. Efficacy of perindopril in reduction of cardiovascular events among patients with stable coronary artery disease: randomised, double-blind, placebo-controlled, multicentre trial (The EUROPA study). Lancet. 2003;362:782–8.
35. Bulpitt CJ, Beckett NS, Cooke J, et al. Results of the pilot study for the Hypertension in the Very Elderly Trial. J Hypertens. 2003;21:2409–17.
36. Marre M, Lievre M, Chatellier G, et al. Effects of low dose ramipril on cardiovascular and renal outcomes in patients with type 2 diabetes and raised excretion of urinary albumin: randomised, double blind, placebo controlled trial (The DIABHYCAR study). DIABHYCAR Study Investigators. BMJ. 2004;328:495.
37. Braunwald E, Domanski MJ, Fowler SE, et al. Angiotensin-converting-enzyme inhibition in stable coronary artery disease. The PEACE Trial Investigators. N Engl J Med. 2004;351:2058–68.
38. Lubsen J, Wagener G, Kirwan BA, de Brouwer S, Poole-Wilson PA. Effect of long-acting nifedipine on mortality and cardiovascular morbidity in patients with symptomatic stable angina and hypertension: the ACTION trial. The ACTION (A Coronary disease Trial Investigating Outcome with Nifedipine GITS) Investigators. J Hypertens. 2005;23:641–8.
39. Suzuki H, Kanno Y, for the Efficacy of Candesartan on Outcome in Saitama Trial (E-COST) Group. Effects of candesartan on cardiovascular outcomes in Japanese hypertensive patients. Hypertens Res. 2005;28:307–14.
40. Liu L, Zhang Y, Liu G, et al., for the FEVER Study Group. The Felodipine Event Reduction (FEVER) study: a randomized long-term placebo-controlled trial in Chinese hypertensive patients. J Hypertens. 2005;23:2157–72.
41. Patel A, and the ADVANCE Collaborative Group. Effects of a fixed combination of perindopril and indapamide on macrovascular and microvascular outcomes in patients with type 2 diabetes mellitus (the ADVANCE trial): a randomised controlled trial. Lancet. 2007;370:829–40.
42. Mochizuki S, Dahlöf B, Shimizu M, et al. Valsartan in a Japanese population with hypertension and other cardiovascular disease (Jikei Heart Study): a randomised, open-label, blinded endpoint morbidity-mortality study. Lancet. 2007;369:1431–9.
43. Beckett NS, Peters R, Fletcher AE, et al. Treatment of hypertension in patients 80 years of age or older. N Engl J Med. 2008;358:1887–98.
44. Yusuf S, for the Telmisartan Randomised Assessment Study in ACE Intolerant Subjects with Cardiovascular Disease (TRANSCEND) Investigators. Effects of the angiotensin-receptor blocker telmisartan on cardiovascular events in high-risk patients intolerant to angiotensin-converting enzyme inhibitors: a randomised controlled trial. Lancet. 2008;371:1174–83.
45. Califf RM, et al., on behalf of The NAVIGATOR Study Group. Effect of valsartan on the incidence of diabetes and cardiovascular events. N Engl J Med. 2010;362:1477–90.
46. Wilhelmsen L, Berglund G, Elmfeldt D, et al. Beta-blockers versus diuretics in hypertensive men: main result from the HAPPHY trial. J Hypertens. 1987;5:560–72.
47. Wikstrand J, Warnold I, Olsson G, et al. Primary prevention with metoprolol in patients with hypertension. Mortality results from the MAPHY study. JAMA. 1988;259:1976–82.
48. Borhani NO, Mercuri M, Borhani PA, et al. Final outcome results of the Multicenter Isradipine Diuretic Atherosclerosis Study (MIDAS): a randomized trial. JAMA. 1996;276:785–91.
49. Agabiti-Rosei E, Dal Palù C, Leonetti G, et al. Clinical results of the Verapamil in Hypertension and Atherosclerosis Study. The VHAS Investigators. J Hypertens. 1997;15:1337–44.

50. Schrier RW, Estacio RO. Additional follow-up from the ABCD Trial in patients with Type 2 diabetes and hypertension [letter]. N Engl J Med. 2000;343:1969.
51. Tatti P, Pahor M, Byington RP, et al. Outcome results of the Fosinopril Amlodipine Cardiovascular Events Randomized Trial (FACET) in patients with hypertension and NIDDM. Diabetes Care. 1998;21:1779–80.
52. Efficacy of atenolol and captopril in reducing the risk of macrovascular and microvascular complications in type 2 diabetes: UKPDS 39. UK Prospective Diabetes Study Group. BMJ. 1998;317:713–20.
53. Hansson L, Lindholm LH, Niskanen L, et al. Effect of angiotensin-converting-enzyme inhibition compared with conventional therapy on cardiovascular morbidity and mortality in hypertension: the Captopril Prevention Project (CAPPP) randomised trial. Lancet. 1999;353:611–6.
54. National Intervention Cooperative Study in Elderly Hypertensives Study Group. Randomized double-blind comparison of a calcium-antagonist and a diuretic in elderly hypertensives. Hypertension. 1999;34:1129–33.
55. Hansson L, Lindholm LH, Ekbom T, et al. Randomised trial of old and new antihypertensive drugs in elderly patients: cardiovascular mortality and morbidity. The Swedish Trial in Old Patients with Hypertension-2 study. Lancet. 1999;354:1751–6.
56. Brown MJ, Palmer CR, Castaigne A, et al. Morbidity and mortality in patients randomised to double-blind treatment with a long-acting calcium-channel blocker or diuretic in the International Nifedipine GITS study: Intervention as a Goal in Hypertension Treatment (INSIGHT). Lancet. 2000;356:366–72.
57. Hansson L, Hedner T, Lund-Johansen P, et al. for the NORDIL Study Group. Randomised trial of effects of calcium antagonists compared with diuretics and β-blockers on cardiovascular morbidity and mortality in hypertension: the Nordic Diltiazem (NORDIL) Study. Lancet. 2000;356:359–65.
58. Agodoa LY, Appel L, Bakris GL, et al. Effect of ramipril vs. amlodipine on renal outcomes in hypertensive nephrosclerosis: a randomized controlled trial. African American Study of Kidney Disease and Hypertension (AASK) Study Group. JAMA. 2001;285:2719–28.
59. Wright Jr JT, Bakris GL, Greene T, et al. Effect of blood pressure lowering and antihypertensive drug class on progression of hypertensive kidney disease: results from the AASK Trial. JAMA. 2002;288:2421–31.
60. Dahlöf B, Devereux RB, Kjeldsen SE, et al. for the LIFE Study group. Cardiovascular morbidity and mortality in the Losartan Intervention For Endpoint reduction in hypertension study (LIFE): a randomised trial against atenolol. Lancet. 2002;359:995–1003.
61. Zanchetti A, Bond M, Hennig M, et al. Calcium-antagonist lacidipine slows down progression of asymptomatic carotid atherosclerosis. Circulation. 2002;106:2422–7.
62. Major outcomes in high-risk hypertensive patients randomized to angiotensin-converting enzyme inhibitor or calcium channel blocker vs. diuretic: the Antihypertensive and Lipid Lowering Treatment to Prevent Heart Attack Trial (ALLHAT). The ALLHAT Officers and Coordinators for the ALLHAT Collaborative Research Group. JAMA. 2002;288:2981–97.
63. Wing LMH, Reid CM, Ryan P, et al. A comparison of outcomes with angiotensin-converting-enzyme inhibitors and diuretics for hypertension in the elderly. Second Australian National Blood Pressure Study Group. N Engl J Med. 2003;348:583–92.
64. Black HR, Elliott WJ, Grandits G, et al., for the CONVINCE Research Group. Principal results of the Controlled ONset Verapamil INvestigation of Cardiovascular Endpoints (CONVINCE) Trial. JAMA. 2003;289:2073–82.
65. Malacco E, Marcia G, Rappelli A, et al. Treatment of isolated systolic hypertension: the SHELL study results. The SHELL Investigators. Blood Press. 2003;12:160–7.
66. Pepine CJ, Handberg EM, Cooper-DeHoff RM, et al. A calcium antagonist vs. a non-calcium antagonist hypertension treatment strategy for patients with coronary artery disease: the International Verapamil-Trandolapril Study (INVEST): a randomized controlled trial. The INVEST Investigators. JAMA. 2003;290:2805–16.
67. Yui Y, Sumiyoshi T, Kodama K, et al. Comparison of nifedipine retard with angiotensin converting enzyme inhibitors in Japanese hypertensive patients with coronary artery disease: the

Japan Multicenter Investigation for Cardiovascular Disease-B (JMIC-B) randomized trial. Hypertens Res. 2004;27:181–91.

68. Julius S, Kjeldsen S, Weber M, et al. Outcomes in hypertensive patients at high cardiovascular risk treated with regimens based on valsartan or amlodipine: the VALUE randomised trial. Lancet. 2004;363:2022–31.

69. Barnett AH, Bain SC, Bouter P, et al. Angiotensin-receptor blockade versus converting-enzyme inhibition in type 2 diabetes and nephropathy. N Engl J Med. 2004;351:1952–61.

70. Dahlöf B, Sever PS, Poulter NR, et al. Prevention of cardiovascular events with an antihypertensive regimen of amlodipine adding perindopril as required versus atenolol adding bendroflumethiazide as required, in the Anglo-Scandinavian Cardiac Outcomes Trial-Blood Pressure Lowering Arm (ASCOT-BPLA): a multicentre randomised controlled trial. Lancet. 2005;366:895–906.

71. Ogihara T, Nakao K, Fukui T, et al., for the Candesartan Antihypertensive Survival Evaluation in Japan Trial Group. Effects of candesartan compared with amlodipine in hypertensive patients with high cardiovascular risks: Candesartan Antihypertensive Survival Evaluation in Japan trial. Hypertension. 2008;51:393–8.

72. Telmisartan, ramipril or both in patients at high risk for vascular events. ONTARGET Investigators. N Engl J Med. 2008;358:1547–9.

73. Jamerson K, Weber MA, Bakris GL, et al., for the ACCOMPLISH Trial Investigators. Benazepril plus amlodipine or hydrochlorothiazide for hypertension in high-risk patients. N Engl J Med. 2008;359:2417–28.

74. Narumi H, Takano H, Shindo S, et al., for the Valsartan Amlodipine Randomized Trial Study Group. Effects of valsartan and amlodipine on cardiorenal protection in Japanese hypertensive patients: the Valsartan Amlodipine Randomized Trial. Hypertens Res. 2011;34:62–9.

75. Matsuzaki M, Ogihara T, Umemoto S, et al., for the Combination Therapy of Hypertension to Prevent Cardiovascular Events Trial Group. Prevention of cardiovascular events with calcium channel blocker-based combination therapies in patients with hypertension: a randomized controlled trial. J Hypertens. 2011;29:1649–59.

76. Muramatsu T, Matsushita K, Yamashita K, et al., for the Nagoya Heart Study Investigators. Comparison between valsartan and amlodipine regarding cardiovascular morbidity and mortality in hypertensive patients with glucose intolerance: Nagoya Heart Study. Hypertension 2012;59:580–6.

77. Staessen JA, Wang J-G, Thijs L. Cardiovascular prevention and blood pressure reduction: a quantitative overview updated until 01 March 2003. J Hypertens. 2003;21:1055–76.

78. Turnbull F, for the Blood Pressure Lowering Treatment Trialists' Collaboration. Effects of different blood-pressure-lowering regimens on major cardiovascular events: results of prospectively-designed overviews of randomised trials. Lancet. 2003;362:1527–35.

79. Verdecchia P, Reboldi G, Angeli F, et al. Angiotensin-converting enzyme inhibitors and calcium channel blockers for coronary heart disease and stroke prevention. Hypertension. 2005;46:386–92.

80. Agabiti-Rosei E, Mancia G, O'Rourke MF, et al. Central blood pressure measurements and antihypertensive therapy: a consensus document. Hypertension. 2007;50:154–60.

81. Williams B, Lacy PS, Thom SM, et al., for the Anglo-Scandinavian Cardiac Outcomes Trial Investigators; CAFÉ Steering Committee and Writing Committee. Differential impact of blood pressure-lowering drugs on central aortic pressure and clinical outcomes: principal results of the Conduit Artery Function Evaluation (CAFE) Study. Circulation. 2005;113:1213–25.

82. Mancia G, De Backer G, Dominiczak A, et al. 2007 Guidelines for the management of arterial hypertension: the Task Force for the Management of Arterial Hypertension of the European Society of Hypertension (ESH) and the European Society of Cardiology (ESC). J Hypertens. 2007;25:1105–87.

83. Wang J-G, Staessen JA, Li Y, et al. Carotid intima-media thickness and antihypertensive treatment: a meta-analysis of randomized controlled trials. Stroke. 2006;37:1933–40.

84. Schrader J, Luders S, Kulschewski A, et al. The ACCESS Study: evaluation of acute candesartan cilexetil therapy in stroke survivors. Stroke. 2003;34:1699–703.

85. Schrader J, Luders S, Kulschewski A, et al. Morbidity and mortality after stroke, eprosartan compared with nitrendipine for secondary prevention: principal results of a prospective randomized controlled study (MOSES). Stroke. 2005;36:1218–26.
86. Yusuf S, Diener H-C, Sacco RL, et al., for the PRoFESS Study Group. Telmisartan to prevent recurrent stroke and cardiovascular events. N Engl J Med. 2008;359:1225–37.
87. Hansson L, Zanchetti A, Carruthers SG, et al. Effects of intensive blood pressure lowering and low-dose aspirin in patients with hypertension: principal results of the Hypertension Optimal Treatment (HOT) randomised trial: the HOT Study Group. Lancet. 1998;351:1755–62.
88. Cushman WC, Evans GW, Byington RP, et al., for the Action to Control Cardiovascular Risk in Diabetes Study Group. Effects of intensive blood-pressure control in type 2 diabetes mellitus. N Engl J Med. 2010;362:1575–85.

Part II
Mechanisms of Hypertension and Hypertension-Related Stroke

Chapter 4
Mechanisms Underlying Essential Hypertension: Neurogenic and Non-neurogenic Contributors

Scott H. Carlson, Sean Stocker, and J. Michael Wyss

Stroke is the fourth leading cause of death in the USA and a leading cause of incapacitation, often leaving individuals permanently impaired and unable to work or live independent lives. One of the leading risk factors for stroke is hypertension, and the risk of stroke is directly proportional to the elevation and duration of high blood pressure [1–3]. Furthermore, hypertension also contributes significantly to cardiovascular disease, which itself increases the risk of stroke. Despite the prevalence of hypertension, its significant negative impacts on health, and nearly a century of research, the mechanisms underlying the chronic increase in arterial pressure in most hypertensive individuals remain elusive. As initially elucidated by Guyton and others, renal factors are a prominent contributor to hypertension in many individuals, but an increasing amount of research indicates that the sympathetic nervous system and its interactions with vasoactive hormones and intracellularly generated substances also contribute to the pathogenesis of hypertension. This chapter reviews the evidence, suggesting that a neurogenic mechanism can chronically elevate peripheral resistance and arterial pressure, and interactions between the sympathetic nervous system and the hormones (e.g., angiotensin and nitric oxide) act synergistically to increase blood pressure. Finally, it reviews the role of intraneuronal reactive oxygen species

S.H. Carlson, Ph.D.
Department of Biology, Luther College, Decorah, IA, USA
e-mail: carlsosc@luther.edu

S. Stocker, Ph.D.
Departments of Cellular and Molecular Physiology and Neural and Behavioral Sciences, Penn State College of Medicine, Hershey, PA, USA
e-mail: sstocker@hmc.psu.edu

J.M. Wyss, Ph.D. (✉)
Departments of Cell Developmental and Integrative Biology and Medicine, University of Alabama at Birmingham, Birmingham, AL, USA
e-mail: jmwyss@uab.edu

© Springer International Publishing Switzerland 2016
V. Aiyagari, P.B. Gorelick (eds.), *Hypertension and Stroke*, Clinical Hypertension and Vascular Diseases, DOI 10.1007/978-3-319-29152-9_4

(ROS) in the modulation of sympathetic activity and the role of the eicosanoid 20-hydroxyeicosatetraenoic acid (20-HETE) in vascular smooth muscle regulation in both hypertension and stroke-induced vasospasm.

The Sympathetic Nervous System and Hypertension

Over the past 40 years, clinical studies and animal research have strongly suggested that sympathetic nervous system overactivity contributes to several forms of essential hypertension [4, 5]. However, what leads to this elevated sympathetic activity is unclear. The rostral ventrolateral medulla (RVLM) is the principal nucleus in the brain that provides the tonic drive to preganglionic neurons in the spinal cord intermediolateral nucleus to support sympathetic nervous system activity. The RVLM neurons are sensitive to baroreceptor feedback to the CNS and spontaneously discharge at a frequency that corresponds to basal sympathetic nervous system activity [6]. The basal activity has been attributed to both autorhythmic pacemaker properties and/or synaptic inputs [7]. Chemical excitation of RVLM neurons increases sympathetic nerve activity and blood pressure, and these neurons mediate acute reflexive changes in sympathetic outflow to a variety of physiological challenges, and more importantly, numerous studies indicate that neurogenic hypertension arises from altered RVLM neuronal properties and/or increased excitatory synaptic input thereby increasing sympathetic nervous system activity, augmenting vasoconstriction and thus elevating arterial pressure (see [5, 8]; Fig. 4.1). Increased excitatory drive (or decreased inhibitory input) in neurogenic hypertension may arise several brain regions including but not limited to: various hypothalamic nuclei including the paraventricular nucleus and dorsomedial hypothalamus, the caudal pressor area in the brain stem [9, 10], chemoreceptor input [11], sodium excitation of neurons in the AV3V region of the forebrain [12], and the inhibitory inputs from baroreceptors and other CNS sites such as the caudal ventrolateral medulla. Published studies by a number of laboratories suggest that modulation of these inputs via increased excitatory or reduced inhibition to the RVLM contributes to neurogenic hypertension [5, 6, 12–15].

Given the role of renal function in cardiovascular homeostasis, much of the research into sympathetic nervous system overactivity has focused on the renal sympathetic nerves and their overactivity. Renal denervation reduces hypertension in several rodent models [16–19] and in non-responsive hypertensive individuals [17, 20]. However, a growing body of evidence indicates that sympathetic control of other vascular regions may also contribute to at least some forms of hypertension. Splanchnic nerve activity is elevated in response to infusion of pressor doses of angiotensin [21], and ablation of the splanchnic nerves attenuates hypertension in Dahl-S [22] and angiotensin-NaCl hypertension [23]. Interestingly, in Dahl-S rats, both renal and splanchnic denervation reduce arterial pressure, while in angiotensin-NaCl treated rats splanchnic, but not renal, denervation attenuates hypertension. Similarly, angiotensin-NaCl rats display an increased splanchnic nerve activity

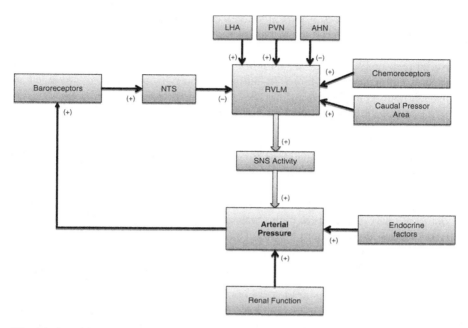

Fig. 4.1 Arterial .pressure is a function of sympathetic nervous system (SNS) activity, circulating endocrine factors, and renal function. SNS activity is regulated by the spontaneous discharge of neurons in the rostral ventrolateral medulla (RVLM), which are regulated by baroreceptor and chemoreceptor input to the nucleus of the solitary tract (NTS) and innervation from the caudal pressor area of the medulla and from hypothalamic regions, e.g., the paraventricular (PVN), lateral hypothalamic area (LHA), and anterior hypothalamic (AHN) nuclei

while renal nerve activity is reduced [24]. These results suggest that sympathetic nervous activity is not uniformly distributed to all organs, and in contrast changes to each region are individually controlled. This concept is supported by a growing number of studies [25–27], and suggests that each form of hypertension may have a unique sympathetic outflow pattern.

Elevated sympathetic nervous system activity may result from impairment of neurohumoral reflexes. Probably the most widely studied feedback systems are the arterial baroreceptors (which respond to changes in arterial pressure), cardiopulmonary receptors (which detect changes in blood volume), and chemoreceptors (which respond to changes in blood gas levels and pH). All of these feedback mechanisms respond to acute changes in the parameters they monitor and alter autonomic nervous system activity to maintain baseline arterial pressure (Fig. 4.1). While impaired sensory feedback can cause acute, large elevations in arterial pressure, the role of such alterations in chronic hypertension remains debatable. Bristow et al. [28] were the first to suggest that arterial baroreceptor imbalance could chronically alter arterial pressure regulation; however, extensive work by Cowley and Guyton demonstrated that in dogs, the elimination of baroreflex feedback increased the lability of blood pressure, but did not increase the average arterial pressure [29]. Subsequent studies demonstrated that in response to sustained increases in arterial pressure, baroreceptors rapidly reset to a new set point and, thereafter, adjusted autonomic nervous system activity to defend the new arterial pressure set point. These findings led to the hypothesis that baroreceptors are only short-term regulators of autonomic activity and are not involved in chronic, neurogenic hypertension (reviewed in Cowley [30]).

In contrast to this common wisdom of earlier decades, a number of recent studies suggest that baroreceptors have a more chronic role in the regulation of autonomic nervous system activity and, therefore, may contribute to elevated sympathetic outflow and sustained hypertension in some individuals. Studies by Thrasher and by Lohmeier suggest that baroreceptors can chronically inhibit the sympathetic nervous system and that imbalances in these reflex feedbacks can lead to sustained hypertension [31–33]. Other studies indicate that while baroreceptor control of heart rate resets to higher pressure, renal sympathetic nerve activity and renal function do not reset [34, 35]. This suggests that, similar to the individual sympathetic outflow patterns discussed above, reflex control of autonomic activity is non-uniform and depends on the specific sensory stimuli. For example, in angiotensin-NaCl rats, heart and splanchnic control have a clearly different time-course [36], and blockade of nitric oxide production in rabbits results in a greater decrease in renal (compared to lumbar) sympathetic activity. In contrast, volume expansion decreases only renal nerve activity, and hypoxia changes both lumbar and renal nerve activity similarly. These findings, along with similar studies [26, 27, 37], indicate that activation of baroreceptors (or other sensory afferents) leads to differential regional control of sympathetic nerve activity, and thus, sympathetic nervous system activity is likely not uniformly reset following sustained changes in arterial pressure. Differential changes in regulation of these distinct sympathetic pathways may lead to imbalances that underlie a chronic role for baroreflexes in hypertension.

Higher Nervous System Regulators of Blood Pressure

In addition to potential alterations in reflex control of autonomic activity, sympathetic overactivity may result from central regulators of arterial pressure. While the RVLM has been extensively studied because of its role as the brain's tonic sympathetic nervous system drive and a dominant acute arterial pressure regulator, higher brain areas coordinate the activity of RVLM and other sympathetic nervous system regulatory neurons. The hypothalamus has emerged as one of the major regulators of this coordinated output to the autonomic nervous system (Fig. 4.1).

Among the areas of the hypothalamus that appear to be important in this regulation are lateral posterior hypothalamus, paraventricular hypothalamic nucleus (PVN), and anterior hypothalamic area nuclei. The lateral hypothalamic area predominantly contains sympathoexcitatory neurons, whereas the anterior and preoptic regions tend to be sympathoinhibitory. In rats made hypertensive by administration of the steroid deoxycorticosterone acetate and a high salt diet, stimulation of the posterior or lateral hypothalamus increases arterial pressure and heart rate, whereas lesions of the posterior hypothalamus reduce arterial pressure [38]. Furthermore, the lateral hypothalamic area, dorsomedial hypothalamus, and the hypothalamic arcuate nucleus respond to circulating leptin levels and thereby play a role in increases of sympathetic activity and blood pressure, and these, at least in part, appear to lead to hypertension that accompanies obesity [39, 40].

In PVN, magnocellular neurons synthesize and release vasopressin into the circulation, while parvocellular neurons project mono- or poly-synaptically to several CNS cardiovascular control nuclei, including the RVLM, area postrema, NTS, and the intermediolateral nucleus of the spinal cord. Through these connections the parvocellular neurons alter cardiovascular function. Conversely, the PVN receives input from a large number of regions in the brain, including those associated with osmotic control (the organum vasculosum of the lamina terminalis, subfornical organ, and median preoptic nuclei), appetite and energy metabolism (lateral hypothalamus, arcuate nucleus), stress and other areas that exert effects on blood pressure [41]. Thus, it is clear that the role of the PVN is to integrate inputs from a variety of sources and modify RVLM activity accordingly.

The anterior hypothalamic region contains several areas that are important in cardiovascular control, including the anteroventral third ventricle, which can contribute to hypertension in several animal models. The median preoptic nucleus appears to underlie many of these cardiovascular effects (*see*, e.g., [42, 43]). Other preoptic nuclei regulate vasopressin release and water balance and contribute, at least indirectly, to arterial pressure control. The anterior hypothalamic nucleus, along with the preoptic area, provides important sympathoinhibitory influences, most of which are mediated by projections to sympathoexcitatory nuclei in the diencephalon and brain stem. An example of their importance is seen in spontaneously hypertensive rats (SHRs), in which diets high in salt exacerbate hypertension, at least in part, by reducing sympathoinhibitory drive from the anterior hypothalamic nucleus [44].

Several cortical regions of the brain also appear to influence blood pressure, especially in relation to volitional [45] or emotional situations [46]. These include the prefrontal cortex [45] and several limbic regions such as the anterior cingulate and insular cortices and the amygdala [47]. Whether these regions contribute to hypertension is not known.

The Renin–Angiotensin System and Hypertension

Circulating endocrine factors contribute significantly to arterial pressure regulation via peripherally mediated actions and may serve as causative factors in hypertension. Of these, the renin–angiotensin–aldosterone system (RAAS) is probably the most thoroughly studied circulating hormone, largely because angiotensin II (AII) exerts potent vasoconstrictor effects and is a powerful regulator of blood volume.

Of the current arsenal of antihypertensive drugs, angiotensin-related pharmaceuticals have emerged as one of the most effective antihypertensives for a majority of patients. Furthermore, several rodent models of hypertension display a strong linkage to circulating AII, including SHRs, TGR mRen2 rats, Dahl salt-sensitive rats, DOCA-salt rats, and renal hypertensive rats [48]. While AII appears to raise arterial pressure in these models, at least in part, through inappropriate volume retention or increased vascular resistance, these models are also characterized by elevated sympathetic activity. This has led researchers to hypothesize that an overactive RAAS may elevate arterial pressure both through its peripheral actions and by directly augmenting sympathetic nervous system activity.

One central action by which AII may modify autonomic outflow is by inhibition of baroreceptor function (Fig. 4.2). Several studies have demonstrated that baroreceptor control of arterial pressure is significantly blunted following AII infusion [49], and this can be blocked by administration of an AII type 1 (AT$_1$) receptor blocker [50]. This effect extends to many hypertensive rat models, including SHR [50], the high renin TGR(mREN2)27 [51], two-kidney one-clip [52, 53], and the Lyon [54]. Conversely, angiotensinogen transgenic rats [TGR (ASrAOGEN)], which are characterized by low levels of AII, demonstrate an enhanced baroreflex response compared to nontransgenic controls, and infusion with AII decreases baroreceptor sensitivity in this model [55].

The observation that circulating AII inhibits baroreflex activity suggests that AII gains access to sites within the CNS to exert this effect. However, AII has traditionally been thought not to cross the intact blood–brain barrier, and act by binding to and stimulating receptors in circumventricular nuclei, where there is no blood–brain

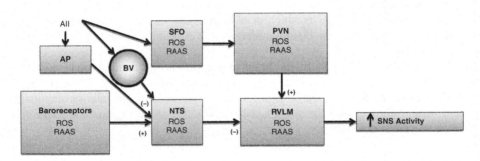

Fig. 4.2 Circulating angiotensin (AII) can bind to circumventricular organs (e.g., the area postrema (AP) or subfornical organ (SFO)), increasing neuronal activity of sympathoexcitatory nuclei or modulating baroreceptor sensitivity. Alternatively, AII stimulation can lead to activation of the intraneuronal renin–angiotensin–aldosterone system (RAAS) and subsequent generation of AII and related metabolites and/or generation of reactive oxygen species (ROS), both of which may alter the neuronal firing rate of cardiovascular regulatory nuclei and increase sympathetic nervous system activity. AII activation of receptors in the blood vessels (BVs) of the brain stem can also alter neuronal activity in the NTS and RVLM through generation of second messengers that cross the blood–brain barrier (e.g., NO and superoxide)

barrier, or binding to cerebrovascular receptors that secondarily transmit a signal to the brain [56]. It is of interest to note that a recent study suggests that blood brain barrier may become permeable in AngII hypertension [57]. The area postrema is likely a circumventricular site for such interactions. It is adjacent to the nucleus tractus solitarius, which is the location of baroreceptor input to the medulla, and it expresses AII receptors [48]. A number of observations support a role for the area postrema in mediating AII-induced inhibition of baroreflexes. Microinjection of angiotensin into the area postrema blunts baroreceptor sensitivity, and microinjection of an angiotensin-converting enzyme (ACE) inhibitor into the area postrema blocks this effect [58]. Ablation of area postrema abolishes AII-induced desensitization of baroreflex in rabbits [49] and eliminates AII-induced hypertension in rats [59]. Furthermore, removal of the area postrema prevents the antihypertensive effects of AII receptor blockade on baroreceptor function in SHR [60]. The subfornical organ (SFO) provides another circumventricular site at which peripheral AII binds to CNS receptors and can alter brain activity.

Research into the role of the RAAS in hypertension has long focused on peripheral actions of AII (for instance, as an enhancer of norepinephrine release) or its central circumventricular-mediated effects. However, over the past 30 years, a growing body of research demonstrates that neurons and glial cells within the CNS contain all RAAS components, including angiotensinogen, renin, angiotensin-converting enzyme, and all angiotensin receptors [48, 61]. This discovery suggested that angiotensin may act as a paracrine neuromodulator or be released as a neurotransmitter. AII receptors are distributed in almost all brain nuclei involved in cardiovascular regulation [61], including PVN, parabrachial nucleus, RVLM, and the NTS [48].

These studies have provided detailed localization of an intrinsic renin–angiotensin system in the central nervous system, but its role is only beginning to be understood. Probably, the most studied region containing an endogenous renin–angiotensin system is the SFO where circulating angiotensin binds to neuronal receptors leading to alterations in drinking and vasopressin release (from the PVN). The SFO neurons not only respond to angiotensin II, but also use the peptide to transmit signals to CNS neurons. Using transgenic mice that express human renin and/or angiotensin genes or have deleted angiotensin system genes in selected areas of the brain [62–65], Sigmund and Davisson demonstrated that expression of the human renin (hREN) or human angiotensinogen (hAGT) induced hypertension in these mice, and intraventricular administration of an AT_1 antagonist blunted this response. Furthermore, their studies using conditional transgenic mice demonstrate that neurons in the CNS utilize angiotensin as a neurotransmitter that regulates blood pressure and other functions. More recently, they modified their double-transgenic strain so that it had a neuronal-specific promoter, ensuring expression only in neural tissue [65]. Compared to nontransgenic mice, these mice display higher arterial pressure. The chronic effects of AII may be mediated by increased endoplasmic reticulum stress [66]. It is noteworthy that recent studies also suggest SFO neurons respond to other circulating factors including but not limited to leptin and sodium concentrations (e.g., [67, 68]) thereby raising the possibility that SFO neurons integrate multiple neurohumoral signals to regulate sympathetic outflow.

One of the major targets of the SFO is PVN, which is a major source of afferents to RVLM. This PVN to RVLM projection also appears to employ angiotensin II to modulate RVLM activity [69]. These results suggest that excitatory synaptic inputs from the PVN to the RVLM are mediated, at least in part, by angiotensin receptors in the RVLM. Together with studies by Chen et al. [70] and others, these results indicate that angiotensin decreases GABAergic inhibition of PVN neurons, thereby increasing their firing rate and leading to excitation of RVLM neurons (Fig. 4.2).

Nitric Oxide and Hypertension

Nitric oxide (NO) is a second circulating agent that has been strongly implicated as a modulator of sympathetic nervous system activity and blood pressure control. NO, which is produced from the amino acid precursor arginine by nitric oxide synthase (NOS), is a potent vasodilator and thus tends to reduce blood pressure when generated in blood vessels, or when its precursor is administered exogenously. Impaired NO-mediated vasorelaxation is observed in most animal and human models of aging and also occurs in age-associated conditions such as hypertension [71]. Chronic inhibition of NOS by L-NAME induces hypertension associated with an increase in peripheral vascular resistance and an enhanced vascular responsiveness to adrenergic stimuli [72]. Furthermore, when a NO donor is coadministered with L-NAME, the hypertension is prevented [72]. Interestingly, L-NAME-induced hypertension appears to involve both the renin–angiotensin system and the sympathetic nervous system [72]. Treatment of rats with an ACE inhibitor prevents the development of hypertension in L-NAME-treated rats [72, 73], at least in part, by reducing sympathetic nervous system activity [72, 74]. These studies suggest that NO may act within the brain to elevate sympathetic nervous system activity.

Although the mechanisms by which central NO modulates neuronal activity are unclear, research suggests that NO may alter neuronal responses to dendritic input from innervating neurons and paracrine factors. One region of interest in this regard is NTS, which is the relay between baroreceptor input and RVLM. Microinjection of glutamate into RVLM simulates a baroreceptor-mediated signal, indicating a transient increase in arterial pressure. This normally elicits a reflex decrease in heart rate and renal sympathetic nerve activity that decreases arterial pressure [13]. Mifflin and colleagues have shown that an RVLM microinjection of the NOS antagonist L-NAME prior to the glutamate injection greatly reduces the reflex response of arterial pressure, heart rate, and renal nerve activity that are normally elicited by the glutamate injection. These results support the hypothesis that within the RVLM, NO facilitates glutamine-mediated feedback from baroreceptors and cardiopulmonary receptors.

Reactive Oxygen Species and Hypertension

While NO and angiotensin play generally opposite roles in the regulation of the sympathetic nervous system in hypertension, both can be responsible for the generation of ROS and thereby elevate arterial pressure. Recent studies have focused on angiotensin-induced generation of ROS, including oxygen ions, free radicals, and peroxides, all of which are natural by-products of the normal metabolism of enzymes such as NADPH-oxidase. As ROS are generated, they are converted by intracellular superoxide dismutase (SOD) into hydrogen peroxide. Since hydrogen peroxide is itself a potent free radical species, it must be quickly degraded by enzymes such as catalase, glutathione peroxidase, and peroxiredoxins.

Recent studies indicate that ROS play a role in hypertension, and ROS have been demonstrated to contribute to neurogenic hypertension by inducing sympathoexcitation. ROS levels are elevated in SHR [75], even prior to the onset of hypertension, and vascular, renal, and cardiac ROS production is also increased in this model [76, 77]. Similarly, stroke-prone SHR (SHR-SP), DOCA, and endothelin-infusion models also display elevated ROS generation [78]. Centrally administered tempol (an SOD mimetic) decreases arterial pressure in these hypertensive models, and it reduces renal sympathetic nerve activity and heart rate [79]. These data support a role for central ROS generation in hypertension.

The mechanism by which excess ROS alter cardiovascular control is unclear. Some effects of ROS clearly occur in the periphery and alter endothelial and renal function. However, recent research has shown that ROS in central cardiovascular nuclei increase sympathetic activity, resulting in neurogenic hypertension. For example, ROS generation is elevated in the RVLM of SHR-SP [80], SHR [81], and one-clip hypertensive rats [80], and microinjection of tempol reduces sympathetic nervous system activity and arterial pressure. Increasing evidence suggests that ROS generation is involved in intracellular signaling pathways, including those utilized by AII. Central infusion of AII increases mean arterial pressure and sympathetic nerve activity, and coadministration of tempol abolishes these AII effects [82]. Similarly, AII-induced pressor and drinking responses are accompanied by increased superoxide production in the SFO, and SOD overexpression in the SFO eliminates these responses [83, 84]. These results suggest that elevated AII can increase arterial pressure by increasing ROS generation within SFO neurons, thereby increasing activation of hypothalamic centers that control sympathetic nervous system activity.

20-HETE

While hypertension may be driven by the central mechanisms described above, vascular factors also act concomitantly to raise blood pressure. One widely studied contributor is the eicosanoid 20-hydroxyeicosatetraenoic acid (20-HETE), which is a by-product of arachidonic acid metabolism by the enzyme cytochrome P450

(CYP). 20-HETE's vascular actions serve to enhance vasoconstrictive responses to both sympathetic input and to vasoactive hormones such as angiotensin and phenylephrine [85]. These actions are mediated by blocking large-conductance calcium-activated potassium channels (BK_{Ca}), leading to the depolarization and contraction of vascular smooth muscle. 20-HETE also serves to increase cytosolic calcium levels by opening protein kinase C-gated L-type Ca^{2+} channels [58, 85], while enhancing calcium sensitivity of myosin in vascular smooth muscle [85].

The vasoactive actions of vascular 20-HETE indicate that it is a prime candidate to contribute to hypertension. Indeed, CYP is overexpressed in several hypertensive models and contributes to the development and maintenance of high blood pressure in these animals. For example, changes in the expression pattern of CYP correspond to the development of high blood pressure in SHRs, and the degree of hypertension can be attenuated by inhibition of the enzyme [86]. CYP overexpression is also observed in angiotensin-induced hypertension [87–89], Lyon rats [90], Dahl salt-sensitive rats [91], androgen-induced hypertension [92], and a reduced uterine perfusion model of preeclampsia [93]. Furthermore, nitric oxide appears to inhibit CYP activity and 20-HETE formation [94], suggesting the possibility that NO-depleted hypertension leads to elevated 20-HETE production and contributes to elevated blood pressure. CYP overexpression also appears to contribute to age-associated increases in blood pressure in normotensive rats. In aged (18-month-old) Sprague Dawley rats, blockade of CYP decreases vascular responsiveness to phenylephrine, while CYP inhibition has no effect on vasoconstrictor response in young (3-month-old) rats [95]. Similar results are observed in aged ovariectomized female rats, and estrogen replacement does not affect the enhanced vasoconstrictor responses [96]. Taken together, these results indicate that alterations in both CYP expression and corresponding 20-HETE levels contribute to multiple forms of hypertension.

In addition to 20-HETE's ability to increase vascular sensitization to exogenous stimuli, research suggests a fundamental role for 20-HETE mediating myogenic autoregulation of resistance arterioles [97]. Changes in transmural pressure of arterioles lead to generation of 20-HETE, which serves to reflexly constrict arterioles by increasing calcium influx via activation of transient receptor potential (TRP) channels and by closing BK_{Ca} channels [97, 98]. This myogenic role of 20-HETE has been demonstrated in multiple vasculatures (e.g., mesenteric, renal, cardiac) [99–101], and blockade of 20-HETE formation impairs autoregulation of both renal and cerebral blood flow in vivo [102].

The second arm of vascular autoregulation is based on the metabolic demands of the perfused regions. Under this model, increases in cell activity lead to the production of vasoactive metabolites, which exert a dilatory influence on precapillary arterioles to increase regional blood flow, thereby matching flow to need. While this metabolic process is seemingly simple, the underlying mechanisms are extremely complex and remain to be fully resolved. An increasing number of studies indicate that astrocytes, glial cells which induce the blood–brain barrier, may respond to changes in extracellular metabolites as well as secreted neurotransmitters and release vasoactive components to modify vascular tone and blood flow [103, 104]. The epoxyeicosatrienoic acids (EETs), which are derived from a different family of

CYP enzymes, have actions opposing those of 20-HETE. Once generated, EETs activate BKCa channels in vascular smooth muscle cells, resulting in hyperpolarization and dilation of the vessels. Thus, EETs have been suggested to serve as endothelium-derived hyperpolarizing factors [105]. EETs are also synthesized by astrocytes within the central nervous system, and have been suggested to function as neurovascular couplers. As such, changes in neuronal activity leads to astrocytic EET formation and corresponding vasodilation [104, 106]. The net effect of EET formation is to match cerebral blood flow to regional metabolic demands. Altered levels of EETs have also been implicated in hypertension and vascular function; in many hypertensive models, the concentration of EETs is decreased through reductions in expression combined with enhanced metabolism of EETs by soluble epoxide hydrolase related to the level of blood pressure; concentrations are decreased (see [105]). Thus, blood pressure may be controlled at the vascular level by the balance of 20-HETE to EET levels.

The role of CYP-derived 20-HETE and EETs in cerebrovasculature regulation has been of particular interest in stroke. Similar to other vasculatures, cerebral blood flow is autoregulated through the balance of two regulatory controls, and under normal conditions this maintains constancy in cerebral blood flow. However, diseased states, such as sustained elevation of blood pressure, can impair cerebral autoregulation, while also inducing vascular remodeling and alterations in endothelial function [85, 104]. These changes may serve to alter the balance of 20-HETE and EET production, thereby enhancing the myogenic constriction and decreasing cerebral blood flow while also increasing the risk of ischemic stroke and cognitive decline [104, 105]. Levels of 20-HETE in cerebrospinal fluid increase hemorrhagic stroke in rats, and increased levels of 20-HETE contribute to associated vasospasms [107]. Administration of a 20-HETE inhibitor prevents ischemic-based reductions in cardiac [108] and cerebral blood flow [109], while also reducing the infarct size. 20-HETE levels are also elevated in the cerebral vasculature of SHR [110] and stroke-prone SHR [111], contributing to oxidative stress, endothelial dysfunction, and the enhanced ischemic damage. Clinical studies have demonstrated a similar association of CYP-derived metabolites with stroke. Acute ischemia patients display elevated CYP expression, higher 20-HETE concentration, and increased levels of arachidonic acid-derived oxidative by-products [112]. Baseline 20-HETE levels were also found to be associated with the lesion size and indices of functionality. Similarly, polymorphisms of CYP genes have linked to ischemic stroke in a variety of ethnic populations (see [113]).

Summary

Based on research in animal models and humans, it is clear that the nervous system plays a significant role in the chronic elevation of arterial pressure. Research is beginning to identify mechanisms by which sympathetic nervous system activity is elevated in these models of hypertension. Increases in RVLM neuronal activity in response to an imbalance in excitatory and inhibitory input, diminished baroreceptor signaling, and enhanced excitatory input from the caudal pressor region of the medulla and PVN all play a role in hypertension. Studies also suggest that the RAAS contributes to sympathoexcitation, through both circulating angiotensin and endogenous neutrally derived angiotensin. Neuronal activity may also be altered by generation of ROS within neurons and/or a reduction in neuronal nitric oxide formation in the brain or periphery. Finally, peripheral actions such as enhanced neuroendocrine signaling through elevated 20-HETE production appear to contribute significantly to hypertension. Future research will more fully elucidate the contribution of each of these factors to chronic hypertension and how they synergize with other factors to exacerbate stroke.

References

1. Mvundura M, McGruder H, Khoury MJ, Valdez R, Yoon PW. Family history as a risk factor for early-onset stroke/transient ischemic attack among adults in the United States. Public Health Genomics. 2010;13:13–20.
2. Collins R, Peto R, Godwin J, MacMahon S. Blood pressure and coronary heart disease. Lancet. 1990;336:370–1.
3. MacMahon S, et al. Blood pressure, stroke, and coronary heart disease. Part 1, Prolonged differences in blood pressure: prospective observational studies corrected for the regression dilution bias. Lancet. 1990;335:765–74.
4. Grassi G, Quarti-Trevano F, Dell'oro R, Mancia G. Essential hypertension and the sympathetic nervous system. Neurol Sci. 2008;29 Suppl 1:S33–6.
5. Guyenet PG. The sympathetic control of blood pressure. Nat Rev Neurosci. 2006;7:335–46.
6. Dampney RA, et al. Medullary and supramedullary mechanisms regulating sympathetic vasomotor tone. Acta Physiol Scand. 2003;177:209–18.
7. Kumagai H, et al. Importance of rostral ventrolateral medulla neurons in determining efferent sympathetic nerve activity and blood pressure. Hypertens Res. 2012;35:132–41.
8. Sved AF, Ito S, Madden CJ, Stocker SD, Yajima Y. Excitatory inputs to the RVLM in the context of the baroreceptor reflex. Ann N Y Acad Sci. 2001;940:247–58.
9. Yajima Y, et al. Enhanced response from the caudal pressor area in spontaneously hypertensive rats. Brain Res. 2008;1227:89–95.
10. Potas JR, Dampney RA. Sympathoinhibitory pathway from caudal midline medulla to RVLM is independent of baroreceptor reflex pathway. Am J Physiol Regul Integr Comp Physiol. 2003;284:R1071–8.
11. Moreira TS, Takakura AC, Colombari E, Guyenet PG. Central chemoreceptors and sympathetic vasomotor outflow. J Physiol. 2006;577:369–86.
12. Simmonds SS, Lay J, Stocker SD. Dietary salt intake exaggerates sympathetic reflexes and increases blood pressure variability in normotensive rats. Hypertension. 2014;64:583–9.
13. Dias AC, Vitela M, Colombari E, Mifflin SW. Nitric oxide modulation of glutamatergic, baroreflex, and cardiopulmonary transmission in the nucleus of the solitary tract. Am J Physiol Heart Circ Physiol. 2005;288:H256–62.
14. Haywood JR, et al. gamma-Aminobutyric acid (GABA)—a function and binding in the paraventricular nucleus of the hypothalamus in chronic renal-wrap hypertension. Hypertension. 2001;37:614–8.
15. Vitela M, Mifflin SW. gamma-Aminobutyric acid(B) receptor-mediated responses in the nucleus tractus solitarius are altered in acute and chronic hypertension. Hypertension. 2001;37:619–22.

16. Pires NM, et al. Blood pressure decrease in spontaneously hypertensive rats following renal denervation or dopamine beta-hydroxylase inhibition with etamicastat. Hypertens Res. 2015;38:605–12.
17. Briasoulis A, Bakris GL. A clinician's perspective of the role of renal sympathetic nerves in hypertension. Front Physiol. 2015;6:75.
18. Khan SA, et al. Obesity depresses baroreflex control of renal sympathetic nerve activity and heart rate in Sprague Dawley rats: role of the renal innervation. Acta Physiol (Oxf). 2015;214:390–401.
19. Hendel MD, Collister JP. Renal denervation attenuates long-term hypertensive effects of Angiotensin II in the rat. Clin Exp Pharmacol Physiol. 2006;33:1225–30.
20. Esler M. The sympathetic nervous system in hypertension: back to the future? Curr Hypertens Rep. 2015;17:11.
21. Luft FC, et al. Angiotensin-induced hypertension in the rat. Sympathetic nerve activity and prostaglandins. Hypertension. 1989;14:396–403.
22. Foss JD, Fink GD, Osborn JW. Reversal of genetic salt-sensitive hypertension by targeted sympathetic ablation. Hypertension. 2013;61:806–11.
23. King AJ, Osborn JW, Fink GD. Splanchnic circulation is a critical neural target in angiotensin II salt hypertension in rats. Hypertension. 2007;50:547–56.
24. Yoshimoto M, Miki K, Fink GD, King A, Osborn JW. Chronic angiotensin II infusion causes differential responses in regional sympathetic nerve activity in rats. Hypertension. 2010;55:644–51.
25. Ramchandra R, Barrett CJ, Guild SJ, Malpas SC. Evidence of differential control of renal and lumbar sympathetic nerve activity in conscious rabbits. Am J Physiol Regul Integr Comp Physiol. 2006;290:R701–8.
26. Yao Y, et al. The effect of losartan on differential reflex control of sympathetic nerve activity in chronic kidney disease. J Hypertens. 2015;33:1249–60.
27. Shi Z, Brooks VL. Leptin differentially increases sympathetic nerve activity and its baroreflex regulation in female rats: role of oestrogen. J Physiol. 2015;593:1633–47.
28. Bristow JD, et al. The influence of ventilation, carbon dioxide and hypoxia on the baroreceptor reflex in man. J Physiol. 1968;198:102; passim-103.
29. Cowley Jr AW, Liard JF, Guyton AC. Role of baroreceptor reflex in daily control of arterial blood pressure and other variables in dogs. Circ Res. 1973;32:564–76.
30. Cowley Jr AW. Long-term control of arterial blood pressure. Physiol Rev. 1992;72:231–300.
31. Thrasher TN. Arterial baroreceptor input contributes to long-term control of blood pressure. Curr Hypertens Rep. 2006;8:249–54.
32. Lohmeier TE, Iliescu R. The baroreflex as a long-term controller of arterial pressure. Physiology (Bethesda). 2015;30:148–58.
33. Iliescu R, Tudorancea I, Lohmeier TE. Baroreflex activation: from mechanisms to therapy for cardiovascular disease. Curr Hypertens Rep. 2014;16:453.
34. Barrett CJ, Guild SJ, Ramchandra R, Malpas SC. Baroreceptor denervation prevents sympathoinhibition during angiotensin II-induced hypertension. Hypertension. 2005;46:168–72.
35. Lohmeier TE. The sympathetic nervous system and long-term blood pressure regulation. Am J Hypertens. 2001;14:147S–54.
36. Kuroki MT, Guzman PA, Fink GD, Osborn JW. Time-dependent changes in autonomic control of splanchnic vascular resistance and heart rate in ANG II-salt hypertension. Am J Physiol Heart Circ Physiol. 2012;302:H763–9.
37. Rahman AA, Shahid IZ, Pilowsky PM. Differential cardiorespiratory and sympathetic reflex responses to microinjection of neuromedin U in rat rostral ventrolateral medulla. J Pharmacol Exp Ther. 2012;341:213–24.
38. Oparil S, Chen YF, Berecek K, Calhoun DA, Wyss JM. The role of the central nervous system in hypertension. In Laragh J.H.M., Brenner, B.M. (eds.), Hypertension: pathophysiology, diagnosis and management. 2nd ed. New York: Raven; 1995.
39. Esler M, et al. Mechanisms of sympathetic activation in obesity-related hypertension. Hypertension. 2006;48:787–96.
40. Dampney RA. Arcuate nucleus—a gateway for insulin's action on sympathetic activity. J Physiol. 2011;589:2109–10.

41. Ferguson AV, Latchford KJ, Samson WK. The paraventricular nucleus of the hypothalamus—a potential target for integrative treatment of autonomic dysfunction. Expert Opin Ther Targets. 2008;12:717–27.
42. Osborn JW, et al. Effect of subfornical organ lesion on the development of mineralocorticoid-salt hypertension. Brain Res. 2006;1109:74–82.
43. Ployngam T, Collister JP. An intact median preoptic nucleus is necessary for chronic angiotensin II-induced hypertension. Brain Res. 2007;1162:69–75.
44. Wyss JM, Yang RH, Oparil S. Lesions of the anterior hypothalamic area increase arterial pressure in NaCl-sensitive spontaneously hypertensive rats. J Auton Nerv Syst. 1990;31:21–9.
45. Shoemaker JK, Norton KN, Baker J, Luchyshyn T. Forebrain organization for autonomic cardiovascular control. Auton Neurosci. 2015;188:5–9.
46. de Morree HM, Szabo BM, Rutten GJ, Kop WJ. Central nervous system involvement in the autonomic responses to psychological distress. Neth Heart J. 2013;21:64–9.
47. Cechetto DF. Cortical control of the autonomic nervous system. Exp Physiol. 2014;99:326–31.
48. Veerasingham SJ, Raizada MK. Brain renin-angiotensin system dysfunction in hypertension: recent advances and perspectives. Br J Pharmacol. 2003;139:191–202.
49. Sanderford MG, Bishop VS. Central mechanisms of acute ANG II modulation of arterial baroreflex control of renal sympathetic nerve activity. Am J Physiol Heart Circ Physiol. 2002;282:H1592–602.
50. Kawano Y, Yoshida K, Matsuoka H, Omae T. Chronic effects of central and systemic administration of losartan on blood pressure and baroreceptor reflex in spontaneously hypertensive rats. Am J Hypertens. 1994;7:536–42.
51. Schiffer S, Pummer S, Witte K, Lemmer B. Cardiovascular regulation in TGR(mREN2)27 rats: 24h variation in plasma catecholamines, angiotensin peptides, and telemetric heart rate variability. Chronobiol Int. 2001;18:461–74.
52. Berenguer LM, Garcia-Estan J, Ubeda M, Ortiz AJ, Quesada T. Role of renin-angiotensin system in the impairment of baroreflex control of heart rate in renal hypertension. J Hypertens. 1991;9:1127–33.
53. Heesch CM, Crandall ME, Turbek JA. Converting enzyme inhibitors cause pressure-independent resetting of baroreflex control of sympathetic outflow. Am J Physiol. 1996;270:R728–37.
54. Lantelme P, Cerutti C, Lo M, Paultre CZ, Ducher M. Mechanisms of spontaneous baroreflex impairment in lyon hypertensive rats. Am J Physiol. 1998;275:R920–5.
55. Baltatu O, et al. Alterations in blood pressure and heart rate variability in transgenic rats with low brain angiotensinogen. Hypertension. 2001;37:408–13.
56. Paton JF, Waki H, Abdala AP, Dickinson J, Kasparov S. Vascular-brain signaling in hypertension: role of angiotensin II and nitric oxide. Curr Hypertens Rep. 2007;9:242–7.
57. Biancardi VC, Son SJ, Ahmadi S, Filosa JA, Stern JE. Circulating angiotensin II gains access to the hypothalamus and brain stem during hypertension via breakdown of the blood-brain barrier. Hypertension. 2014;63:572–9.
58. Tan PS, Killinger S, Horiuchi J, Dampney RA. Baroreceptor reflex modulation by circulating angiotensin II is mediated by AT1 receptors in the nucleus tractus solitarius. Am J Physiol Regul Integr Comp Physiol. 2007;293:R2267–78.
59. Fink GD, Bruner CA, Mangiapane ML. Area postrema is critical for angiotensin-induced hypertension in rats. Hypertension. 1987;9:355–61.
60. Matsumura K, Averill DB, Ferrario CM. Role of AT1 receptors in area postrema on baroreceptor reflex in spontaneously hypertensive rats. Brain Res. 1999;850:166–72.
61. Parsons KK, Coffman TM. The renin-angiotensin system: it's all in your head. J Clin Invest. 2007;117:873–6.
62. Davisson RL, et al. The brain renin-angiotensin system contributes to the hypertension in mice containing both the human renin and human angiotensinogen transgenes. Circ Res. 1998;83:1047–58.
63. Sinnayah P, et al. Genetic ablation of angiotensinogen in the subfornical organ of the brain prevents the central angiotensinergic pressor response. Circ Res. 2006;99:1125–31.

64. Doobay MF, et al. Differential expression of neuronal ACE2 in transgenic mice with overexpression of the brain renin-angiotensin system. Am J Physiol Regul Integr Comp Physiol. 2007;292:R373–81.
65. Sakai K, et al. Local production of angiotensin II in the subfornical organ causes elevated drinking. J Clin Invest. 2007;117:1088–95.
66. Young CN, et al. ER stress in the brain subfornical organ mediates angiotensin-dependent hypertension. J Clin Invest. 2012;122:3960–4.
67. Dai L, Smith PM, Kuksis M, Ferguson AV. Apelin acts in the subfornical organ to influence neuronal excitability and cardiovascular function. J Physiol. 2013;591:3421–32.
68. Young CN, Morgan DA, Butler SD, Mark AL, Davisson RL. The brain subfornical organ mediates leptin-induced increases in renal sympathetic activity but not its metabolic effects. Hypertension. 2013;61:737–44.
69. Tagawa T, Dampney RA. AT(1) receptors mediate excitatory inputs to rostral ventrolateral medulla pressor neurons from hypothalamus. Hypertension. 1999;34:1301–7.
70. Chen Q, Pan HL. Signaling mechanisms of angiotensin II-induced attenuation of GABAergic input to hypothalamic presympathetic neurons. J Neurophysiol. 2007;97:3279–87.
71. Walsh T, Donnelly T, Lyons D. Impaired endothelial nitric oxide bioavailability: a common link between aging, hypertension, and atherogenesis? J Am Geriatr Soc. 2009;57:140–5.
72. Torok J. Participation of nitric oxide in different models of experimental hypertension. Physiol Res. 2008;57:813–25.
73. Pechanova O, Bernatova I, Pelouch V, Simko F. Protein remodelling of the heart in NO-deficient hypertension: the effect of captopril. J Mol Cell Cardiol. 1997;29:3365–74.
74. Zicha J, Dobesova Z, Kunes J. Antihypertensive mechanisms of chronic captopril or N-acetylcysteine treatment in L-NAME hypertensive rats. Hypertens Res. 2006;29:1021–7.
75. Kimura Y, et al. Overexpression of inducible nitric oxide synthase in rostral ventrolateral medulla causes hypertension and sympathoexcitation via an increase in oxidative stress. Circ Res. 2005;96:252–60.
76. Zhang F, et al. Decreased levels of cytochrome P450 2E1-derived eicosanoids sensitize renal arteries to constrictor agonists in spontaneously hypertensive rats. Hypertension. 2005;45:103–8.
77. Zalba G, et al. Vascular NADH/NADPH oxidase is involved in enhanced superoxide production in spontaneously hypertensive rats. Hypertension. 2000;35:1055–61.
78. Callera GE, Tostes RC, Yogi A, Montezano AC, Touyz RM. Endothelin-1-induced oxidative stress in DOCA-salt hypertension involves NADPH-oxidase-independent mechanisms. Clin Sci (Lond). 2006;110:243–53.
79. Paravicini TM, Touyz RM. NADPH oxidases, reactive oxygen species, and hypertension: clinical implications and therapeutic possibilities. Diabetes Care. 2008;31 Suppl 2:S170–80.
80. Hirooka Y, et al. Amlodipine-induced reduction of oxidative stress in the brain is associated with sympatho-inhibitory effects in stroke-prone spontaneously hypertensive rats. Hypertens Res. 2006;29:49–56.
81. Bolad I, Delafontaine P. Endothelial dysfunction: its role in hypertensive coronary disease. Curr Opin Cardiol. 2005;20:270–4.
82. Campese VM, Shaohua Y, Huiquin Z. Oxidative stress mediates angiotensin II-dependent stimulation of sympathetic nerve activity. Hypertension. 2005;46:533–9.
83. Zimmerman MC, et al. Superoxide mediates the actions of angiotensin II in the central nervous system. Circ Res. 2002;91:1038–45.
84. Zimmerman MC, Lazartigues E, Sharma RV, Davisson RL. Hypertension caused by angiotensin II infusion involves increased superoxide production in the central nervous system. Circ Res. 2004;95:210–6.
85. Hoopes SL, Garcia V, Edin ML, Schwartzman ML, Zeldin DC. Vascular actions of 20-HETE. Prostaglandins Other Lipid Mediat. 2015;120:9–16.
86. Capdevila JH, Falck JR, Imig JD. Roles of the cytochrome P450 arachidonic acid monooxygenases in the control of systemic blood pressure and experimental hypertension. Kidney Int. 2007;72:683–9.

87. Alonso-Galicia M, Maier KG, Greene AS, Cowley Jr AW, Roman RJ. Role of 20-hydroxyeicosatetraenoic acid in the renal and vasoconstrictor actions of angiotensin II. Am J Physiol Regul Integr Comp Physiol. 2002;283:R60–8.

88. Moreno C, Maier KG, Hoagland KM, Yu M, Roman RJ. Abnormal pressure-natriuresis in hypertension: role of cytochrome P450 metabolites of arachidonic acid. Am J Hypertens. 2001;14:90S–7.

89. Muthalif MM, et al. Angiotensin II-induced hypertension: contribution of Ras GTPase/mitogen-activated protein kinase and cytochrome P450 metabolites. Hypertension. 2000;36:604–9.

90. Messer-Letienne I, Bernard N, Roman RJ, Sassard J, Benzoni D. 20-Hydroxyeicosatetraenoic acid and renal function in Lyon hypertensive rats. Eur J Pharmacol. 1999;378:291–7.

91. Hoagland KM, Maier KG, Roman RJ. Contributions of 20-HETE to the antihypertensive effects of Tempol in Dahl salt-sensitive rats. Hypertension. 2003;41:697–702.

92. Singh H, Schwartzman ML. Renal vascular cytochrome P450-derived eicosanoids in androgen-induced hypertension. Pharmacol Rep. 2008;60:29–37.

93. Llinas MT, Alexander BT, Capparelli MF, Carroll MA, Granger JP. Cytochrome P-450 inhibition attenuates hypertension induced by reductions in uterine perfusion pressure in pregnant rats. Hypertension. 2004;43:623–8.

94. Miyata N, Roman RJ. Role of 20-hydroxyeicosatetraenoic acid (20-HETE) in vascular system. J Smooth Muscle Res. 2005;41:175–93.

95. Berezan DJ, Dunn KM, Falck JR, Davidge ST. Aging increases cytochrome P450 4A modulation of alpha1-adrenergic vasoconstriction in mesenteric arteries. J Cardiovasc Pharmacol. 2008;51:327–30.

96. Berezan DJ, Xu Y, Falck JR, Kundu AP, Davidge ST. Ovariectomy, but not estrogen deficiency, increases CYP4A modulation of alpha(1)-adrenergic vasoconstriction in aging female rats. Am J Hypertens. 2008;21:685–90.

97. Bubb KJ, et al. Activation of neuronal transient receptor potential vanilloid 1 channel underlies 20-hydroxyeicosatetraenoic acid-induced vasoactivity: role for protein kinase A. Hypertension. 2013;62:426–33.

98. Toth P, et al. Role of 20-HETE, TRPC channels, and BKCa in dysregulation of pressure-induced Ca2+ signaling and myogenic constriction of cerebral arteries in aged hypertensive mice. Am J Physiol Heart Circ Physiol. 2013;305:H1698–708.

99. Harder DR, et al. Formation and action of a P-450 4A metabolite of arachidonic acid in cat cerebral microvessels. Am J Physiol. 1994;266:H2098–107.

100. Imig JD, Zou AP, Ortiz de Montellano PR, Sui Z, Roman RJ. Cytochrome P-450 inhibitors alter afferent arteriolar responses to elevations in pressure. Am J Physiol. 1994;266:H1879–85.

101. Frisbee JC, Roman RJ, Murali Krishna U, Falck JR, Lombard JH. Altered mechanisms underlying hypoxic dilation of skeletal muscle resistance arteries of hypertensive versus normotensive Dahl rats. Microcirculation. 2001;8:115–27.

102. Gebremedhin D, et al. Production of 20-HETE and its role in autoregulation of cerebral blood flow. Circ Res. 2000;87:60–5.

103. Gordon GR, Mulligan SJ, MacVicar BA. Astrocyte control of the cerebrovasculature. Glia. 2007;55:1214–21.

104. Imig JD, Simpkins AN, Renic M, Harder DR. Cytochrome P450 eicosanoids and cerebral vascular function. Expert Rev Mol Med. 2011;13, e7.

105. Tacconelli S, Patrignani P. Inside epoxyeicosatrienoic acids and cardiovascular disease. Front Pharmacol. 2014;5:239.

106. Metea MR, Newman EA. Signalling within the neurovascular unit in the mammalian retina. Exp Physiol. 2007;92:635–40.

107. Cambj-Sapunar L, Yu M, Harder DR, Roman RJ. Contribution of 5-hydroxytryptamine1B receptors and 20-hydroxyeicosatetraenoic acid to fall in cerebral blood flow after subarachnoid hemorrhage. Stroke. 2003;34:1269–75.

108. Yousif MH, Benter IF, Roman RJ. Cytochrome P450 metabolites of arachidonic acid play a role in the enhanced cardiac dysfunction in diabetic rats following ischaemic reperfusion injury. Auton Autacoid Pharmacol. 2009;29:33–41.

109. Renic M, et al. Effect of 20-HETE inhibition on infarct volume and cerebral blood flow after transient middle cerebral artery occlusion. J Cereb Blood Flow Metab. 2009;29:629–39.
110. Toth P, et al. Treatment with the cytochrome P450 omega-hydroxylase inhibitor HET0016 attenuates cerebrovascular inflammation, oxidative stress and improves vasomotor function in spontaneously hypertensive rats. Br J Pharmacol. 2013;168:1878–88.
111. Dunn KM, et al. Elevated production of 20-HETE in the cerebral vasculature contributes to severity of ischemic stroke and oxidative stress in spontaneously hypertensive rats. Am J Physiol Heart Circ Physiol. 2008;295:H2455–65.
112. Ward NC, et al. Cytochrome P450 metabolites of arachidonic acid are elevated in stroke patients compared with healthy controls. Clin Sci (Lond). 2011;121:501–7.
113. Deng S, et al. CYP4F2 gene V433M polymorphism is associated with ischemic stroke in the male Northern Chinese Han population. Prog Neuropsychopharmacol Biol Psychiatry. 2010;34:664–8.

Chapter 5
The Effects of Hypertension and Stroke on the Cerebral Vasculature

Anne M. Dorrance

Cerebral blood flow must be tightly regulated to ensure that the metabolic demands of the neurons are always met [1]. This exquisite control is facilitated by two physiological mechanisms, neurovascular coupling and autoregulation. This chapter will discuss these mechanisms and how they are perturbed by hypertension and cerebral ischemia. Arterial resistance also contributes to the regulation of cerebral blood flow. Hypertension causes structural alterations in cerebral arteries that increase arterial resistance and the damage caused by cerebral ischemia. The mechanisms responsible for this cerebral artery remodeling will also be discussed. Ischemic strokes are the most common in the population; thus the discussion here will be largely limited to this stroke subtype. The cerebral blood vessels control the duration and depth of the ischemia experienced during a stroke, thus their structure and function are important determinants of the magnitude of the final infarct and the clinical outcome [2].

Cerebral Artery Anatomy

Prior to discussing the effects on hypertension on cerebral arteries it is worth pausing to describe some basic physiology of the cerebral circulation. The cerebral arteries are highly specialized to prevent reductions in blood flow to the parenchyma in the event of an ischemic insult [3, 4]. The circle of Willis is a ring of connected arteries at the base of the brain (Fig. 5.1a). This structure allows for cross perfusion of the cerebral hemispheres, and blood flow within the circle of Willis can be reversed to

A.M. Dorrance, Ph.D. (✉)
Department of Pharmacology and Toxicology, Michigan State University,
East Lansing, MI, USA
e-mail: dorranc3@msu.edu

© Springer International Publishing Switzerland 2016
V. Aiyagari, P.B. Gorelick (eds.), *Hypertension and Stroke*, Clinical
Hypertension and Vascular Diseases, DOI 10.1007/978-3-319-29152-9_5

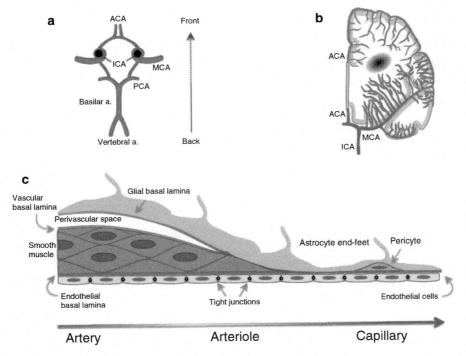

Fig. 5.1 Cerebral blood supply. (**a**) Depicts the major cerebral arteries including the circle of Willis, the middle cerebral artery, and the basilar artery. (**b**) Depicts the blood supply to the deep white matter. The penetrating arterioles branch from the pial arteries and dive into the brain parenchyma. (**c**) Depicts the structure of the artery/arteriole/capillary wall. *ACA* anterior cerebral artery, *ICA* internal carotid artery, *MCA* middle cerebral artery, *PCA* posterior cerebral artery. (From Iadecola, C., The pathobiology of vascular dementia. Neuron, 2013. **80**(4): p. 844-66, with permission)

circumvent an ischemic occlusion in a constituent artery. The pial arteries that cover the surface of the brain also provide protection from ischemia. A large number of anastomoses connect the arteries branching from the posterior and middle cerebral arteries and the anterior and middle cerebral arteries [5]. These connections provide collateral blood flow in the event that a small surface artery is occluded [6–8]. The pial arteries are innervated by the peripheral nervous system [9], and the sympathetic and parasympathetic nerves help regulate vascular tone by releasing neurotransmitters that cause vasoconstriction (norepinephrine and neuropeptide Y) and vasodilation (acetylcholine and nitric oxide), respectively [9–11].

The penetrating (or parenchymal) arteries and arterioles branch from the pial arteries and dive into the parenchyma to perfuse the cortex and regulate flow to the microcirculation (Fig. 5.1b) [12]. When they enter the brain the penetrating arteries are bathed in cerebrospinal fluid in the Virchow-Robin space. As they dive further into the parenchyma, the penetrating arteries and arterioles are surrounded by astrocytic end-feet and neuronal axon endings (Figs. 5.1c and 5.2) [9]. Unlike the

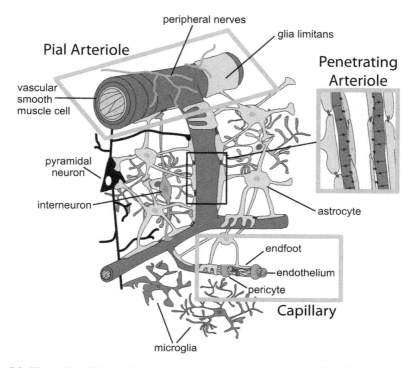

Fig. 5.2 Illustration of the cerebral arteries and the neurovascular unit. The diagram shows the pial arteries on the surface of the brain including the extrinsic innervation. The penetrating arterioles are also depicted; these arterioles contain endothelial cells and one layer of vascular smooth muscle cells. The penetrating arterioles are surrounded by astrocytes, neurons, and pericytes (not illustrated here) and they receive intrinsic innervation from within the neuropil. The capillaries consist of a layer of endothelial cells sounded by pericytes, neurons, and astrocytes. (Adapted from Filosa, J.A., et al., Beyond neurovascular coupling, role of astrocytes in the regulation of vascular tone. Neuroscience, 2015., doi:10.1016/j.neuroscience.2015.03.064, with permission)

pial arteries the penetrating arterioles have very few branches, thus occluding one penetrating arteriole causes significant injury to the surrounding cortex [13]. Flow through the penetrating arterioles is partly regulated by intrinsic innervation from within the neuropil (Fig. 5.2) [9]. Most of the nerves involved in this regulation target the astrocytes surrounding the artery and not the artery itself, thus the astrocytes relay signals from active neurons to arterioles to increase perfusion in times of high metabolic demand [14, 15].

A dense network of cerebral capillaries arises from the penetrating arterioles [16], and there is significant redundancy in this system to provide protection from cerebral ischemia [17]. The capillaries are surrounded by pericytes which have classically been thought to constrict and relax to regulate perfusion [18]. However, more recent studies show that pericytes do not contain the contractile protein alpha smooth muscle actin, and they do not regulate blood flow in response to neuronal stimulation or spreading depression [19]. However, the high pericyte density observed in the cerebral vasculature compared to other organs suggests these cells play an important physiological role in the brain [20, 21]. The pericytes are part of the neurovascular unit, which also contains vascular smooth muscle cells, endothelial cells, astrocytes, and neurons (Fig. 5.2). The pericytes may act as a conduit for relaying information between the neural and vascular compartment in the brain [19]. Stroke causes a breakdown in communication between the cells in the neurovascular unit [22] that dysregulates cerebral blood flow control and blood brain barrier (BBB) function [23, 24].

Neurovascular Coupling

Neurovascular coupling links the metabolic demands of the neurons to cerebral perfusion [13]. This requires rapid integrated signaling between neurons, interneurons, perivascular nerves, glia, and the cells in the vasculature [25, 26]. Active neurons [27], interneurons, and astrocytes [28] release vasodilators that cause localized dilation, or functional hyperemia, in penetrating arterioles and pial arteries supplying them [13]. Neurovascular coupling requires the activity of the three key vasodilator pathways: nitric oxide (NO) [29, 30], cyclooxygenase (COX)-2 metabolites [31], and epoxyeicosatrienoic acids (EETs) [32]. For a detailed description of the signaling mechanisms involved in neurovascular coupling please see [25].

Effects of Hypertension on Neurovascular Coupling

Studies of the effects of hypertension on neurovascular coupling in humans are limited. One study showed that increases in regional perfusion in response to a memory test were impaired in patients with untreated hypertension [33]. It should be noted that the patients in this study were only mildly hypertensive (systolic/diastolic 144.2/84.4 mmHg). It is possible that patients with more malignant hypertension will exhibit more marked impairments in neurovascular coupling.

In laboratory studies utilizing rodents, neurovascular coupling is assessed by measuring increased perfusion or vasodilation in response to a sensory stimulus such as whisker stimulation. Several of these studies have utilized the angiotensin II model of hypertension. Both chronic and acute angiotensin II administration reduces the blood flow response to whisker stimulation in mice [34]. Interestingly, in the chronic studies impaired neurovascular coupling preceded development of hypertension [35]. This suggests angiotensin II may have direct effects on the cerebral vasculature that are unrelated to the increase in blood pressure it mediates. The argument for direct vascular effects of angiotensin II is strengthened by studies showing that the application of angiotensin II directly to the cerebral cortex impairs the blood flow response to whisker stimulation without altering blood pressure [35]. Subsequent studies suggest that this direct effect of angiotensin II occurs via activation of the type 1 angiotensin receptor and requires reactive oxygen species generation [36].

The finding of a direct vascular effect of angiotensin II on neurovascular coupling makes it difficult to determine how much of the suppressed neurovascular coupling observed in angiotensin II treated mice is due to the elevation in blood pressure per se. Studies using genetically hypertensive rats such as the spontaneously hypertensive rat (SHR) could help solve this problem, but there are surprisingly few studies of neurovascular coupling using this type of model. The only available study suggests that neurovascular coupling is impaired in SHR. Normalizing the blood pressure with losartan, an angiotensin receptor blocker (ARB), had no beneficial effect on neurovascular coupling, suggesting that the impaired neurovascular coupling observed in SHR is not angiotensin II dependent [37]. It also suggests that the impaired neurovascular coupling is not blood pressure dependent. This study is clearly at odds with the previously described studies in mice with angiotensin II dependent hypertension. The rats treated with losartan were quite old (30 weeks) and these rats would have been hypertensive for at least two-thirds of their life. Therefore, it is possible that the drug was ineffective because the vascular injury mediated by the prolonged hypertension could not be reversed.

The Effects of Stroke on Neurovascular Coupling

Studies of neurovascular coupling in humans post-stroke have yielded variable results. Positron emission tomography (PET) scanning has been used to measure the blood flow response to bilateral motor activation in patients with unilateral internal carotid artery or middle cerebral artery (MCA) steno-occlusive lesions. Functional hyperemia was intact in both somatosensory cortices where the neuronal activation was occurring. This suggests that in these patients neurovascular coupling is intact. Interestingly, administration of a potent cerebral artery dilator, acetazolamide, did not increase blood flow in the ipsilateral somatosensory cortex. Acetazolamide is used to measure cerebrovascular reserve capacity, or the maximal possible perfusion in the brain. This study suggests that ischemia reduces cerebrovascular reserve capacity without impairing neurovascular coupling, thus the dilator mechanisms employed by neurovascular coupling appear to be able to overcome the hemodynamic impairments in the brain post-ischemia. In these studies the PET scans were conducted at least 2 months after the ischemic insult, therefore they do not provide information about blood flow control in the acute and subacute time points post-stroke. It should be noted that in these studies the neurological dysfunction was mild. Although all of the patients had a confirmed occlusion only 60 % of them had an abnormal neurological exam [38].

Other studies using PET scanning and visual stimulation have been conducted in patients with internal carotid artery steno-occlusive disease. Visual stimulation of both eyes caused an increase in perfusion to both visual cortices in all patients. Perfusion of the regions around the visual cortex was highly variable. Most patients exhibited reduced blood flow in the damaged hemisphere when compared to the contralateral hemisphere. The reduced blood flow in the regions surrounding the visual cortex may be the result of a redistribution of blood flow in the brain, i.e., the increase in blood flow to the visual cortex may steal blood from the surrounding areas [39].

There are many potential variables in human studies that make the interpretation of the results difficult. For this reason animal studies can provide valuable information. One of the benefits of rodent studies is that the acute effects of stroke can be easily studied in a controlled manner. Laboratory studies show that neurovascular coupling is impaired after both global and focal cerebral ischemia. Impaired neurovascular coupling was observed in Wistar rats 5 days after the induction of focal cerebral ischemia. The impaired neurovascular response was observed in a location remote to the infarct itself but within the same hemisphere. It is of note that in this particular study overall brain function may have been depressed post-stroke because glucose utilization was also reduced [40]; this would reduce the need for enhanced regional blood flow giving the appearance of impaired neurovascular coupling. However, later studies where brain function was normal also suggest that neurovascular coupling is impaired acutely after a short period of transient focal ischemia induced by MCA occlusion [41]. Studies of global ischemia induced by occluding the vertebral and carotid arteries also suggest that neurovascular coupling is impaired by ischemia. Three hours after the ischemic insult a marked reduction in cerebral perfusion in response to neural stimulation was detected, and this occurred without a significant change in neural activity. This study clearly suggests that in the aftermath of ischemia the communication between the active neurons and the vasculature to stimulate hyperemia is impaired [42]. This basic finding was confirmed by Baker et al. [43] who also showed that the magnitude of the ischemic insult was important. As one might expect, more severe ischemic insults produce larger impairments in neurovascular coupling [43, 44]. These studies were conducted in normotensive rats; it is not clear how hypertension affects the neurovascular response to stroke. It is possible that the impairments in neurovascular coupling observed post-stroke will be of a greater magnitude in hypertensive populations.

Cerebral Artery Autoregulation

Before discussing the effects of hypertension and stroke on cerebral autoregulation it is important that we define two key terms: myogenic tone and myogenic reactivity. Myogenic tone is an intrinsic property of arteries and arterioles to maintain an active contractile force in the smooth muscle cells of the vascular wall. Myogenic tone is regulated by several factors including the intraluminal pressure, the resting potassium conductance, calcium channel activity, and the

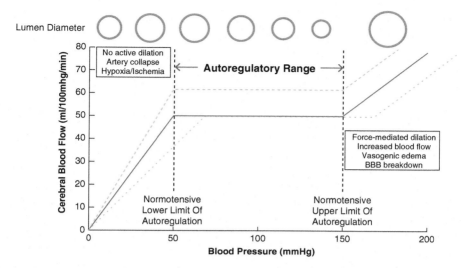

Fig. 5.3 Cerebral autoregulation. The lower and upper limits of autoregulation are indicated by the *dotted vertical lines*. The *solid line* depicts normal cerebral blood flow, the *dashed* and *dotted lines* depict two of the proposed effects of hypertension on the autoregulatory response. The *red circles* at the *top* of the figure provide an indication of the effects of intraluminal pressure on the lumen diameter of the cerebral arteries. The *Text boxes* describe the effects of intralumenal pressures that rise above or fall below the limits of autoregulation

sensitivity of the contractile signaling pathways to calcium. The generation of tone is initiated purely by the vascular smooth muscle cells, but the endothelium can regulate myogenic tone [45, 46] through the production of NO [47], prostacyclin [48], and endothelium derived hyperpolarizing factor (EDHF) [49]. The term myogenic reactivity describes a more active process; myogenic reactivity is the ability of the artery to change tone in response to fluctuations in intralumenal pressure while keeping blood flow constant. These myogenic mechanisms are responsible for much of the basal vascular tone that regulates cerebrovascular resistance [50].

Cerebral artery autoregulation, or the Bayliss effect, contributes to the brain's ability to maintain a constant blood flow while the perfusion pressure is fluctuating (Fig. 5.3). In most adults, cerebral arteries autoregulate over a range of mean arterial pressures from approximately 60 to 150 mmHg [51]. When blood pressure increases within the autoregulatory range cerebral arteries constrict and when pressure falls the arteries dilate. This pattern of constriction and dilation allows for the maintenance of constant cerebral blood flow [52, 53]. At high perfusion pressures the contribution of myogenic reactivity to cerebral autoregulation is particularly important because arteries must constrict to prevent an increase in blood flow [52]. At pressures above and below the limits of autoregulation blood flow is directly proportional to the intraluminal pressure. Breaching the upper limit of autoregulation causes increased perfusion and vasogenic edema. When the intralumenal pressure in an artery falls below the lower limit of autoregulation, hypoperfusion and ischemic injury ensue [6]. Several factors have been associated with the control of cerebral autoregulation, these include neuronal NO production [51, 54–56], blood flow itself [57], sympathetic nervous system mediated vasoconstriction [58], and cholinergic vasodilation [59].

Effect of Hypertension on Myogenic Tone Generation and Autoregulation

Studies of the effects of hypertension on autoregulation and myogenic reactivity in rodent models of hypertension have yielded differing results. Some studies suggest that arteries from SHR autoregulate over a higher range of pressures than arteries from normotensive Wistar Kyoto (WKY) rats (65–190 vs. 40–150 mmHg) [60, 61]. Other studies suggest the autoregulatory range is the same between SHR and WKY rats but myogenic tone generation is affected by hypertension such that for a given arterial pressure arteries from SHR are relatively more constricted than those from WKY rats [62]. Sex differences in the control of autoregulation have also been reported. The myogenic response in middle cerebral arteries from male stroke prone spontaneously hypertensive rats (SHRSP) are similar to those from WKY rats, but the middle cerebral arteries from female SHRSPs exhibit more myogenic constriction than arteries from female WKY rats [63]. SHRSPs are a widely used model of human essential hypertension and their cerebral vasculature has been extensively studied [64, 65].

Recent studies focusing on the penetrating arterioles show that their myogenic tone is significantly higher in SHRSP than in WKY rats. This increased tone was reduced by administration of antihypertensive therapy (hydralazine, hydrochlorothiazide, and reserpine) beginning after the development of hypertension. The increased tone observed in the SHRSP was largely dependent on the activity of the L-type voltage gated calcium channel [66].

Too much myogenic tone in the large cerebral arteries could impede cerebral blood flow, but a complete loss of tone is also detrimental. Loss of myogenic tone in the larger arteries puts the small arterioles and capillaries at risk of rupture if blood pressure increases. SHRSPs exhibit a complete loss of myogenic tone when fed a high salt or stroke prone diet [67]. SHRSP fed this diet from weaning develop hemorrhagic strokes within 10 weeks, at this time the cerebral arteries have lost the ability to generate tone and cerebral perfusion is largely regulated by blood pressure [68]. This loss of tone generation may be a consequence of the malignant hypertension that is observed in salt-loaded SHRSP [69, 70]. At present it is not clear if humans with uncontrolled malignant hypertension also exhibit impaired myogenic tone generation.

Aging influences myogenic mechanisms and their response to hypertension. Studies comparing young (3-month-old) or old (24-month-old) angiotensin II treated mice suggest that myogenic reactivity is lost when hypertension is superimposed on a background of aging. This loss of the contractile response to increased intraluminal pressure was associated with reduced production of the vasoconstrictor 20-hydroxye-icosatetraenoic acid (20-HETE) [71] and a reduced sensitivity of the smooth muscle cells to 20-HETE [72]. The activity of the transient receptor potential (TRP) channel canonical 6 (TRPC6) was also reduced in the old hypertensive mice [71]. TRPC6 has been proposed to be a mechanosensor in cerebral arteries responsible for linking pressure and stretch to constriction [73].

Although the studies directly measuring the effects of hypertension on tone and reactivity are conflicting, the biochemical pathways that regulate tone certainly suggest that tone should be increased by hypertension. For example, endothelial NO synthase (eNOS) expression is reduced in cerebral microvessels from hypertensive rats [74]; this would reduce dilation and increase tone generation. Increased superoxide production could also impair NO-mediated dilation in arteries from hypertensive subjects because superoxide reacts with NO to reduce its bioavailability [75, 76]. EDHF is also an important determinant of cerebrovascular tone and reactivity [77]. EDHF mediated dilation requires the activation of calcium-activated K^+ channels, the small- and intermediate-conductance Ca^{2+}-activated K^+ channels (SK_{Ca} and IK_{Ca}, respectively) [78, 79]. IK_{Ca} knockout mice are hypertensive and they exhibit impaired endothelium dependent dilation and this could increase tone generation [80]. TRP channels also regulate endothelial function in cerebral arteries [81, 82]. Activation of TRPC3 causes vasoconstriction [83]. TRPC3 expression is increased in carotid and mesenteric arteries from SHR compared to normotensive rats and this is linked to augmented contractility [84]. Unfortunately TRPC3 expression has not been studied in cerebral arteries. EETs cause cerebral artery dilation by activating TRPV4 [85, 86]. 11,12-EET production is reduced in cerebral arteries from SHR [87], and this could increase vascular tone. EETs are inactivated by soluble epoxide hydrolase (sEH) [88, 89], and sEH inhibitors are used experimentally to increase EETs levels. sEH inhibition does not lower blood pressure in SHRSP, but it does reduce the damage caused by cerebral ischemia through a combination of vascular and neuroprotective effects [88, 89]. Additional studies are required to elucidate if any of these pathways are important for the regulation of tone in the hypertensive population.

Effect of Stroke on Myogenic Tone Generation and Autoregulation

The effects of cerebral ischemia on cerebral artery autoregulation have been well studied using animal models of focal ischemic stroke [90]. It is generally accepted that cerebral artery function is impaired by cerebral ischemia and that this can increase the initial ischemic injury and contribute to secondary injuries including edema and hemorrhagic transformation [90]. Cerebral arteries dilate, or lose tone, in response to an ischemic insult; this is partly the result of a build-up of vasoactive metabolites including lactic acid and carbon dioxide in the parenchyma [2]. Myogenic dilation is also important for post-stroke dilation. When any artery is occluded the perfusion pressure in the downstream arteries is reduced and this causes myogenic dilation. In general the vascular response to ischemia/reperfusion injury is hyperemia [91–94]; this occurs in almost 50 % of stroke patients within 3 days of the initial insult [94, 95]. This post-stroke hyperemia increases the damage caused by the initial insult because it causes BBB breakdown and edema formation [95, 96].

In animal studies hyperemia increases the size of the ischemic infarct and this leads to a worsening of the neurodeficits observed after the stroke [97, 98]. During reactive hyperemia the arteries are essentially maximally dilated; in this situation the lumen diameter of the arteries is a critical determinant of cerebral perfusion. The effects of hypertension on the lumen diameter of the cerebral arteries will be discussed further later in this chapter. It is important to note that artery dilation does not occur if the intraluminal pressure falls below the lower limit of autoregulation. In this situation the blood flow will be proportional to the intralumenal pressure and in some cases the arteries will collapse, exacerbating the ischemic injury. The hyperemic response to ischemia is impaired in SHRSP. In normotensive rats the anastomoses between the pial arteries dilate quickly in response to an ischemic insult; this dilator mechanism is impaired in SHRSP [99]. The inability to increase perfusion to the ischemic zone through the pial arteries increases the ischemic injury observed in the event of a stroke in SHRSP [100].

Impaired myogenic tone generation and myogenic reactivity also contribute to the hyperemia observed post-stroke. After 2 h of ischemia followed by 1 min of reperfusion myogenic tone is normal in the MCA, but after prolonged reperfusion (24 h) myogenic tone and reactivity are significantly impaired [101]. Shorter durations of ischemia have similar effects on tone measured between 6 and 24 h after the initial ischemic insult [102, 103]. The MCA on the contralateral side of the brain is also impaired by cerebral ischemia/reperfusion, suggesting that a circulating factor released post-stroke may have detrimental effects on the ability of the cerebral arteries as a whole to autoregulate [103]. This circulating factor does not appear to be a reactive oxygen species as potent antioxidants do not reverse the effects of ischemia/reperfusion injury on myogenic tone generation [98, 104]. Others have reported similar effects of stroke on the contralateral hemisphere. In one study the impaired myogenic tone was associated with increased artery stiffness 1 h and 15 min after the initial ischemic insult. The authors linked this to an increase in protein nitration associated with post-reperfusion oxidative stress [105]. This result is difficult to reconcile with the finding that preventing oxidative stress had no effect on the reduction in myogenic tone generation post-stroke.

There is a general consensus that ischemia followed by reperfusion causes a reduction in myogenic tone generation in normotensive rats. The same cannot be said for hypertensive rats where 2 h of ischemia followed by 22 h of reperfusion had no effect on the active lumen diameter of the MCA that was occluded and no effect on the generation of myogenic tone [106]. This is in keeping with the studies showing that post-stroke hyperemia does not occur in SHRSP.

The mechanisms responsible for the loss of myogenic tone and the impaired myogenic reactivity post-stroke in normotensive rats have not been completely elucidated, but it seems that the loss of filamentous actin in the vascular smooth muscle cells is an important step in the process [102]. It is also likely that the build-up of vasoactive metabolites that occurs post-stroke could decrease myogenic tone. This cannot be the only explanation for the reduced tone post-stroke because reduced tone can also be observed in organ bath studies where the vasoactive metabolites are not present. The loss of myogenic tone post-stroke may also be a consequence of an increased release of dilator agents post-stroke. After ischemia/reperfusion injury the response of the MCA to agonists that cause NO mediated dilation is impaired, but the response to agonists that produce EDHF mediated dilation is enhanced by ischemia/reperfusion injury [107].

The studies described above were conducted in middle cerebral arteries, and the penetrating arterioles respond to ischemia with reperfusion injury differently. In general tone is higher in the penetrating arterioles than it is in the MCA, and ischemia with reperfusion does not reduce tone generation in the penetrating arteries [108, 109]. Their high basal tone [110, 111] and lack of braches makes the penetrating arterioles a bottleneck in the perfusion of the cortex and microcirculation [12, 17, 112, 113]. The absence of a dilator response to ischemia could protect the small downstream vessels from damage in the event of fluctuations in flow and pressure, but it could also be detrimental because it could limit perfusion of the microcirculation when reperfusion occurs.

Recent studies have attempted to understand the mechanism responsible for the maintenance of tone in the penetrating arterioles post-stroke. This study suggests that the balance on vasoconstriction and dilation is important, and that both are altered in the penetrating arterioles with reperfusion. Like the middle cerebral arteries [114, 115] endothelium derived hyperpolarization mediated dilation is increased in penetrating arterioles post-stroke [116]. Conversely, endothelin-1 mediated constriction was enhanced and this constriction counteracts the enhanced dilation to maintain tone at the pre-stroke level. This enhanced endothelin-1 mediated constriction occurs through activation of the endothelin B receptor and this was dependent on peroxynitrite production [116].

In humans reperfusion or recanalization can be spontaneous or it can be induced mechanically or chemically. Chemical induction of reperfusion requires the administration of recombinant tissue plasminogen activator (rTPA), and rTPA has detrimental effects of the cerebral arteries. In middle cerebral arteries that underwent ischemia followed by reperfusion, rTPA caused a significant reduction in myogenic tone generation and myogenic reactivity. Ischemia and rTPA independently reduced endothelium dependent dilation, and the effects of ischemia and rTPA were additive. Interestingly, ischemia and rTPA also caused an impairment in the contractile response of the arteries to serotonin, which could enhance cerebral perfusion and potentially cause hyperemia.

A handful of studies have accessed cerebral autoregulation in humans post-stroke. These relied on the analysis of cerebral blood flow in conjunction with blood pressure lowering to assess the autoregulatory capacity of the cerebral arteries. One study by Powers et al. assessed global cerebral blood flow and peri-clot flow after intracerebral hemorrhage. Blood flow was similar in both regions before and after the administration of nicardipine or labetalol to reduce blood pressure. This suggests that during the first 24 h after a cerebral hemorrhage autoregulation is intact [117]. Similar protocols have been utilized to study the effect of focal ischemia on autoregulation. Seven of the nine individuals studied had intact cerebral autoregulation in the infracted region, the peri-infract region, and the contralateral hemisphere. In two individuals blood flow was reduced in response to blood pressure lowering, but this was observed in all the regions studied and was deemed to be an effect of chronic hypertension in the affected patients [118].

Cerebral Artery Structure

In the absence of a stroke cerebral blood flow is influenced by cerebrovascular resistance, which is elevated in hypertension as a result of artery rarefaction and remodeling. Both of these pathological conditions have the potential to impact the outcome of stroke by impairing blood flow to the ischemic region when the vasculature is maximally dilated.

Artery Rarefaction

Cerebral artery rarefaction has been widely studied in rodent models of hypertension. Hypertension reduces the number of intracerebral capillaries [119, 120]. In SHR the reduction in capillary number is blood pressure dependent; rarefaction is present in adult SHR that have hypertension, but rarefaction was not observed in young SHR with developing hypertension [121]. Beyond its potential detrimental effects on stroke outcome this reduction in capillary number could reduce perfusion and increase the risk of developing vascular dementia.

The effects of hypertension on the pial arteries are more controversial. Elegant studies have shown that the number of collateral arteries between the middle cerebral and anterior cerebral arteries is similar in SHRSP, SHR, and normotensive rats, suggesting the pial artery rarefaction does not occur in these models of essential hypertension [122, 123]. The picture is less clear in models of secondary hypertension where pial artery rarefaction was reported in one study [119] but not in another [124]. Notably, these studies were conducted in relatively young rats; aging itself causes rarefaction and we do not know how hypertension and aging interact.

There are surprisingly few studies of artery rarefaction in hypertensive patients. Hypertension causes skin artery rarefaction [125–127], and this may be predictive of stroke outcome. A significant association between skin artery rarefaction and impaired cerebrovascular reserve capacity has been observed [128]. Together these studies suggest that the cerebrovascular reserve capacity will be reduced in hypertensive patients, and could have detrimental effects on the outcome of cerebral ischemia.

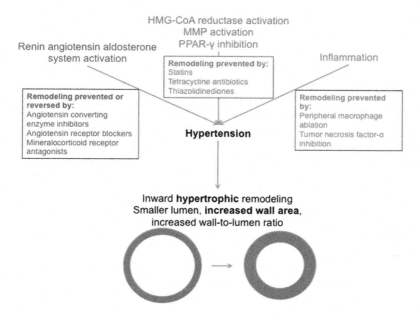

Fig. 5.4 Hypertensive artery remodeling. The figure depicts most commonly observed effects of hypertension on cerebral artery structure, a normotensive artery is shown on the *left*, and hypertensive artery undergoing hypertrophic inward remodeling is shown on the *right*. The *text boxes* describe some of the clinically relevant mechanisms to prevent or reverse cerebral artery remodeling

Cerebral Artery Remodeling

Artery remodeling refers to a situation where artery structure differs between two groups of test subjects. Remodeling is described as inward when the lumen diameter is reduced and outward when the lumen diameter is increased (Fig. 5.4). Remodeling can also affect the artery wall; wall area is increased during hypertrophic remodeling and reduced during hypotrophic remodeling [129]. Hypertensive cerebral artery remodeling has been described in several recent reviews [130–134].

In 1973 Folkow first hypothesized that artery remodeling increases cerebrovascular resistance in hypertensive rats [135]. Artery remodeling is generally described as a detrimental process, but it begins as an adaptive process that protects the cerebral microvessels from the elevated blood pressure and prevents microhemorrhages, vasogenic edema, and BBB breakdown [13, 136–138]. This protective remodeling process becomes maladaptive when hypertension is sustained and cerebral artery function is impaired. Initially remodeling normalizes flow by increasing vascular resistance [33, 139]. However, as hypertensive subjects age the remodeling process becomes deleterious; older hypertensive patients have reduced blood flow in the occipitotemporal and prefrontal cortex, and the hippocampus

[140]. Also, as patients with poorly controlled blood pressure age, they exhibit lower total cerebral blood flow compared to age matched normotensive controls. This hypoperfusion occurs independently of atherosclerosis [141], and is likely the result of artery remodeling and impaired control of constriction and dilation. Aging is a risk factor for cerebrovascular disease independent of hypertension, but approximately 70 % of the elderly population is hypertensive [142], which makes separating these two risk factors difficult. Aging itself causes artery remodeling and this has been linked to the development of dementia [143, 144].

One of the most commonly used metrics of artery remodeling is the wall-to-lumen ratio, and elevations in this predict end-organ damage [145] and stroke risk [146]. In hypertension this frequently observed remodeling pattern is associated with an increase in artery wall thickness and reduction in the lumen diameter [131, 147]. This type of remodeling has been observed in the middle cerebral arteries [148, 149] and pial arteries [150] from SHR and SHRSP compared to normotensive WKY rats. It has also been observed in several models of secondary hypertension [151–155].

As one might expect, aging has significant effects on artery structure in SHRSP. Young SHRSP (6 weeks) already have marked hypertension but blood pressure in this strain continues to increase for several more weeks and begins to plateau at 12 weeks of age [156]. Pial artery structure changes during the time that blood pressure is increased and not changing. Pial arteries from 3-month-old SHRSP are normal when compared to WKY rats, but with aging an inward remodeling is observed such that the lumen diameter is reduced [150, 157]. It seems that early structural changes in the larger cerebral arteries, like the MCA, may protect the pial arteries in the young SHRSP. The middle cerebral arteries from young SHRSP exhibit marked remodeling including a smaller lumen and an increased wall-to-lumen ratio when compared to WKY rats [148, 149, 158]. Thus it is likely that the different segments of the cerebrovascular tree respond to hypertension in a temporally distinct manner; remodeling begins in the larger arteries and progresses to the small arteries with sustained hypertension. This is in keeping with studies showing that vascular resistance increases in the small arteries during sustained hypertension [159].

It is not clear if the penetrating arteries follow the same temporal pattern of remodeling. 18-week-old SHRSP have marked and sustained hypertension and the penetrating arteries from these rats exhibit a marked remodeling that includes a reduction in the lumen diameter, an increase in the wall thickness and in the wall-to-lumen ratio [66]. Penetrating arterioles from 18-week-old female SHR also exhibit inward remodeling when compared to arterioles from WKY rats [160].

The cerebral artery remodeling observed in SHRSP is associated with changes in the orientation of the smooth muscle cells in the artery wall. Normally smooth muscle cells in the artery wall are arranged such that the long axis of the cell is perpendicular to the direction of flow. This organization is lost in several regions of the basilar artery wall in SHSRP [161, 162]. The regions of vascular smooth muscle cell disorganization are associated with a thinner adventitia, thus these areas might be weak spots in the artery that could cause hemorrhages [161].

The mechanisms responsible for cerebral artery remodeling are still being investigated. The hemodynamic effects of hypertension are a large stimulus for remodeling, but circulating factors associated with the development and maintenance of hypertension also contribute to the process. In the following paragraphs several potential mechanisms for artery remodeling will be described. A focus has been placed on mechanisms where interventional drugs already exist, although not all of these drugs are antihypertensive therapies.

The Renin-Angiotensin-Aldosterone-System

Drugs that interrupt the renin-angiotensin-aldosterone-system (RAAS) are widely used clinically and therefore have been the focus of many studies of artery structure in hypertension. Studies comparing the effectiveness of angiotensin converting enzyme (ACE) inhibitors, ARBs, and β-blockers led to the discovery that blood pressure lowering alone is not sufficient to prevent the effects of hypertension on the pial arteries. All the drugs lowered blood pressure but only the drugs that inhibited the effects of the RAAS also prevented the hypertension induced pial [163–166] and MCA remodeling [74, 167] in SHR or SHRSP. The lack of an effect of β-blockers is surprising given that these drugs reduce plasma renin activity and angiotensin II levels [168]. Not surprisingly these studies found that cerebral perfusion increased when the lumen diameter of the cerebral arteries was increased [166, 169, 170]. Interestingly a recent study has shown that artery remodeling in penetrating arteries from SHRSP can be improved with antihypertensive treatments that do not directly interfere with the RAAS [66].

Interrupting the RAAS appears to correct the hypertension associated artery remodeling fairly rapidly in adult hypertensive rats. Ten days of telmisartan treatment reduced the blood pressure and increased the pial artery lumen diameter in SHR compared to WKY rats. The authors of this study propose that the beneficial effects of telmisartan occur through a peroxisome proliferator-activated receptor γ (PPARγ) dependent mechanism. Candesartan also lowered blood pressure in this study but had no effect on artery structure [171]. The effects of direct PPARγ activation on artery remodeling will be described in more detail later. Telmisartan had no effect on the structure of the middle cerebral arteries [172] in rats undergoing the same treatment regime. This differential effect of ARBs on the middle cerebral and pial arteries is interesting, but at present unexplained.

A role of angiotensin II in artery remodeling is supported by studies using angiotensinogen knockout mice that do not produce angiotensin II. This study focused on the collateral arteries connecting the anterior and middle cerebral arteries. The lumen diameter of these arteries was increased in the angiotensinogen knockout compared to wild-type mice, but the number of anastomoses was similar between the strains. The angiotensinogen knockout mice also had lower blood pressure and that may have affected artery structure [173].

The timing of the treatments in laboratory studies is an area of concern, in many studies the drug treatments were administered while the hypertension was developing. With this treatment paradigm, effective drugs are preventing, not reversing artery remodeling. Clinically, it is more important to identify treatments to improve artery structure and function after the hypertension and artery remodeling has developed. ACE inhibitors have been found to do this effectively in SHR that were 1-year-old when the treatment began [170].

Aldosterone, the last signaling molecule produced by the RAAS, activates the mineralocorticoid receptor and its effects on cerebral arteries can be inhibited with mineralocorticoid receptor antagonists. Spironolactone treatment of SHRSP both prevents [149] and reverses [174] MCA remodeling. Spironolactone also reduces the damage caused by cerebral ischemia [175]. Interestingly, spironolactone did not lower the blood pressure in either study, thus the effects of mineralocorticoid receptor antagonism is this strain are blood pressure independent. Similarly recent studies have shown that mineralocorticoid receptor antagonists improve the structure of the penetrating arterioles in rats with established hypertension. Eplerenone increased penetrating artery lumen diameter and reduced the wall-to-lumen ratio compared to placebo treated SHRSP [66]. Mineralocorticoid receptor activation has also been implicated in the endothelial dysfunction that occurs in cerebral arteries from hypertensive rats. This effect of aldosterone on the basilar artery appears to be the result of increased oxidative stress [176].

The molecular mechanisms responsible for angiotensin II and aldosterone induced artery remodeling have not been completely elucidated. Angiotensin II and aldosterone both increase NADPH oxidase mediated reactive oxygen species generation [177, 178]. This increases superoxide levels and may drive the cerebral artery remodeling process. Treatment of SHRSP with tempol, a superoxide dismutase mimetic, prevents the reduction in the MCA lumen diameter normally observed in SHRSP with the development of hypertension [179].

Tetracycline Antibiotics

Artery remodeling requires extracellular matrix breakdown and reorganization. In eutrophic inward remodeling this allows the smooth muscle cells to rearrange themselves around a smaller lumen. In hypertrophic remodeling extracellular matrix breakdown is needed to accommodate smooth muscle cell hypertrophy or hyperplasia. The matrix metalloproteinase (MMP) family of enzymes cause extracellular matrix breakdown, and these enzymes may be involved in the artery remodeling process [180]. Inhibiting MMPs with doxycycline reduces the development of hypertension-associated MCA remodeling. Doxycycline had no effect on blood pressure suggesting its ability to prevent artery remodeling occurs through a blood pressure-independent mechanism. Importantly the improvement in artery structure was associated with a reduction in the damage caused by cerebral ischemia and an improvement in pial artery blood perfusion [158]. In this study doxycycline was withdrawn several days before the stroke was induced; thus the reduction in infarct size observe with doxycycline was not the result of acute MMP inhibition at the time of the stroke. This is important because clinical studies showed that tetracycline antibiotics have acute beneficial effects post-stroke [181, 182]; these effects do not appear to be vascular in nature. Interestingly MMP expression is modulated by RAAS activation [174, 183], thus this could be a potential mechanism for the effects of ACE inhibitors, ARBs, and mineralocorticoid receptor blockers.

Peroxisome Proliferator-Activated Receptor γ and HMG-CoA Reductase

Inhibiting the production of NO causes hypertension and these rats develop inward remodeling of the large cerebral arteries. Rosiglitazone, a PPARγ activator, reverses this remodeling without lowering blood pressure [184]. New Zealand hypertensive rats have basilar arteries with thicker walls than control rats and pioglitazone, another PPARγ activator, reduces the wall thickness in this strain. Pioglitazone also reduces the blood pressure, making it impossible to separate the effects of PPARγ activation and blood pressure lowering [185]. It is not clear why rosiglitazone and pioglitazone have different effects on blood pressure, but this may be a consequence of different models of hypertension being used. HMG-CoA reductase inhibitors (statins) also improve the basilar artery structure in New Zealand hypertensive rats by reducing the wall thickness and increasing the lumen diameter [186]. The role of blood pressure in this beneficial effect remains unclear because the statin therapy caused a marked reduction in blood pressure.

Inflammation

Hypertension and cardiovascular diseases have a clear inflammatory component (for reviews see [187–189]), and T cells [189–191] and macrophages [192–194] have been implicated in hypertension-associated peripheral vascular injury. The effects of T cells on cerebral arteries have not been described, but macrophage infiltration into the cerebral arteries appears to be an important determinant of the development of MCA remodeling in SHRSP. Peripheral macrophage depletion, during the time when blood pressure was increasing rapidly, reduced the number of perivascular macrophages in the brain by 50 %. The MCA lumen diameter was increased and the wall thickness and wall-to-lumen ratio were reduced by macrophage depletion. Macrophage depletion did not affect tone generation, or 5-HT induced contraction, but it did improve NO mediated endothelium dependent dilation. These changes occurred without a significant reduction in blood pressure [195]. The authors propose that as hypertension develops, perivascular macrophages accumulate within the brain and these macrophages contribute to the artery remodeling process.

Macrophages release cytokines including tumor necrosis factor (TNF)-α which has been implicated in hypertension associated renal injury [196, 197]. Etanercept, a TNF-α inhibitor, improves the MCA structure in SHRSP. Rats were treated from 6 to 12 weeks so that the actions of TNF-α were being inhibited as the hypertension developed. TNF-α inhibition significantly increased the lumen diameter and reduced the wall thickness and wall-to-lumen ratio of the MCA. Combined, these changes in artery structure were associated with an improvement in pial artery perfusion [198].

Effects of Ischemia on Artery Structure

It is becoming increasingly clear that ischemia also alters the structure of the cerebral arteries. At present only laboratory studies using rats are available, and all of these studies rely on models involving ischemia followed by reperfusion.

Two hours of ischemia followed by 1 h of reperfusion increases the distensibility of the MCA. After 24 h of reperfusion the artery distensibility was normal, but the wall thickness was increased, and this increase in wall thickness may be an adaptive mechanism to correct for the change in distensibility [101]. Interestingly, later studies by the same group have shown that ischemia followed by 24 h of reperfusion causes an increase in the stiffness of the MCA that was ischemic [199].

Some studies have compared the effects of ischemia and reperfusion injury in hypertensive and normotensive rats. In WKY rats the outer diameter of the MCA increases in response to ischemia/reperfusion injury, this was associated with an increase in the wall area and wall-to-lumen ratio. These structural changes were associated with a reduction in the wall stress in the MCA and in this case the artery wall was less stiff. Arteries from SHR rats did not show the expected increase in the outer diameter, and the wall area and wall-to-lumen ratio were both reduced by ischemia/reperfusion injury. Wall stress was increased in the middle cerebral arteries from SHR post-stroke [106]. The author of this study linked the normotensive artery remodeling to an increase in the number of cells present in the arteries adventitia [106].

The oxidative stress that occurs with ischemia/reperfusion injury may mediate some of the effects on artery structure. CR-6 is a derivative of vitamin E and a potent antioxidant. CR-6 was administered to the rats after ischemia at the time of reperfusion and this reduced the area of injury caused by ischemia. It also reduced the previously observed increase in wall thickness and wall area post-ischemia and increased the wall stress [104]. Recent studies have confirmed this finding using a different antioxidant, uric acid [98]. This study also investigated the effects of post-ischemic hyperemia on artery structure. As mentioned above, 50 % of stroke patients exhibit hyperemia following their ischemic event [94, 95]. The incidence of hyperemia in rats was similar to that in humans, with 56 % of the rats studied exhibiting hyperemia. Uric acid only reduced the cerebral infarct size in rats that exhibited hyperemia; it had no effects in rats that had normal blood flow post-stroke. Only the rats that exhibited hyperemia had significant changes in their artery structure that were similar to those described above, an increase in the outer diameter and an increase in the artery wall thickness and cross-sectional area. Wall stress was also reduced in the rats that had a stroke followed by hyperemia. The authors linked these structural changes to increased inflammation driven by the hyperemia because there was increased monocyte and macrophage infiltration into the cerebral arteries in the rats that exhibited hyperemia.

Conclusions and Outstanding Questions

Hypertension and stroke both have detrimental effects on the cerebral arteries. Stroke impairs myogenic tone generation and the regulation of blood flow. It also alters the structure of the cerebral arteries such that the lumen diameter of the ischemic artery increases after ischemia/reperfusion injury. Hypertension also causes artery remodeling but this results in a reduction in the lumen diameter of the arteries that could increase the risk of cerebral ischemia and the damage caused by it. Hypertension is a leading risk factor for stroke. Given the increasing interest in the vasculature as a therapeutic target for acute ischemic stroke, it would seem important that we develop a better understanding of the combined effects of hypertension and stroke on the cerebral arteries.

Studies of cerebrovascular structure and function in humans are limited. Much of what we know about the effects of these two conditions has come from rat and mouse studies. The use of young rats and mice to study conditions that do not develop in humans until old age is therefore a serious concern. The rodent studies have also largely utilized male rats, and there is an urgent need to consider the effects of hypertension and stroke in males and females separately.

References

1. Vander AJ, Sherman JH, Luciano DS. Human physiology: the mechanisms of body function. 5th ed. New York: McGraw-Hill; 1990.
2. Hossmann KA. Pathophysiology and therapy of experimental stroke. Cell Mol Neurobiol. 2006;26(7–8):1057–83.
3. del Zoppo GJ, Hallenbeck JM. Advances in the vascular pathophysiology of ischemic stroke. Thromb Res. 2000;98(3):73–81.
4. Hirsch S, et al. Topology and hemodynamics of the cortical cerebrovascular system. J Cereb Blood Flow Metab. 2012;32(6):952–67.
5. Coyle P. Dorsal cerebral collaterals of stroke-prone spontaneously hypertensive rats (SHRSP) and Wistar Kyoto rats (WKY). Anat Rec. 1987;218(1):40–4.
6. Cipolla MJ. The cerebral circulation. San Rafael: Morgan & Claypool Life Sciences; 2009.
7. Schaffer CB, et al. Two-photon imaging of cortical surface microvessels reveals a robust redistribution in blood flow after vascular occlusion. PLoS Biol. 2006;4(2), e22.

8. Baran U, Li Y, Wang RK. Vasodynamics of pial and penetrating arterioles in relation to arteriolo-arteriolar anastomosis after focal stroke. Neurophotonics. 2015;2(2):025006.

9. Hamel E. Perivascular nerves and the regulation of cerebrovascular tone. J Appl Physiol. 2006;100(3):1059–64.

10. Edvinsson L, Krause DN. Cerebral blood flow and metabolism. Philadelphia: Lippincott, Williams & Wilkins; 2002.

11. Ayata C, et al. L-NA-sensitive rCBF augmentation during vibrissal stimulation in type III nitric oxide synthase mutant mice. J Cereb Blood Flow Metab. 1996;16(4):539–41.

12. Nishimura N, et al. Penetrating arterioles are a bottleneck in the perfusion of neocortex. Proc Natl Acad Sci U S A. 2007;104(1):365–70.

13. Iadecola C, Davisson RL. Hypertension and cerebrovascular dysfunction. Cell Metab. 2008;7(6):476–84.

14. Cohen Z, Molinatti G, Hamel E. Astroglial and vascular interactions of noradrenaline terminals in the rat cerebral cortex. J Cereb Blood Flow Metab. 1997;17(8):894–904.

15. Filosa JA, et al. Beyond neurovascular coupling, role of astrocytes in the regulation of vascular tone. Neuroscience. 2015. doi:10.1016/j.neuroscience.2015.03.064.

16. Gobel U, Theilen H, Kuschinsky W. Congruence of total and perfused capillary network in rat brains. Circ Res. 1990;66(2):271–81.

17. Shih AY, et al. Robust and fragile aspects of cortical blood flow in relation to the underlying angioarchitecture. Microcirculation. 2015;22:204–18.

18. Sa-Pereira I, Brites D, Brito MA. Neurovascular unit: a focus on pericytes. Mol Neurobiol. 2012;45(2):327–47.

19. Hill RA, et al. Regional blood flow in the normal and ischemic brain is controlled by arteriolar smooth muscle cell contractility and not by capillary pericytes. Neuron. 2015;87(1):95–110.

20. Dalkara T, Gursoy-Ozdemir Y, Yemisci M. Brain microvascular pericytes in health and disease. Acta Neuropathol. 2011;122(1):1–9.

21. Shepro D, Morel NM. Pericyte physiology. FASEB J. 1993;7(11):1031–8.

22. Dirnagl U. Pathobiology of injury after stroke: the neurovascular unit and beyond. Ann N Y Acad Sci. 2012;1268:21–5.

23. Hawkins BT, Davis TP. The blood-brain barrier/neurovascular unit in health and disease. Pharmacol Rev. 2005;57(2):173–85.

24. Koehler RC, Gebremedhin D, Harder DR. Role of astrocytes in cerebrovascular regulation. J Appl Physiol (1985). 2006;100(1):307–17.

25. Dunn KM, Nelson MT. Neurovascular signaling in the brain and the pathological consequences of hypertension. Am J Physiol Heart Circ Physiol. 2014;306(1):H1–14.

26. Bloch S, Obari D, Girouard H. Angiotensin and neurovascular coupling: beyond hypertension. Microcirculation. 2015;22(3):159–67.

27. Iliff JJ, et al. Epoxyeicosanoids as mediators of neurogenic vasodilation in cerebral vessels. Am J Physiol Heart Circ Physiol. 2009;296(5):H1352–63.

28. Harder DR, et al. Functional hyperemia in the brain: hypothesis for astrocyte-derived vasodilator metabolites. Stroke. 1998;29(1):229–34.

29. Dirnagl U, et al. Coupling of cerebral blood flow to neuronal activation: role of adenosine and nitric oxide. Am J Physiol. 1994;267(1 Pt 2):H296–301.

30. Lindauer U, et al. Nitric oxide: a modulator, but not a mediator, of neurovascular coupling in rat somatosensory cortex. Am J Physiol. 1999;277(2 Pt 2):H799–811.

31. Niwa K, et al. Cyclooxygenase-2 contributes to functional hyperemia in whisker-barrel cortex. J Neurosci. 2000;20(2):763–70.

32. Roman RJ. P-450 metabolites of arachidonic acid in the control of cardiovascular function. Physiol Rev. 2002;82(1):131–85.

33. Jennings JR, et al. Reduced cerebral blood flow response and compensation among patients with untreated hypertension. Neurology. 2005;64(8):1358–65.

34. Kazama K, et al. Angiotensin II attenuates functional hyperemia in the mouse somatosensory cortex. Am J Physiol Heart Circ Physiol. 2003;285(5):H1890–9.

35. Capone C, et al. The cerebrovascular dysfunction induced by slow pressor doses of angiotensin II precedes the development of hypertension. Am J Physiol Heart Circ Physiol. 2011;300(1):H397–407.
36. Kazama K, et al. Angiotensin II impairs neurovascular coupling in neocortex through NADPH oxidase-derived radicals. Circ Res. 2004;95(10):1019–26.
37. Calcinaghi N, et al. Multimodal imaging in rats reveals impaired neurovascular coupling in sustained hypertension. Stroke. 2013;44(7):1957–64.
38. Inao S, et al. Neural activation of the brain with hemodynamic insufficiency. J Cereb Blood Flow Metab. 1998;18(9):960–7.
39. Yamauchi H, et al. Altered patterns of blood flow response during visual stimulation in carotid artery occlusive disease. Neuroimage. 2005;25(2):554–60.
40. Ginsberg MD, et al. Acute thrombotic infarction suppresses metabolic activation of ipsilateral somatosensory cortex: evidence for functional diaschisis. J Cereb Blood Flow Metab. 1989;9(3):329–41.
41. Kunz A, et al. Neurovascular protection by ischemic tolerance: role of nitric oxide and reactive oxygen species. J Neurosci. 2007;27(27):7083–93.
42. Ueki M, Linn F, Hossmann KA. Functional activation of cerebral blood flow and metabolism before and after global ischemia of rat brain. J Cereb Blood Flow Metab. 1988;8(4):486–94.
43. Baker WB, et al. Neurovascular coupling varies with level of global cerebral ischemia in a rat model. J Cereb Blood Flow Metab. 2013;33(1):97–105.
44. Shen Q, et al. Functional, perfusion and diffusion MRI of acute focal ischemic brain injury. J Cereb Blood Flow Metab. 2005;25(10):1265–79.
45. Geary GG, Krause DN, Duckles SP. Estrogen reduces mouse cerebral artery tone through endothelial NOS- and cyclooxygenase-dependent mechanisms. Am J Physiol Heart Circ Physiol. 2000;279(2):H511–9.
46. Cipolla MJ, Porter JM, Osol G. High glucose concentrations dilate cerebral arteries and diminish myogenic tone through an endothelial mechanism. Stroke. 1997;28(2):405–10; discussion 410–1.
47. Faraci FM, Brian Jr JE. Nitric oxide and the cerebral circulation. Stroke. 1994;25(3):692–703.
48. Malomvolgyi B, et al. Relaxation by prostacyclin (PGI2) and 7-oxo-PGI2 of isolated cerebral, coronary and mesenteric arteries. Acta Physiol Acad Sci Hung. 1982;60(4):251–6.
49. Gonzales RJ, Krause DN, Duckles SP. Testosterone suppresses endothelium-dependent dilation of rat middle cerebral arteries. Am J Physiol Heart Circ Physiol. 2004;286(2):H552–60.
50. Faraci FM, Baumbach GL, Heistad DD. Myogenic mechanisms in the cerebral circulation. J Hypertens Suppl. 1989;7(4):S61–4; discussion S65.
51. Paulson OB, Strandgaard S, Edvinsson L. Cerebral autoregulation. Cerebrovasc Brain Metab Rev. 1990;2(2):161–92.
52. Osol G, et al. Myogenic tone, reactivity, and forced dilatation: a three-phase model of in vitro arterial myogenic behavior. Am J Physiol Heart Circ Physiol. 2002;283(6):H2260–7.
53. Bayliss WM. On the local reactions of the arterial wall to changes of internal pressure. J Physiol. 1902;28(3):220–31.
54. Talman WT, Nitschke Dragon D. Neuronal nitric oxide mediates cerebral vasodilatation during acute hypertension. Brain Res. 2007;1139:126–32.
55. Duchemin S, et al. The complex contribution of NOS interneurons in the physiology of cerebrovascular regulation. Front Neural Circuits. 2012;6:51.
56. Jones SC, et al. Cortical NOS inhibition raises the lower limit of cerebral blood flow-arterial pressure autoregulation. Am J Physiol. 1999;276(4 Pt 2):H1253–62.
57. Koller A, Toth P. Contribution of flow-dependent vasomotor mechanisms to the autoregulation of cerebral blood flow. J Vasc Res. 2012;49(5):375–89.
58. Hamner JW, et al. Sympathetic control of the cerebral vasculature in humans. Stroke. 2010;41(1):102–9.

59. Hamner JW, et al. Cholinergic control of the cerebral vasculature in humans. J Physiol. 2012;590(Pt 24):6343–52.
60. Osol G, Halpern W. Myogenic properties of cerebral blood vessels from normotensive and hypertensive rats. Am J Physiol. 1985;249(5 Pt 2):H914–21.
61. Barry DI. Cerebral blood flow in hypertension. J Cardiovasc Pharmacol. 1985;7(2):S94–8.
62. Jarajapu YP, Knot HJ. Relative contribution of Rho kinase and protein kinase C to myogenic tone in rat cerebral arteries in hypertension. Am J Physiol Heart Circ Physiol. 2005;289(5):H1917–22.
63. Ibrahim J, et al. Sex-specific differences in cerebral arterial myogenic tone in hypertensive and normotensive rats. Am J Physiol Heart Circ Physiol. 2006;290(3):H1081–9.
64. Yamori Y, et al. Pathogenetic similarity of strokes in stroke-prone spontaneously hypertensive rats and humans. Stroke. 1976;7(1):46–53.
65. Yamori Y, et al. Cerebral stroke and myocardial lesions in stroke-prone SHR. Jpn Heart J. 1978;19(4):609–11.
66. Pires PW, Jackson WF, Dorrance AM. Regulation of myogenic tone and structure of parenchymal arterioles by hypertension and the mineralocorticoid receptor. Am J Physiol Heart Circ Physiol. 2015;309(1):H127–36.
67. Izzard AS, et al. Myogenic and structural properties of cerebral arteries from the stroke-prone spontaneously hypertensive rat. Am J Physiol Heart Circ Physiol. 2003;285(4):H1489–94.
68. Smeda JS, VanVliet BN, King SR. Stroke-prone spontaneously hypertensive rats lose their ability to auto-regulate cerebral blood flow prior to stroke. J Hypertens. 1999;17(12 Pt 1):1697–705.
69. Ishizuka T, et al. Involvement of thromboxane A2 receptor in the cerebrovascular damage of salt-loaded, stroke-prone rats. J Hypertens. 2007;25(4):861–70.
70. Griffin KA, et al. Differential salt-sensitivity in the pathogenesis of renal damage in SHR and stroke prone SHR. Am J Hypertens. 2001;14(4 Pt 1):311–20.
71. Toth P, et al. Age-related autoregulatory dysfunction and cerebromicrovascular injury in mice with angiotensin II-induced hypertension. J Cereb Blood Flow Metab. 2013;33(11):1732–42.
72. Toth P, et al. Role of 20-HETE, TRPC channels, and BKCa in dysregulation of pressure-induced Ca2+ signaling and myogenic constriction of cerebral arteries in aged hypertensive mice. Am J Physiol Heart Circ Physiol. 2013;305(12):H1698–708.
73. Welsh DG, et al. Transient receptor potential channels regulate myogenic tone of resistance arteries. Circ Res. 2002;90(3):248–50.
74. Yamakawa H, et al. Normalization of endothelial and inducible nitric oxide synthase expression in brain microvessels of spontaneously hypertensive rats by angiotensin II AT1 receptor inhibition. J Cereb Blood Flow Metab. 2003;23(3):371–80.
75. Touyz RM, Briones AM. Reactive oxygen species and vascular biology: implications in human hypertension. Hypertens Res. 2011;34(1):5–14.
76. Paravicini TM, Sobey CG. Cerebral vascular effects of reactive oxygen species: recent evidence for a role of NADPH-oxidase. Clin Exp Pharmacol Physiol. 2003;30(11):855–9.
77. Bryan Jr RM, et al. Endothelium-derived hyperpolarizing factor: a cousin to nitric oxide and prostacyclin. Anesthesiology. 2005;102(6):1261–77.
78. Stankevicius E, et al. Opening of small and intermediate calcium-activated potassium channels induces relaxation mainly mediated by nitric-oxide release in large arteries and endothelium-derived hyperpolarizing factor in small arteries from rat. J Pharmacol Exp Ther. 2011;339(3):842–50.
79. Marrelli SP, Eckmann MS, Hunte MS. Role of endothelial intermediate conductance KCa channels in cerebral EDHF-mediated dilations. Am J Physiol Heart Circ Physiol. 2003;285(4):H1590–9.
80. Si H, et al. Impaired endothelium-derived hyperpolarizing factor-mediated dilations and increased blood pressure in mice deficient of the intermediate-conductance Ca2+-activated K+ channel. Circ Res. 2006;99(5):537–44.

81. Earley S, Brayden JE. Transient receptor potential channels and vascular function. Clin Sci (Lond). 2010;119(1):19–36.
82. Venkatachalam K, Montell C. TRP channels. Annu Rev Biochem. 2007;76:387–417.
83. Reading SA, et al. TRPC3 mediates pyrimidine receptor-induced depolarization of cerebral arteries. Am J Physiol Heart Circ Physiol. 2005;288(5):H2055–61.
84. Noorani MM, Noel RC, Marrelli SP. Upregulated TRPC3 and downregulated TRPC1 channel expression during hypertension is associated with increased vascular contractility in Rat. Front Physiol. 2011;2:42.
85. Earley S, et al. TRPV4 forms a novel Ca2+ signaling complex with ryanodine receptors and BKCa channels. Circ Res. 2005;97(12):1270–9.
86. Earley S. Endothelium-dependent cerebral artery dilation mediated by transient receptor potential and Ca2+-activated K+ channels. J Cardiovasc Pharmacol. 2011; 57(2):148–53.
87. Dunn KM, et al. Elevated production of 20-HETE in the cerebral vasculature contributes to severity of ischemic stroke and oxidative stress in spontaneously hypertensive rats. Am J Physiol Heart Circ Physiol. 2008;295(6):H2455–65.
88. Dorrance AM, et al. An epoxide hydrolase inhibitor, 12-(3-adamantan-1-yl-ureido)dodecanoic acid (AUDA), reduces ischemic cerebral infarct size in stroke-prone spontaneously hypertensive rats. J Cardiovasc Pharmacol. 2005;46(6):842–8.
89. Simpkins AN, et al. Soluble epoxide inhibition is protective against cerebral ischemia via vascular and neural protection. Am J Pathol. 2009;174(6):2086–95.
90. Palomares SM, Cipolla MJ. Vascular protection following cerebral ischemia and reperfusion. J Neurol Neurophysiol. 2011;2011:S1-004.
91. Gourley JK, Heistad DD. Characteristics of reactive hyperemia in the cerebral circulation. Am J Physiol. 1984;246(1 Pt 2):H52–8.
92. Sundt Jr TM, Waltz AG. Cerebral ischemia and reactive hyperemia. Studies of cortical blood flow and microcirculation before, during, and after temporary occlusion of middle cerebral artery of squirrel monkeys. Circ Res. 1971;28(4):426–33.
93. Hayakawa T, Waltz AG, Hansen T. Relationships among intracranial pressure, blood pressure, and superficial cerebral vasculature after experimental occlusion of one middle cerebral artery. Stroke. 1977;8(4):426–32.
94. Skinhoj E, et al. Regional cerebral blood flow and its autoregulation in patients with transient focal cerebral ischemic attacks. Neurology. 1970;20(5):485–93.
95. Olsen TS, et al. Focal cerebral hyperemia in acute stroke. Incidence, pathophysiology and clinical significance. Stroke. 1981;12(5):598–607.
96. Macfarlane R, et al. The role of neuroeffector mechanisms in cerebral hyperperfusion syndromes. J Neurosurg. 1991;75(6):845–55.
97. Perez-Asensio FJ, et al. Antioxidant CR-6 protects against reperfusion injury after a transient episode of focal brain ischemia in rats. J Cereb Blood Flow Metab. 2010;30(3):638–52.
98. Onetti Y, et al. Middle cerebral artery remodeling following transient brain ischemia is linked to early postischemic hyperemia: a target of uric acid treatment. Am J Physiol Heart Circ Physiol. 2015;308(8):H862–74.
99. Coyle P, Heistad DD. Blood flow through cerebral collateral vessels in hypertensive and normotensive rats. Hypertension. 1986;8(6 Pt 2):II67–71.
100. Coyle P, Jokelainen PT. Differential outcome to middle cerebral artery occlusion in spontaneously hypertensive stroke-prone rats (SHRSP) and Wistar Kyoto (WKY) rats. Stroke. 1983;14(4):605–11.
101. Cipolla MJ, et al. Reperfusion decreases myogenic reactivity and alters middle cerebral artery function after focal cerebral ischemia in rats. Stroke. 1997;28(1):176–80.
102. Cipolla MJ, et al. Threshold duration of ischemia for myogenic tone in middle cerebral arteries: effect on vascular smooth muscle actin. Stroke. 2001;32(7):1658–64.
103. Cipolla MJ, Curry AB. Middle cerebral artery function after stroke: the threshold duration of reperfusion for myogenic activity. Stroke. 2002;33(8):2094–9.

104. Jimenez-Altayo F, et al. Participation of oxidative stress on rat middle cerebral artery changes induced by focal cerebral ischemia: beneficial effects of 3,4-dihydro-6-hydroxy-7-methoxy-2,2-dimethyl-1(2H)-benzopyran (CR-6). J Pharmacol Exp Ther. 2009; 331(2):429–36.
105. Coucha M, et al. Protein nitration impairs the myogenic tone of rat middle cerebral arteries in both ischemic and nonischemic hemispheres after ischemic stroke. Am J Physiol Heart Circ Physiol. 2013;305(12):H1726–35.
106. Jimenez-Altayo F, et al. Transient middle cerebral artery occlusion causes different structural, mechanical, and myogenic alterations in normotensive and hypertensive rats. Am J Physiol Heart Circ Physiol. 2007;293(1):H628–35.
107. Marrelli SP, et al. P2 purinoceptor-mediated dilations in the rat middle cerebral artery after ischemia-reperfusion. Am J Physiol. 1999;276(1 Pt 2):H33–41.
108. Cipolla MJ, et al. SKCa and IKCa Channels, myogenic tone, and vasodilator responses in middle cerebral arteries and parenchymal arterioles: effect of ischemia and reperfusion. Stroke. 2009;40(4):1451–7.
109. Cipolla MJ, Bullinger LV. Reactivity of brain parenchymal arterioles after ischemia and reperfusion. Microcirculation. 2008;15(6):495–501.
110. Cipolla MJ, Li R, Vitullo L. Perivascular innervation of penetrating brain parenchymal arterioles. J Cardiovasc Pharmacol. 2004;44(1):1–8.
111. Dabertrand F, Nelson MT, Brayden JE. Acidosis dilates brain parenchymal arterioles by conversion of calcium waves to sparks to activate BK channels. Circ Res. 2012;110(2):285–94.
112. Nishimura N, et al. Limitations of collateral flow after occlusion of a single cortical penetrating arteriole. J Cereb Blood Flow Metab. 2010;30(12):1914–27.
113. Shih AY, et al. The smallest stroke: occlusion of one penetrating vessel leads to infarction and a cognitive deficit. Nat Neurosci. 2013;16(1):55–63.
114. Marrelli SP. Altered endothelial Ca2+ regulation after ischemia/reperfusion produces potentiated endothelium-derived hyperpolarizing factor-mediated dilations. Stroke. 2002;33(9):2285–91.
115. Marrelli SP, et al. PLA2 and TRPV4 channels regulate endothelial calcium in cerebral arteries. Am J Physiol Heart Circ Physiol. 2007;292(3):H1390–7.
116. Cipolla MJ, et al. Mechanisms of enhanced basal tone of brain parenchymal arterioles during early postischemic reperfusion: role of ET-1-induced peroxynitrite generation. J Cereb Blood Flow Metab. 2013;33(10):1486–92.
117. Powers WJ, et al. Autoregulation of cerebral blood flow surrounding acute (6 to 22 hours) intracerebral hemorrhage. Neurology. 2001;57(1):18–24.
118. Powers WJ, et al. Autoregulation after ischaemic stroke. J Hypertens. 2009;27(11): 2218–22.
119. Sokolova IA, et al. Rarefication of the arterioles and capillary network in the brain of rats with different forms of hypertension. Microvasc Res. 1985;30(1):1–9.
120. Suzuki K, et al. Pathologic evidence of microvascular rarefaction in the brain of renal hypertensive rats. J Stroke Cerebrovasc Dis. 2003;12(1):8–16.
121. Paiardi S, et al. Immunohistochemical evaluation of microvascular rarefaction in hypertensive humans and in spontaneously hypertensive rats. Clin Hemorheol Microcirc. 2009;42(4):259–68.
122. Coyle P, Heistad DD. Blood flow through cerebral collateral vessels one month after middle cerebral artery occlusion. Stroke. 1987;18(2):407–11.
123. Harper SL, Bohlen HG. Microvascular adaptation in the cerebral cortex of adult spontaneously hypertensive rats. Hypertension. 1984;6(3):408–19.
124. Werber AH, et al. No rarefaction of cerebral arterioles in hypertensive rats. Can J Physiol Pharmacol. 1990;68(4):476–9.
125. Noon JP, et al. Impaired microvascular dilatation and capillary rarefaction in young adults with a predisposition to high blood pressure. J Clin Invest. 1997;99(8):1873–9.

126. Serne EH, et al. Impaired skin capillary recruitment in essential hypertension is caused by both functional and structural capillary rarefaction. Hypertension. 2001;38(2):238–42.
127. Serne EH, et al. Capillary recruitment is impaired in essential hypertension and relates to insulin's metabolic and vascular actions. Cardiovasc Res. 2001;49(1):161–8.
128. Nazzaro P, et al. Effect of clustering of metabolic syndrome factors on capillary and cerebrovascular impairment. Eur J Intern Med. 2013;24(2):183–8.
129. Mulvany MJ, et al. Vascular remodeling. Hypertension. 1996;28(3):505–6.
130. Baumbach GL, Chillon JM. Effects of angiotensin-converting enzyme inhibitors on cerebral vascular structure in chronic hypertension. J Hypertens Suppl. 2000;18(1):S7–11.
131. Heagerty AM, et al. Small artery structure in hypertension. Dual processes of remodeling and growth. Hypertension. 1993;21(4):391–7.
132. Heistad DD, et al. Impaired dilatation of cerebral arterioles in chronic hypertension. Blood Vessels. 1990;27(2-5):258–62.
133. Mulvany MJ. Small artery remodelling in hypertension. Basic Clin Pharmacol Toxicol. 2012;110(1):49–55.
134. Pires PW, et al. The effects of hypertension on the cerebral circulation. Am J Physiol Heart Circ Physiol. 2013;304(12):H1598–614.
135. Folkow B, et al. Importance of adaptive changes in vascular design for establishment of primary hypertension, studied in man and in spontaneously hypertensive rats. Circ Res. 1973;32(1):2–16.
136. Hayashi K, Naiki T. Adaptation and remodeling of vascular wall; biomechanical response to hypertension. J Mech Behav Biomed Mater. 2009;2(1):3–19.
137. Baumbach GL, Heistad DD. Cerebral circulation in chronic arterial hypertension. Hypertension. 1988;12(2):89–95.
138. Laurent S, Boutouyrie P, Lacolley P. Structural and genetic bases of arterial stiffness. Hypertension. 2005;45(6):1050–5.
139. Kety SS, Hafkenschiel JH, et al. The blood flow, vascular resistance, and oxygen consumption of the brain in essential hypertension. J Clin Invest. 1948;27(4):511–4.
140. Beason-Held LL, et al. Longitudinal changes in cerebral blood flow in the older hypertensive brain. Stroke. 2007;38(6):1766–73.
141. Muller M, et al. Hypertension and longitudinal changes in cerebral blood flow: the SMART-MR study. Ann Neurol. 2012;71(6):825–33.
142. Go AS, et al. Heart disease and stroke statistics--2014 update: a report from the American Heart Association. Circulation. 2014;129(3):e28–292.
143. Tomonaga M, et al. Clinicopathologic study of progressive subcortical vascular encephalopathy (Binswanger type) in the elderly. J Am Geriatr Soc. 1982;30(8):524–9.
144. Furuta A, et al. Medullary arteries in aging and dementia. Stroke. 1991;22(4):442–6.
145. Izzard AS, et al. Small artery structure and hypertension: adaptive changes and target organ damage. J Hypertens. 2005;23(2):247–50.
146. De Ciuceis C, et al. Structural alterations of subcutaneous small-resistance arteries may predict major cardiovascular events in patients with hypertension. Am J Hypertens. 2007;20(8):846–52.
147. Mulvany MJ. Small artery remodeling and significance in the development of hypertension. News Physiol Sci. 2002;17:105–9.
148. Dorrance AM, et al. A high-potassium diet reduces infarct size and improves vascular structure in hypertensive rats. Am J Physiol Regul Integr Comp Physiol. 2007;292(1):R415–22.
149. Rigsby CS, Pollock DM, Dorrance AM. Spironolactone improves structure and increases tone in the cerebral vasculature of male spontaneously hypertensive stroke-prone rats. Microvasc Res. 2007;73(3):198–205.
150. Baumbach GL, Heistad DD. Remodeling of cerebral arterioles in chronic hypertension. Hypertension. 1989;13(6 Pt 2):968–72.
151. Deutsch C, et al. Diet-induced obesity causes cerebral vessel remodeling and increases the damage caused by ischemic stroke. Microvasc Res. 2009;78(1):100–6.

152. Osmond JM, et al. Obesity increases blood pressure, cerebral vascular remodeling, and severity of stroke in the Zucker rat. Hypertension. 2009;53(2):381–6.
153. Dorrance AM, Rupp NC, Nogueira EF. Mineralocorticoid receptor activation causes cerebral vessel remodeling and exacerbates the damage caused by cerebral ischemia. Hypertension. 2006;47(3):590–5.
154. Osmond JM, Dorrance AM. 11Beta-hydroxysteroid dehydrogenase type II inhibition causes cerebrovascular remodeling and increases infarct size after cerebral ischemia. Endocrinology. 2009;150(2):713–9.
155. Moreau P, et al. Structure and function of the rat basilar artery during chronic nitric oxide synthase inhibition. Stroke. 1995;26(10):1922–8; discussion 1928–9.
156. Davidson AO, et al. Blood pressure in genetically hypertensive rats. Influence of the Y chromosome. Hypertension. 1995;26(3):452–9.
157. Baumbach GL, et al. Mechanics of cerebral arterioles in hypertensive rats. Circ Res. 1988;62(1):56–64.
158. Pires PW, et al. Doxycycline, a matrix metalloprotease inhibitor, reduces vascular remodeling and damage after cerebral ischemia in stroke-prone spontaneously hypertensive rats. Am J Physiol Heart Circ Physiol. 2011;301(1):H87–97.
159. Bohlen HG. The microcirculation in hypertension. J Hypertens Suppl. 1989;7(4):S117–24.
160. Chan SL, Sweet JG, Cipolla MJ. Treatment for cerebral small vessel disease: effect of relaxin on the function and structure of cerebral parenchymal arterioles during hypertension. FASEB J. 2013;27(10):3917–27.
161. Arribas SM, et al. Functional reduction and associated cellular rearrangement in SHRSP rat basilar arteries are affected by salt load and calcium antagonist treatment. J Cereb Blood Flow Metab. 1999;19(5):517–27.
162. Arribas SM, et al. Confocal microscopic characterization of a lesion in a cerebral vessel of the stroke-prone spontaneously hypertensive rat. Stroke. 1996;27(6):1118–22; discussion 1122–3.
163. Hajdu MA, Heistad DD, Baumbach GL. Effects of antihypertensive therapy on mechanics of cerebral arterioles in rats. Hypertension. 1991;17(3):308–16.
164. Chillon JM, Baumbach GL. Effects of an angiotensin-converting enzyme inhibitor and a beta-blocker on cerebral arterioles in rats. Hypertension. 1999;33(3):856–61.
165. Clozel JP, Kuhn H, Hefti F. Effects of cilazapril on the cerebral circulation in spontaneously hypertensive rats. Hypertension. 1989;14(6):645–51.
166. Dupuis F, et al. Comparative effects of the angiotensin II receptor blocker, telmisartan, and the angiotensin-converting enzyme inhibitor, ramipril, on cerebrovascular structure in spontaneously hypertensive rats. J Hypertens. 2005;23(5):1061–6.
167. Kumai Y, et al. Protective effects of angiotensin II type 1 receptor blocker on cerebral circulation independent of blood pressure. Exp Neurol. 2008;210(2):441–8.
168. Blumenfeld JD, et al. Beta-adrenergic receptor blockade as a therapeutic approach for suppressing the renin-angiotensin-aldosterone system in normotensive and hypertensive subjects. Am J Hypertens. 1999;12(5):451–9.
169. Dupuis F, et al. Effects of suboptimal doses of the AT1 receptor blocker, telmisartan, with the angiotensin-converting enzyme inhibitor, ramipril, on cerebral arterioles in spontaneously hypertensive rat. J Hypertens. 2010;28(7):1566–73.
170. Dupuis F, et al. Captopril improves cerebrovascular structure and function in old hypertensive rats. Br J Pharmacol. 2005;144(3):349–56.
171. Foulquier S, et al. Differential effects of short-term treatment with two AT1 receptor blockers on diameter of pial arterioles in SHR. PLoS One. 2012;7(9), e42469.
172. Foulquier S, Lartaud I, Dupuis F. Impact of short-term treatment with Telmisartan on cerebral arterial remodeling in SHR. PLoS One. 2014;9(10), e110766.
173. Maeda K, et al. Larger anastomoses in angiotensinogen-knockout mice attenuate early metabolic disturbances after middle cerebral artery occlusion. J Cereb Blood Flow Metab. 1999;19(10):1092–8.

174. Rigsby CS, et al. Effects of spironolactone on cerebral vessel structure in rats with sustained hypertension. Am J Hypertens. 2011;24(6):708–15.
175. Dorrance AM, et al. Spironolactone reduces cerebral infarct size and EGF-receptor mRNA in stroke-prone rats. Am J Physiol Regul Integr Comp Physiol. 2001;281(3):R944–50.
176. Chrissobolis S, et al. Chronic aldosterone administration causes Nox2-mediated increases in reactive oxygen species production and endothelial dysfunction in the cerebral circulation. J Hypertens. 2014;32(9):1815–21.
177. Touyz RM, Tabet F, Schiffrin EL. Redox-dependent signalling by angiotensin II and vascular remodelling in hypertension. Clin Exp Pharmacol Physiol. 2003;30(11):860–6.
178. Queisser N, Fazeli G, Schupp N. Superoxide anion and hydrogen peroxide-induced signaling and damage in angiotensin II and aldosterone action. Biol Chem. 2010; 391(11):1265–79.
179. Pires PW, et al. Tempol, a superoxide dismutase mimetic, prevents cerebral vessel remodeling in hypertensive rats. Microvasc Res. 2010;80(3):445–52.
180. Galis ZS, Khatri JJ. Matrix metalloproteinases in vascular remodeling and atherogenesis: the good, the bad, and the ugly. Circ Res. 2002;90(3):251–62.
181. Switzer JA, et al. Minocycline prevents IL-6 increase after acute ischemic stroke. Transl Stroke Res. 2012;3(3):363–8.
182. Switzer JA, et al. Matrix metalloproteinase-9 in an exploratory trial of intravenous minocycline for acute ischemic stroke. Stroke. 2011;42(9):2633–5.
183. Patel VB, et al. Angiotensin-converting enzyme 2 is a critical determinant of angiotensin II-induced loss of vascular smooth muscle cells and adverse vascular remodeling. Hypertension. 2014;64(1):157–64.
184. Cipolla MJ, et al. PPAR{gamma} activation prevents hypertensive remodeling of cerebral arteries and improves vascular function in female rats. Stroke. 2010;41(6):1266–70.
185. Ledingham JM, Laverty R. Effects of glitazones on blood pressure and vascular structure in mesenteric resistance arteries and basilar artery from genetically hypertensive rats. Clin Exp Pharmacol Physiol. 2005;32(11):919–25.
186. Ledingham JM, Laverty R. Effect of simvastatin given alone and in combination with valsartan or enalapril on blood pressure and the structure of mesenteric resistance arteries and the basilar artery in the genetically hypertensive rat model. Clin Exp Pharmacol Physiol. 2005;32(1-2):76–85.
187. Schiffrin EL. Immune mechanisms in hypertension and vascular injury. Clin Sci (Lond). 2014;126(4):267–74.
188. Crowley SD. The cooperative roles of inflammation and oxidative stress in the pathogenesis of hypertension. Antioxid Redox Signal. 2014;20(1):102–20.
189. Schiffrin EL. The immune system: role in hypertension. Can J Cardiol. 2013;29(5):543–8.
190. Kassan M, et al. CD4+CD25+Foxp3 regulatory T cells and vascular dysfunction in hypertension. J Hypertens. 2013;31(10):1939–43.
191. Schiffrin EL. Immune modulation of resistance artery remodelling. Basic Clin Pharmacol Toxicol. 2012;110(1):70–2.
192. Knorr M, Munzel T, Wenzel P. Interplay of NK cells and monocytes in vascular inflammation and myocardial infarction. Front Physiol. 2014;5:295.
193. Shen JZ, Young MJ. Corticosteroids, heart failure, and hypertension: a role for immune cells? Endocrinology. 2012;153(12):5692–700.
194. Luft FC, Dechend R, Muller DN. Immune mechanisms in angiotensin II-induced target-organ damage. Ann Med. 2012;44(1):S49–54.
195. Pires PW, et al. Improvement in middle cerebral artery structure and endothelial function in stroke-prone spontaneously hypertensive rats after macrophage depletion. Microcirculation. 2013;20(7):650–61.
196. Elmarakby AA, et al. Tumor necrosis factor alpha blockade increases renal Cyp2c23 expression and slows the progression of renal damage in salt-sensitive hypertension. Hypertension. 2006;47(3):557–62.

197. Elmarakby AA, et al. TNF-alpha inhibition reduces renal injury in DOCA-salt hypertensive rats. Am J Physiol Regul Integr Comp Physiol. 2008;294(1):R76–83.
198. Pires PW, et al. Tumor necrosis factor-alpha inhibition attenuates middle cerebral artery remodeling but increases cerebral ischemic damage in hypertensive rats. Am J Physiol Heart Circ Physiol. 2014;307(5):H658–69.
199. Coulson RJ, et al. Effects of ischemia and myogenic activity on active and passive mechanical properties of rat cerebral arteries. Am J Physiol Heart Circ Physiol. 2002;283(6): H2268–75.

Chapter 6
Pathophysiology and Mechanisms Whereby Hypertension May Cause Stroke

Beom Joon Kim, Hee-Joon Bae, and Lawrence K.S. Wong

The association between hypertension and stroke has been known since the nineteenth century. Although a number of vascular risk factors have been identified since, it is estimated that 51 % of stroke death may be attributable to elevated systolic blood pressure. The powerful effect of hypertension on the incidence and mortality of stroke has repeatedly been documented regardless of region or ethnic background [1].

Hypertension is the most important modifiable risk factor for stroke. The prevalence of hypertension in ischemic stroke patients ranges from two-thirds to as much as 80 % [2]. The degree of elevation of blood pressure is tightly correlated with the risk of stroke. The risk curve is a continuum without any clear point separating the stroke-prone from the non-stroke-prone subjects [3–5]. Hypertension plays a key role in the pathogenesis of large artery atherosclerosis, which in turn causes ischemic stroke due to thrombotic arterial occlusion, artery-to-artery embolism, or a combination of these factors. In the microscopic level of small arteries or arterioles, hypertension also generates specific vasculopathies such as lipohyalinosis and thus causing lacunar infarctions. Hypertension does not seem to directly cause cardioembolic stroke through generation of intracardiac thrombus, but such thrombophilic cardiac conditions including atrial fibrillation or ischemic cardiomyopathy are strongly under the influence of chronically elevated blood pressure. Additionally, hypertension is a major risk factor for intracerebral hemorrhage (ICH) and subarachnoid hemorrhage (SAH), two major subtypes of hemorrhagic stroke.

B.J. Kim, M.D., Ph.D. • H.-J. Bae, M.D., Ph.D. (✉)
Department of Neurology, Seoul National University Bundang Hospital,
Gyeonggi-do, South Korea
e-mail: braindoc@snu.ac.kr

L.K.S. Wong, M.D.
Departments of Medicine and Therapeutics, Chinese University of Hong Kong,
Hong Kong Special Administrative Region, Hong Kong, China

© Springer International Publishing Switzerland 2016
V. Aiyagari, P.B. Gorelick (eds.), *Hypertension and Stroke*, Clinical
Hypertension and Vascular Diseases, DOI 10.1007/978-3-319-29152-9_6

Microscopic and biological mechanisms contributed by hypertension on the cerebral vasculature will be discussed in other chapters. In this chapter, we will discuss clinical issues related to chronically elevated blood pressure in relation to ischemic or hemorrhagic strokes.

Mechanisms of Ischemic Stroke or Tia in Relation to Hypertension

Large Artery Disease

Artherosclerotic Stroke

Atherosclerosis may involve multiple arteries throughout the body, including the aorta, coronary arteries, peripheral blood vessels, and cerebral blood vessels. Fatty streaks, fibrous plaques, and complicated plaques are the pathologic hallmarks of atherosclerosis. Atherosclerotic lesions begin with an inflammatory reaction followed by smooth muscle proliferation and thickening of the arterial wall. Hypertension, endothelial dysfunction, shear stress, elevated low-density lipoproteins, free radicals, and chronic inflammatory response are closely associated with the process of atherosclerosis [6]. The common locations of atherosclerosis include the bifurcation of the common carotid artery, origin and intracavernous portion of the internal carotid artery (ICA), first segment of the middle cerebral artery (MCA), origin and the distal portion of the vertebral artery, and mid-portion of the basilar artery. Vulnerable plaques in the coronary artery tend to have a thin fibrous cap and a large lipid core. Autopsy findings and histopathological examination of surgical endarterectomy specimens suggest that intraplaque hemorrhage, reparative neovascularization, and ulceration are the factors leading to plaque instability in the carotid artery [7–9]. Atherosclerosis of the MCA most commonly affects the M1 segment, which extends from the origin of the artery to the insula. The lenticulostriate arteries arise from this section, and the origins of these vessels can be affected by the development of atherosclerotic plaque, which may result in an isolated small subcortical infarct. Hemorrhage, ulceration, and calcification are less common in intracranial atherosclerotic plaques compared to extracranial plaques. An autopsy study from Hong Kong found that luminal stenosis caused by atherosclerotic plaque, percentage of lipid in the lesions, and the presence of intraplaque neovasculature in the MCA are independent risk factors for MCA infarcts [10].

Recent development of imaging modalities including high-resolution MRI, enhanced doppler technology, and the combination of PET-MRI scans provide deeper insights into the characteristics of atherosclerotic plaques. Atherosclerotic plaques are largely divided into stable or vulnerable plaques, and the former usually grow slowly and thus causing hemodynamic insufficiency of the perfused territory due to intraluminal narrowing. However, the vulnerable plaques, characterized by thin fibrous cap over the necrotic core with high density of inflammation, have a tendency to rupture and cause sudden formation of intraluminal thrombus with distal embolization or vascular occlusions in situ [11].

Age, hypertension, diabetes mellitus, smoking, and hyperlipidemia are well-known risk factors for atherosclerosis. Large artery atherosclerosis is the most common type of vascular pathology, in which fibrous and muscular tissues proliferate in the subintima of the vessel wall, and fatty materials form plaques that can impinge on the vessel lumen. Platelets then adhere to plaque and form clumps that serve as a nidus for the deposition of fibrin, thrombi, and clot [12]. Acute thrombosis begins with fissuring of the fibrous cap of the atherosclerotic plaque, and the release of tissue factors promotes the development of a clot adjacent to the plaque. Local occlusion can then lead to a significant decrease in blood flow and oxygen supply, which may cause ischemic brain damage.

In contrast to Caucasians, intracranial occlusive disease is common in persons of Asian and African ancestry [13–16]. Intracranial atherosclerosis accounts for 33–50 % of stroke in Asians [13], and up to 10 % of stroke or TIA in the USA are caused by intracranial artery stenosis [17]. Age, hypertension, diabetes mellitus, and probably the metabolic syndrome are the most consistent risk factors for intracranial atherosclerosis [18]. And a higher incidence of hypertension in populations of African and Asian ancestry may explain their higher prevalence of intracranial atherosclerosis. Severity of stenosis is widely accepted as the major prognostic risk factor in patients with symptomatic and asymptomatic ICA disease [19, 20], and has been reported to increase the risk of ischemic stroke in the territory of symptomatic intracranial arterial stenosis [21]. Furthermore, progression of MCA occlusion as assessed by an increase of flow velocity on TCD is associated with an increased risk of further cardiovascular events [22].

Peculiarity of Intracranial Artery Atherosclerosis

Intracranial artery stenosis is an interesting topic, which deserves a separate discussion. Asian and African-American patients have disproportionately higher rates of intracranial atherosclerosis than Caucasian populations [23–25]. In a postmortem study from China, severe intracranial atherosclerosis was found in 30 % of subjects in their 60s and 70s and around 50 % in elderly patients aged ≥80. Such ethnic disproportion has not been clearly elaborated but it may originate from differences in genetic background or in the profile of vascular risk factors. Interestingly, South Korea, which has entered into a modern industrialized society within a short time period of 20–30 years, had significant changes in the proportion of intracranial stenosis over extracranial stenosis which supports a role of nutritional and environmental factors [26].

Intracranial atherosclerosis shares basic pathological components with extracranial atherosclerosis; intimal necrosis and proliferative fibrosis of intima and adventitia with extension of vasa vasorum into the vascular media. However, two major characteristics distinguish intracranial and extracranial atherosclerosis; the later onset and the more stable plaque phenotype in intracranial arteries [18].

The above two features may be explained by the distinct characteristics of the intracranial arteries, including (1) thicker, denser internal elastic lamina and no external elastic lamina; (2) vasa vasorum only in large intracranial arteries surrounded by CSF; (3) distinct vessel wall metabolism; (4) presence of tight Junctions between endothelial cells; (5) reduced endothelial permeability; (6) relative insensitivity to sympathomimetic and histamine stimulations compared with systemic vessels; (7) enhanced protective mechanisms against oxidative stress; and (8) flow characteristics determined by circle of Willis anatomy [18]. Thus far, the larger antioxidant response of intracranial compared with extracranial arteries is the single reported functional characteristic that may contribute to the reported later onset and steep increase in intracranial atherosclerosis in the sixth decade.

Clinical issues related to intracranial atherosclerosis may be summarized by the following points: (1) occlusion of small perforator branches in middle cerebral arteries or basilar arteries. Such ischemic stroke from branched artery occlusion may occur long before any noticeable luminal narrowing develops. (2) When the cross-sectional area of intracranial arteries became smaller, hemodynamic insufficiency and related pathological changes may develop before a typical atherosclerotic pathology accumulates. However, it is relatively not uncommon that the extent of any irreversible infarction became relatively smaller due to leptomeningeal collaterals from posterior cerebral arteries or extracarotid arterial channels. (3) Intracranial arteries intermittently pose technical hurdles for endovascular interventions.

Artery-to-Artery Embolism

Artery-to-artery embolism is another important stroke mechanism in patients with extracranial large artery disease. Emboli are composed of clot, platelet clumps, or fragments of plaques that break off from the proximal vessels [27]. Proximal ICA and extracranial vertebral artery atherosclerosis is an important source of embolism. High-intensity transient signals (HITS) recorded over the MCA with TCD monitoring can be used to detect artery-to-artery embolism in patients with proximal artery disease [21].

Artery-to-artery embolism is also an important but less well-recognized mechanism of stroke among patients with intracranial artery disease. Wong et al. [22] reported that among stroke patients with multiple acute infarcts and MCA stenosis, unilateral, deep, chainlike border-zone infarcts were the most common pattern. However, the number of microembolic signals predicted the number of acute infarcts, which suggested an embolic mechanism for this pattern of stroke. A possible explanation is that emboli in the trunk of the MCA may simultaneously occlude several of the lenticulostriate perforating vessels.

Branch Atheromatous Disease

Atheromatous plaque, often referred to as microatheroma, can obstruct the orifices of penetrating arteries and occlude the lumen, causing an isolated small subcortical infarct. Pathological features of microatheroma include microdissection, plaque

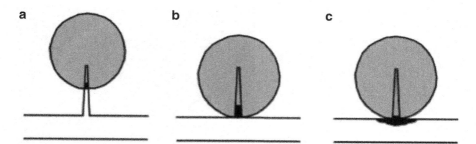

Fig. 6.1 Classification of SSSI according to the lesion extension and the presence of PAD. (**a**) Distal SSSI without PAD; (**b**) proximal SSSI without PAD; (**c**) SSSI associated with PAD. *SSSI* indicates single small subcortical infarction and *PAD* parent artery disease. (From Nah H-W, Kang D-W, Kwon SU, Kim JS. Diversity of Single Small Subcortical Infarctions According to Infarct Location and Parent Artery Disease Analysis of Indicators for Small Vessel Disease and Atherosclerosis. Stroke; a journal of cerebral circulation. 2010;41(12):2822-7, with permission)

hemorrhage, and deposition of platelet-fibrin materials [28]. Branch atheromatous disease was first described in pontine infarction caused by basilar branch occlusion, but its concept can be applied to infarcts in the territory of lenticulostriate branches, thalamogeniculate branches, anterior choroidal artery, Huebner's artery, and thalamoperforating artery branches [29]. This pathogenic mechanism of stroke has been underappreciated in the past [29–31]. However, recent studies have demonstrated that in patients with MCA stenosis, occlusion of a single penetrating artery to produce a small subcortical lacune-like infarct is relatively common [32, 33].

Technological development of MRI permitted the acquisition of high-resolution images on intracranial vascular wall pathologies. Such MRI techniques visualized that a part of intracranial arteries, previously considered as conspicuous but undisturbed vascular lesions, have spread atherosclerotic plaques alongside the curves of vascular lumen and thus occluding the orifice of parenchymal perforators. In this context, detailed classification has been proposed as following [34] (Fig. 6.1). The traditional lacunar infarction pathology, mainly composed of lipohyalinosis and fibrinoid necrosis of microscopic arteriolar walls, may locate at the inside of brain parenchyma thus causing small and confined infarction (Fig. 6.1a). However, atherosclerotic pathologies involving vascular walls of intracranial arteries may involve the opening of direct and long perforators (Fig. 6.1c). Such occlusion may result in a vertically elongated lesion from basal ganglia to corona radiata in the lenticulostriate artery territory or stretched lesion involving basal surface of the pons or midbrain in the brainstem.

Likewise, a recent report supported the concept. The authors classified so-called traditional lacunar infarction with axial diameter less than 1.5 cm into branch atheromatous diseases and lacunar infarctions by involvement of the basal surface of brainstem or elongated lesions in lenticulostriate artery territories. Early neurological deterioration, defined as any new neurological symptom/signs within 3 weeks from the index stroke, occurred more frequently in a group of branch atheromatous disease than in a lacunar infarction group [35].

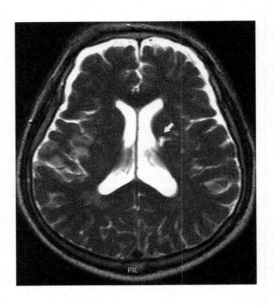

Fig. 6.2 Lacunar infarction. *White arrow* indicates a small lacunar infarction in left corona radiata

Small Vessel Occlusion

The classical example of small vessel disease is the occlusion of a single, non-branching penetrating end artery (usually smaller than 500 μm in diameter), which causes small subcortical lacunar infarcts (1–20 mm in diameter) (Fig. 6.2). There are a number of potential causes of small vessel occlusive disease, e.g., embolism and vasospasm; however, lipohyalinosis and atherosclerosis remain the two major pathologies.

Fibrinoid necrosis is caused by the insudation of plasma proteins, i.e., fibrin, into the arteriolar wall, which is common in hypertensive brains. The affected area is deeply eosinophilic and structureless, or very finely granular (Fig. 6.3). In hypertensive individuals, the vessel wall may also be eosinophilic and structureless due to degeneration of muscle and collagen (hyalinization). Hyalinization is considered as a "mundane" change because it does not cause the rupture of the blood vessels. However, on light microscopy, it may be difficult to distinguish between hyalinization and fibrinoid necrosis. Special stains such as the Putz stain may help in differentiating between fibrinoid and hyaline material [36]. Immunohistochemistry and electron microscopy have established that the fibrinoid areas do indeed contain fibrin, and electron microscopy clearly distinguishes fibrin with its characteristic periodicity from areas of hyalinization which contain only degenerated collagen and smooth muscle and unidentified amorphous material [36, 37]. Fibrinoid deposition may be very segmental so that the material appears only at widely separated points along the length of arterioles or only in a portion of its circumference. In a study combining light microscopy with electron microscopy, fibrinoid necrosis occurred in vessels that also displayed hyalinization with no suggestion that fibrinoid necrosis preceded hyalinization [38].

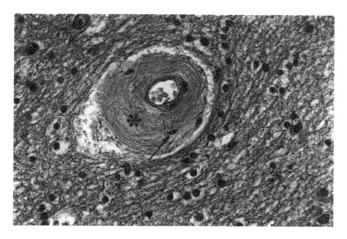

Fig. 6.3 Hyaline arteriosclerosis, roughly concentric vessel wall thickening by hyaline collagenous material (*asterisk*), with occasional surviving smooth muscle cell nuclei (*arrow*). (From Lammie GA. Pathology of small vessel stroke. Br Med Bull. 2000;56:296–306, with permission [39])

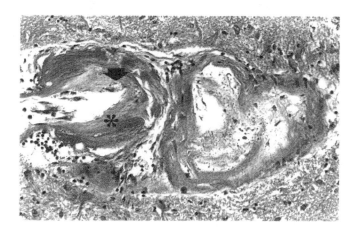

Fig. 6.4 Lipohyalinosis, an asymmetrically thickened, disorganized vessel wall with focal fibrosis (*asterisk*) and foam cell infiltration (*thick arrow*). (From Lammie GA. Pathology of small vessel stroke. Br Med Bull. 2000;56:296–306, with permission.)

Lipohyalinosis, formerly considered the most frequent cause of lacunes, shares some of the histochemical, electron microscopic, and immunofluorescent characteristics of fibrinoid necrosis [40]. Lipohyalinosis has been thought to be an intermediate stage between fibrinoid necrosis of severe hypertension and microatheroma associated with more long standing hypertension. Although often considered identical, lipohyalinosis and fibrinoid necrosis differ histochemically in that fibrinoid necrosis stains strongly for phosphotungstic acid hematoxylin, whereas lipohyalinosis does not (Fig. 6.4) [41, 42]. Lipohyalinosis is found most commonly in a setting of chronic, nonmalignant hypertension, whereas fibrinoid necrosis is said to be found uncommonly with extreme blood pressure elevation such as those that occur in hypertensive encephalopathy and eclampsia [40]. Original Fisher's description was that vascular lesions involved small arteries of 40–200 µm diameter and caused correspondingly small, often asymptomatic, cerebral infarcts, particularly in the striatocapsule [43, 44]. He chose the term lipohyalinosis instead of fibrinoid necrosis just because he perceived that the affected arteriolar segments also contained lipid. Owing to his huge influence in this area, the term lipohyalinosis has come into widespread use, while fibrinoid necrosis has become the less-used term.

The most common locations for lacunes are the putamen and the pallidum, followed by the pons, thalamus, caudate nucleus, internal capsule, and corona radiate [44]. The incidence of cerebral lacunes has declined since the introduction of antihypertensive therapy, an indication that antihypertensive therapy is effective in the prevention of this type of stroke [44]. Initially, lipohyalinosis was thought to be the main cause of lacunar stroke. However, with recent advances in modern neuroimaging, microatheroma is now thought to be the most common mechanism of small vessel occlusion, especially in Asian populations with high prevalence of large intracranial artery stenosis [45]. The culprit atheromatous plaques are often seen in the proximal portion of the perforating artery (microatheroma), at its origin (junctional atheroma), or in the parent artery itself (mural atheroma). Infarcts are related to stenotic or occlusive plaques, some but not all of which may be complicated by overlying thrombus [44]. Subcortical infarcts caused by atheromatous disease are larger in size, usually more than 5 mm in diameter, and associated with a more unstable clinical course than those caused by lipohyalinosis [45].

Cardioembolism

In cardioembolic stroke, the embolus most commonly originates from the heart valves, endocardium, and atrial or ventricular cavities. Other clots may originate in systematic veins and then travel to the brain through cardiac defects, such as a patent foramen ovale, a process termed paradoxical embolism. A larger infarct is more common in cardioembolic stroke when compared to an artery-to-artery embolic stroke because the clots are larger and there is insufficient time to develop an effective collateral circulation. Atrial fibrillation is the most common cardiac source of brain embolism. Atrial fibrillation is more likely to develop in hypertensive patients with left ventricular hypertrophy and an increased left atrial size. A recent study also showed that regression of left ventricular hypertrophy with antihypertensive therapy reduced the risk of developing atrial fibrillation [46]. Hence, better blood pressure control in addition to anticoagulation may further reduce the risk of embolic stroke.

Hemodynamic Stroke

Cardiac failure and systemic hypotension are the two major causes of systemic hypoperfusion. Systemic hypoperfusion is more generalized than cerebral arterial thrombosis or embolism and usually affects both cerebral hemispheres. Recent studies have demonstrated an association between blood pressure and heart failure. In a US study of over 48,000 patients admitted with acute heart failure, patients in the lowest quartile of systolic pressure (<120 mmHg) had the highest in-hospital and 3-month postdischarge mortality rate [47]. A prospective community-based study found that nondipping of nocturnal blood pressure conferred an additional risk of developing chronic heart failure beyond conventional blood pressure measurement [48]. Therefore, we speculate that good control of blood pressure may lower the risk of developing cardiac failure and thereby lower the risk of cerebral hypoperfusion.

Additionally, chronic hypertension leads to atherosclerosis and increased peripheral vascular resistance, which may further reduce the collateral reserve and result in severe ischemia distal to an arterial occlusion [49]. The border-zone areas between vascular territories are usually vulnerable to hypoperfusion, and when there is a profound decrease in systemic blood pressure, watershed infarcts occur in these areas.

Hypoperfusion caused by a process occurring at a distance from the brain (i.e., the heart or extracranial arteries) rarely produces major brain infarction. In contrast, decreased blood flow caused by a lesion directly at the site of brain tissue is not so benign. Occlusion of penetrating arteries often causes an infarct in the territory supplied by the obstructed artery. In addition, severe intracranial arterial disease also seems more likely to cause brain infarction than extracranial occlusive disease [50].

Traditionally, hypoperfusion and embolism are considered independent mechanisms of stroke in patients with arterial occlusive disease. Caplan proposed that they often coexist in patients with severe occlusive disease [51, 52]. Arterial luminal narrowing and endothelial abnormalities promote clot formation and subsequent embolization, whereas reduced perfusion limits clearance of emboli, especially in the border zones. Impaired washout is an important mechanism that combines hypoperfusion, embolization, and brain infarction [51, 52].

Stroke and the Variability of Blood Pressure

Blood pressure tends to fluctuate over time. Such variability is thought to reflect normal physiology of the autonomic nervous system, cardiac cycle and changes in body posture as well as external environmental change, psychological stress and circadian rhythm [53].

Short-term variability of blood pressure, usually referring to beat-to-beat variability over the 24 h of a single circadian cycle, represents an adaptive response of body regulatory systems to the internal and external environment. Short-term variability is usually summarized as an average of standard deviation or a coefficient of variation but is only modestly associated with cardiovascular complications [54, 55]. Long-term variability usually refers to the variation of blood pressure readings between clinic visits, over seasons and years. Surprisingly, long-term blood pressure variability shows only a weak correlation with short-term fluctuations and may be affected by environmental changes between each measurement and the exposure to BP-lowering medications [56–58].

Until recently published pivotal papers, fluctuations in blood pressure were mostly dismissed and not included in analyses. However, a series of papers published in 2010 demonstrated that such variability is important and may influence certain vascular outcomes after stroke, for example, and certain classes of blood pressure lowering medication may modify blood pressure variability better than other classes of blood pressure lowering medication. Rothwell and colleagues selected recent ischemic stroke or transient ischemic attack patients with more than seven measurements of office blood pressure over at least a 4-month interval. They discovered there is a significant variation in the blood pressure readings over the long period of follow-up, and the blood pressure variability showed noticeable correlation with recurrent stroke events [59]. In a parallel paper, they reported that visit-to-visit variability was more evident in a beta-blocker treated group than in a calcium channel blocker treated group. This suggested that blood pressure variability itself may be mitigated [56].

Earlier, Swedish investigators documented that blood pressure lowering medication may protect against stroke by lowering variability of blood pressure as well as by decreasing the level of blood pressure [60]. In a large cohort of 16,000 hypertensive patients with a follow-up duration up to 35 years, the investigators detect a consistent association between long-term blood pressure variability and the risk of cardiovascular diseases and vascular mortality [61]. Diaz and colleagues reported a meta-analysis of seven cohort studies and noted that for each 5 mmHg higher standard deviation of systolic blood pressure, the risk of cardiovascular diseases were increased by 17 % for stroke, by 27 % for coronary heart disease, by 12 % for all cardiovascular diseases, and by 22 % for all-cause mortality [62]. The strength of association was moderate, and detailed indices of BP variability were not analyzed.

Mechanisms of Intracranial Hemorrhages in Relation to Hypertension

Intracranial hemorrhages involve the brain parenchyma or subarachnoid space, or both. Approximately 15 % of strokes are hemorrhagic. While this accounts for a small proportion of stroke, hemorrhagic stroke has a higher mortality rate compared to ischemic stroke. Hypertension and ruptured cerebral aneurysms are two major causes of intracranial hemorrhage, which are discussed subsequently.

Hypertensive Intracerebral Hemorrhage

Traditionally, hypertension has been considered the predominant cause of ICH [63]. Hypertension-related ICH often leads to subcortical hemorrhage, such as in the putamen (Fig. 6.5) and adjacent internal capsule, thalamus, pons, and cerebellum. However, the importance of hypertension in the etiology of lobar hemorrhage should also be recognized. A study by Broderick and colleagues found that

Fig. 6.5 Intracerebral hemorrhage. A small hypertensive intracerebral hemorrhage in *left* basal ganglia

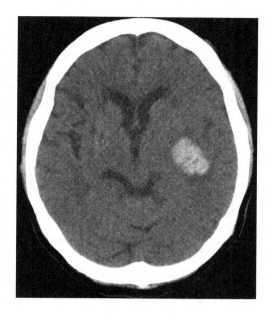

hypertension is nearly as common in primary lobar hemorrhage as in deep hemispheric, cerebellar, and pontine hemorrhages, and its association with lobar hemorrhage does not diminish with advancing age [64]. In this study, 67 % of 66 patients with lobar ICH had hypertension, compared to 77 patients with deep hemispheric (73 %), 11 with cerebellar (73 %), and 9 with pontine (78 %) hemorrhages.

There are two important mechanisms that result in hypertensive ICH: (a) rupture of small penetrating arteries damaged by chronic hypertension and aging and (b) acute elevation of blood pressure leading to rupture of normal arterioles and capillaries.

Chronic Hypertension

Chronic hypertension produces arteriolar changes consisting of fibrinoid necrosis, lipohyalinosis, medial degeneration, and microaneurysm formation, all of which make the vessel susceptible to rupture. The rupture usually occurs in the middle or distal portions of penetrating arteries at or very near to bifurcations. The role of microaneurysms in causing ICH was first proposed by Charcot and Bouchard in 1868, but has been debated over a century. There is accumulating evidence against the theory that the spontaneous ICH is due to a rupture of Charcot–Bouchard microaneurysms as it has never been clearly identified as the definite cause of spontaneous cerebral hematomas. Challa et al. [65] failed to demonstrate microaneurysms in hypertensive patients with spontaneous ICH. An electron microscopic study of ruptured arteries in hypertensive ICH showed severe degenerative changes in 46 of 48 ruptured arteries, but ruptured microaneurysms were found only in two cases [66]. These studies indicated that degenerative changes caused by age and hypertension can predispose to ICH, but it is not certain that a ruptured microaneurysm is the cause of the bleeding.

Acute Hypertension

In clinical practice, many patients with ICH have no prior history of hypertension. In addition, pathologic evidence of chronic hypertension, such as left ventricular hypertrophy or other cardiac and renal changes, is often not found. Bahemuka et al. [67] found only 46 % of fatal cases of spontaneous ICH had chronic hypertension or left ventricular hypertrophy. Similarly, in a case series of 154 patients with spontaneous ICH during 1 year, only 45 % had a history of hypertension [68]. In these two studies, the location of hematoma, increased blood pressure on admission, and absence of other etiologies suggest that the ICH is often caused by an acute elevation of blood pressure. Evidence also indicates that an acute increase in blood pressure and blood flow can precipitate rupture of normal arterioles and capillaries unprotected from these changes in the absence of prior hypertension. Usually, the more sudden and the more severe the change, the higher the risk of rupture.

The combination of a significant increase in cerebral blood flow and blood pressure may also lead to ICH following carotid endarterectomy or carotid artery stenting. A retrospective review of 4494 patients who underwent carotid endarterectomy or carotid artery stenting found that strict control of postoperative blood pressure prevents ICH caused by cerebral hyperperfusion syndrome after CEA [69]. A more recent study also demonstrated that comprehensive management of hypertension can lower the incidence of ICH and hyperperfusion syndrome in high-risk patients following carotid artery stenting [70].

ICH has been frequently associated with the use of illicit drugs, especially cocaine and amphetamine, which are known to have sympathomimetic effects. Cocaine-induced hypertension is a long-recognized risk factor of ICH. Some patients may also develop a hypertensive encephalopathy with multiple ICH and brain edema [71]. The exact mechanism by which these drugs cause ICH is not yet clear. One possible explanation is that the sudden elevation of blood pressure that occurs immediately after using drugs may cause an existing aneurysm or arteriovenous malformation in the brain to rupture. Interestingly, a higher frequency of an underlying vascular malformation has been noted in cocaine-related hemorrhage compared to amphetamine-related hemorrhage [71, 72].

What is interesting in the issue of blood pressure and ICH is that blood pressure variability measured with the maximal systolic blood pressure and the standard deviation of systolic blood pressure in both hyperacute and acute periods of ICH was well correlated with poor clinical outcomes [73].

Aneurysmal Subarachnoid Hemorrhage

SAH (Fig. 6.6) occurs when a blood vessel near the brain surface leaks, leading to extravasation of blood into the subarachnoid space. SAH is most often caused by rupture of a saccular aneurysm. Saccular aneurysms are most commonly seen at the ICA–posterior communicating artery junction, anterior communicating artery–ACA junction, the apex of basilar artery, and the MCA bifurcation. Histopathologic

Fig. 6.6 Subarachnoid hemorrhage. Extensive blood clots occupy basal and perimesencephalic cisterns and both sylvian fissures

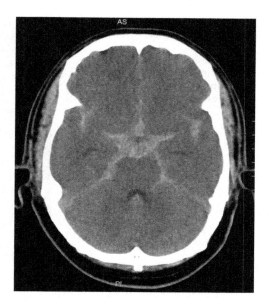

features of aneurysms include degenerative changes, thinning of the media, inflammatory changes, atherosclerosis, and presence of medial and elastic defects of the aneurysmal wall [74].

The mechanism of the origin, growth, and rupture of saccular intracranial aneurysm is largely unknown. Intracranial arteries are more susceptible to aneurysm formation than extracranial arteries because intracranial vessels are thinner, with less elastin; the external elastic lamina is absent; and vessels in the subarachnoid space lack surrounding supporting tissue. A congenital deficit in the arterial media may be a weak spot through which the inner layers of the arterial wall bulge and is a possible explanation for aneurysmal formation. Focal deficits are often located at arterial bifurcations. Reduced production of type III collagen has also been reported to be associated with familial intracranial aneurysms [75]. In addition, acquired changes in the arterial wall are also likely to be important since hypertension, smoking, and alcohol abuse are known risk factors for SAH. These conditions lead to local thickening of the intimal layer of the arterial wall. This, in turn, may increase strain on the more elastic portions of the vessel wall [76].

In animal models, saccular aneurysms can be produced by combining experimental renal hypertension and ligation of a carotid artery to alter hemodynamic stress in the circle of Willis. However, the administration of beta-aminopropionitrile alone, a potent irreversible inhibitor of lysyl oxidase which initiates cross-linkage formation in elastin and collagen, without the presence of hypertension does not induce aneurysm formation, which indicates that a vascular lesion and hemodynamic stress are both important in the pathogenesis of aneurysm formation [49]. In addition, abnormalities in structural proteins of the extracellular matrix have been identified in the arterial wall at a distance from the aneurysm itself [77].

Fig. 6.7 White matter
lesions. Extensive white
matter changes
(leukoaraiosis) are
observed in both
periventricular and
subcortical white matter

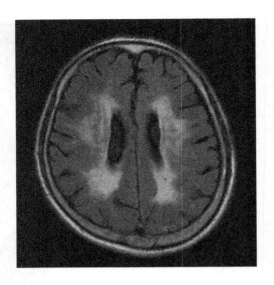

Stress on the vessel wall increases as the radius of the aneurysm enlarges. When the wall stress exceeds the wall strength, aneurysms rupture. Evidence indicates that aneurysms larger than 10 mm in diameter are more likely to rupture [78]. Aneurysms may rupture at any time, but are more prone to do so when blood pressure or blood flow increases during strenuous activity.

Mechanisms of Silent Brain Lesions in Relation to Hypertension

White Matter Lesions

White matter lesions (WMLs) (Fig. 6.7) are considered present if visible as hyperintense lesions on proton-density and T2-weighted images, without prominent hypointensity on T1-weighted scans [79]. WMLs are strongly associated with increasing age. However, in most studies, white matter changes are more common in hypertensive than in normotensive individuals, especially in the young. A population-based study showed that the duration of hypertension was associated with both periventricular and subcortical WMLs. Furthermore, subjects with successfully treated hypertension had only moderately increased subcortical and periventricular WMLs compared with normotensive subjects [80]. The importance of WMLs as a predictor of stroke risk [79, 81] and vascular dementia [80] has been demonstrated in previous studies.

The pathology of WML is heterogeneous, including small infarction, gliosis, demyelination, vascular ectasia, and dilated perivascular spaces, all of which are also commonly seen in the experimental hypertension model [82]. The exact mechanism of WMLs is unclear, but hypertension-related arteriolosclerosis appears to be the most important causative factor, and the extent of WMLs is thought to reflect the extent of brain arteriolosclerosis [83].

Silent Infarctions: Old Lacunar Infarcts and Microinfarcts

Silent infarcts may be divided into two comparable categories: old lacunar infarctions and microinfarcts. Old lacunar infarcts are defined as focal hyperintensities on T2-weighted images, 3 mm in size or larger, with corresponding prominent hypointensities on T1-weighted images [79]. Old lacunar infarcts and WMLs are thought to have similar vascular origin. However, the majority of silent infarcts are lacunar infarcts which may be caused by either large or small vessel disease, whereas WMLs reflect mainly small vessel disease. In terms of clinical outcome, studies indicate that both community-based normal elderly people [79, 84] and stroke patients [81, 85] with old lacunar infarcts and WMLs are at a strongly increased risk of stroke, which cannot be explained by other stroke risk factors. Microinfarcts are typically undetected by conventional structural MRI and can be detected only by microscopic histological examinations, although the largest acute microinfarcts can be detected by diffusion-weighted imaging [86, 87]. This category of silent, or at least subclinical, lesions has been associated with macroscopic infarcts and commonly coexists with Alzheimer disease pathology [88, 89].

Cerebral Microbleeds

Microbleeds (MBs) (Fig. 6.8) are defined as punctate, homogeneous, rounded, lesions less than 0.5 cm in size, with signal loss or hypointensity on gradient echo MRI. The pathology of microbleeds is perivascular deposits of hemosiderin in the

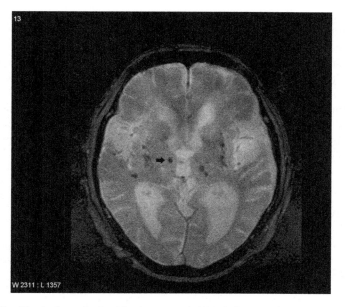

Fig. 6.8 Microbleeds. Several microbleeds are seen in both thalamus and basal ganglia. The *black arrow* indicates one of them. (*Sources*: Figs. 5, 6, 7, and 8 from Dr Bae's collections)

brain, which is regarded as evidence of previous rupture of small vessels [90, 91]. MBs have been found in patients with both ICHs and ischemic stroke. The presence of MBs predicts the recurrence of ICH in patients with primary lobar ICH and is associated with aspirin-associated ICH [92]. Hence, antiplatelet medications should be used with caution in patients with diffuse MBs. Various studies have shown that microbleeds are related with subsequent cerebral bleeding among patients with ischemic stroke including acute hemorrhagic transformation after thrombolysis [93], although there is also some evidence against the importance of MBs as a predictor of hemorrhagic transformation [94]. Lobar microbleeds detected in the elderly are often attributed to amyloid angiopathy and associated with Alzheimer's disease.

The mechanism of microbleedsMicrobleeds (MBs) is largely unknown. MBs have been found to be associated with increased age, hypertension, WMLs, lacunar infarcts, and ICH [95, 96]. One recent study found that there were linear associations between MBs, WMLs, and lacunar infarcts. With increasing number of lacunar infarcts or severity of WMLs, the frequency and the number of MBs increased in parallel [90]. This finding indicates that microbleeds, white matter changes, and lacunar infarcts most probably share the same pathogenesis of advanced microangiopathy.

Conclusions

Hypertension has deleterious effects on the cerebral circulation. Hypertension alters the structure of blood vessels by producing vascular hypertrophy and remodeling and by promoting atherosclerosis in large cerebral arteries and lipohyalinosis in penetrating arterioles. In addition, hypertension also impairs endothelium-dependent relaxation and alters cerebrovascular autoregulation and neurovascular coupling. With these functional and structural alternations, hypertension facilitates vascular occlusions or degenerative change that is prone to rupture and bleeding, thereby causing both ischemic and hemorrhagic stroke. Recently it has been shown that short-term and also long-term blood pressure variability can play a role in the pathogenesis of stroke.

Better understanding of these underlying mechanisms may provide new insights into stroke management and prevention. Since hypertension is one of the modifiable risk factors of cerebrovascular disease, optimal blood pressure control may significantly lower the risk of stroke.

References

1. Gaciong Z, Siński M, Lewandowski J. Blood pressure control and primary prevention of stroke: summary of the recent clinical trial data and meta-analyses. Curr Hypertens Rep. 2013; 15(6):559–74.
2. Kim BJ, Park JM, Kang K, Lee SJ, Ko Y, Kim JG, et al. Case characteristics, hyperacute treatment, and outcome information from the clinical research center for stroke-fifth division registry in South Korea. J Stroke. 2015;17(1):38–53.

3. Kannel WB, Wolf PA, Verter J, McNamara PM. Epidemiologic assessment of the role of blood pressure in stroke. The Framingham study. JAMA. 1970;214(2):301–10.
4. Whisnant JP. Epidemiology of stroke: emphasis on transient cerebral ischemia attacks and hypertension. Stroke. 1974;5(1):68–70.
5. Ohkubo T, Asayama K, Kikuya M, Metoki H, Obara T, Saito S, et al. Prediction of ischaemic and haemorrhagic stroke by self-measured blood pressure at home: the Ohasama study. Blood Press Monit. 2004;9(6):315–20.
6. Ross R. Atherosclerosis—an inflammatory disease. N Engl J Med. 1999;340(2):115–26.
7. Fisher M, Paganini-Hill A, Martin A, Cosgrove M, Toole JF, Barnett HJ, et al. Carotid plaque pathology: thrombosis, ulceration, and stroke pathogenesis. Stroke. 2005;36(2):253–7.
8. Bornstein NM, Krajewski A, Lewis AJ, Norris JW. Clinical significance of carotid plaque hemorrhage. Arch Neurol. 1990;47(9):958–9.
9. Bornstein NM, Norris JW. The unstable carotid plaque. Stroke. 1989;20(8):1104–6.
10. Chen XY, Wong KS, Lam WW, Zhao HL, Ng HK. Middle cerebral artery atherosclerosis: histological comparison between plaques associated with and not associated with infarct in a postmortem study. Cerebrovasc Dis. 2008;25(1–2):74–80.
11. Bodle JD, Feldmann E, Swartz RH, Rumboldt Z, Brown T, Turan TN. High-resolution magnetic resonance imaging: an emerging tool for evaluating intracranial arterial disease. Stroke. 2013;44(1):287–92.
12. Caplan LR. Basic pathology, anatomy, and pathophysiology of stroke. In: Caplan LR, editor. Caplan's stroke: a clinical approach. 3rd ed. Woburn: Butterworth-Heinemann; 2000. p. 17–50.
13. Wong LKS. Global burden of intracranial atherosclerosis. Int J Stroke. 2006;1:158–9.
14. Bang OY, Kim JW, Lee JH, Lee MA, Lee PH, Joo IS, et al. Association of the metabolic syndrome with intracranial atherosclerotic stroke. Neurology. 2005;65(2):296–8.
15. Nam HS, Han SW, Lee JY, Ahn SH, Ha JW, Rim SJ, et al. Association of aortic plaque with intracranial atherosclerosis in patients with stroke. Neurology. 2006;67(7):1184–8.
16. Suh DC, Lee SH, Kim KR, Park ST, Lim SM, Kim SJ, et al. Pattern of atherosclerotic carotid stenosis in Korean patients with stroke: different involvement of intracranial versus extracranial vessels. AJNR Am J Neuroradiol. 2003;24(2):239–44.
17. Nishimaru K, McHenry Jr LC, Toole JF. Cerebral angiographic and clinical differences in carotid system transient ischemic attacks between American Caucasian and Japanese patients. Stroke. 1984;15(1):56–9.
18. Ritz K, Denswil NP, Stam O, van Lieshout JJ. Cause and mechanisms of intracranial atherosclerosis. Circulation. 2014;130(16):1407–14.
19. Norris JW, Zhu CZ, Bornstein NM, Chambers BR. Vascular risks of asymptomatic carotid stenosis. Stroke. 1991;22(12):1485–90.
20. Streifler JY, Eliasziw M, Benavente OR, Harbison JW, Hachinski VC, Barnett HJ, et al. The risk of stroke in patients with first-ever retinal vs hemispheric transient ischemic attacks and high-grade carotid stenosis. North American Symptomatic Carotid Endarterectomy Trial. Arch Neurol. 1995;52(3):246–9.
21. Kasner SE, Chimowitz MI, Lynn MJ, Howlett-Smith H, Stern BJ, Hertzberg VS, et al. Predictors of ischemic stroke in the territory of a symptomatic intracranial arterial stenosis. Circulation. 2006;113(4):555–63.
22. Wong KS, Li H, Lam WW, Chan YL, Kay R. Progression of middle cerebral artery occlusive disease and its relationship with further vascular events after stroke. Stroke. 2002;33(2):532–6.
23. Kieffer SA, Takeya Y, Resch JA, Amplatz K. Racial differences in cerebrovascular disease. Angiographic evaluation of Japanese and American populations. Am J Roentgenol Radium Ther Nucl Med. 1967;101(1):94–9.
24. Caplan LR, Gorelick PB, Hier DB. Race, sex and occlusive cerebrovascular disease: a review. Stroke. 1986;17(4):648–55.
25. Waddy SP, Cotsonis G, Lynn MJ, Frankel MR, Chaturvedi S, Williams JE, et al. Racial differences in vascular risk factors and outcomes of patients with intracranial atherosclerotic arterial stenosis. Stroke. 2009;40(3):719–25.
26. Hachinski V. Stroke in Korean. Stroke. 2008;39(4):1067.

27. Fisher CM. Observations of the fundus oculi in transient monocular blindness. Neurology. 1959;9(5):333–47.
28. Lhermitte F, Gautier JC, Derouesne C. Nature of occlusions of the middle cerebral artery. Neurology. 1970;20(1):82–8.
29. Caplan LR. Intracranial branch atheromatous disease: a neglected, understudied, and under-used concept. Neurology. 1989;39(9):1246–50.
30. Kang SY, Kim JS. Anterior cerebral artery infarction: stroke mechanism and clinical-imaging study in 100 patients. Neurology. 2008;70(24 Pt 2):2386–93.
31. Vemmos KN, Spengos K, Tsivgoulis G, Manios E, Zis V, Vassilopoulos D. Aetiopathogenesis and long-term outcome of isolated pontine infarcts. J Neurol. 2005;252(2):212–7.
32. Wong KS, Gao S, Chan YL, Hansberg T, Lam WW, Droste DW, et al. Mechanisms of acute cerebral infarctions in patients with middle cerebral artery stenosis: a diffusion-weighted imaging and microemboli monitoring study. Ann Neurol. 2002;52(1):74–81.
33. Lee DK, Kim JS, Kwon SU, Yoo SH, Kang DW. Lesion patterns and stroke mechanism in atherosclerotic middle cerebral artery disease: early diffusion-weighted imaging study. Stroke. 2005;36(12):2583–8.
34. Nah H-W, Kang D-W, Kwon SU, Kim JS. Diversity of single small subcortical infarctions according to infarct location and parent artery disease analysis of indicators for small vessel disease and atherosclerosis. Stroke. 2010;41(12):2822–7.
35. Jeong H-G, Kim BJ, Yang MH, Han M-K, Bae H-J. Neuroimaging markers for early neuro-logic deterioration in single small subcortical infarction. Stroke. 2015;46(3):687–91.
36. Rosenblum WI. Fibrinoid necrosis of small brain arteries and arterioles and miliary aneurysms as causes of hypertensive hemorrhage: a critical reappraisal. Acta Neuropathol. 2008;116(4):361–9.
37. Amano S. Vascular changes in the brain of spontaneously hypertensive rats: hyaline and fibri-noid degeneration. J Pathol. 1977;121(2):119–28.
38. Wiener J, Spiro D, Lattes RG. The cellular pathology of experimental hypertension. II. Arteriolar hyalinosis and fibrinoid change. Am J Pathol. 1965;47:457–85.
39. Lammie GA. Pathology of small vessel stroke. Br Med Bull. 2000;56:296–306.
40. Marti-Vilalta JLAA, Arborix A, Mohr JP. Microangiopathies (Lacunes). In: Mohr JP, Wolf PA, Grotta JC, Moskowitz MA, Mayberg MR, von Kummer R, editors. Stroke: pathophysiology, diagnosis, and management. 5th ed. Philadelphia: Elsevier; 2011. p. 485–515.
41. Hanaway J, Young RR. Localization of the pyramidal tract in the internal capsule of man. J Neurol Sci. 1977;34(1):63–70.
42. Gies J. The pathogenesis of hypertensive vascular disease. Dan Med Bull. 1967;14:259.
43. Fisher CM. Pathological observations in hypertensive cerebral hemorrhage. J Neuropathol Exp Neurol. 1971;30(3):536–50.
44. Fisher CM. Lacunar strokes and infarcts: a review. Neurology. 1982;32(8):871–6.
45. Bang OY, Heo JH, Kim JY, Park JH, Huh K. Middle cerebral artery stenosis is a major clinical determinant in striatocapsular small, deep infarction. Arch Neurol. 2002;59(2):259–63.
46. Okin PM, Wachtell K, Devereux RB, Harris KE, Jern S, Kjeldsen SE, et al. Regression of electrocardiographic left ventricular hypertrophy and decreased incidence of new-onset atrial fibrillation in patients with hypertension. JAMA. 2006;296(10):1242–8.
47. Lee DS, Austin PC, Rouleau JL, Liu PP, Naimark D, Tu JV. Predicting mortality among patients hospitalized for heart failure: derivation and validation of a clinical model. JAMA. 2003;290(19):2581–7.
48. Ingelsson E, Bjorklund-Bodegard K, Lind L, Arnlov J, Sundstrom J. Diurnal blood pressure pattern and risk of congestive heart failure. JAMA. 2006;295(24):2859–66.
49. Johansson BB. Hypertension mechanisms causing stroke. Clin Exp Pharmacol Physiol. 1999;26(7):563–5.
50. Wong KS, Caplan LR, Kim JS. Stroke mechanisms. In: Kim JS, Caplan LR, Wong KS, editors. Intracranial atherosclerosis. 1st ed. West Sussex: Wiley-Blackwell; 2008. p. 57–68.
51. Caplan LR, Hennerici M. Impaired clearance of emboli (washout) is an important link between hypoperfusion, embolism, and ischemic stroke. Arch Neurol. 1998;55(11):1475–82.
52. Caplan LR, Wong KS, Gao S, Hennerici MG. Is hypoperfusion an important cause of strokes? If so, how? Cerebrovasc Dis. 2006;21(3):145–53.

53. Nagai M, Kario K. Visit-to-visit blood pressure variability, silent cerebral injury, and risk of stroke. Am J Hypertens. 2013;26(12):1369–76.
54. Parati G, Liu X, Ochoa JE, Bilo G. Prognostic relevance of blood pressure variability: role of long-term and very long-term blood pressure changes. Hypertension. 2013;62(4):682–4.
55. Stolarz-Skrzypek K, Thijs L, Li Y, Hansen TW, Boggia J, Kuznetsova T, et al. Short-term blood pressure variability in relation to outcome in the International Database of Ambulatory blood pressure in relation to Cardiovascular Outcome (IDACO). Acta Cardiol. 2011;66(6):701–6.
56. Kannel WB, Dawber TR, Sorlie P, Wolf PA. Components of blood pressure and risk of athero-thrombotic brain infarction: the Framingham study. Stroke. 1976;7(4):327–31.
57. Mancia G, Bombelli M, Facchetti R, Madotto F, Corrao G, Trevano FQ, et al. Long-term prognostic value of blood pressure variability in the general population: results of the Pressioni Arteriose Monitorate e Loro Associazioni Study. Hypertension. 2007;49(6):1265–70.
58. Muntner P, Shimbo D, Diaz KM, Newman J, Sloan RP, Schwartz JE. Low correlation between visit-to-visit variability and 24-h variability of blood pressure. Hypertens Res. 2013;36(11):940–6.
59. Rothwell PM, Howard SC, Dolan E, et al. Prognostic significance of visit-to-visit variability, maximum systolic blood pressure, and episodic hypertension. Lancet. 2010;375(9718):895–905.
60. Ekbom T, Dahlöf B, Hansson L, Lindholm LH, Odén A, Scherstén B, et al. The stroke preventive effect in elderly hypertensives cannot fully be explained by the reduction in office blood pressure—insights from the Swedish Trial in Old Patients with Hypertension (STOP-Hypertension). Blood Press. 1992;1(3):168–72.
61. Hastie CE, Jeemon P, Coleman H, McCallum L, Patel R, Dawson J, et al. Long-term and ultra long-term blood pressure variability during follow-up and mortality in 14,522 patients with hypertension. Hypertension. 2013;62(4):698–705.
62. Diaz KM, Tanner RM, Falzon L, Levitan EB. Visit-to-visit variability of blood pressure and cardiovascular disease and all-cause mortality a systematic review and meta-analysis. Hypertension. 2014;64(5):965–82.
63. Ariesen MJ, Claus SP, Rinkel GJ, Algra A. Risk factors for intracerebral hemorrhage in the general population: a systematic review. Stroke. 2003;34(8):2060–5.
64. Broderick J, Brott T, Tomsick T, Leach A. Lobar hemorrhage in the elderly. The undiminishing importance of hypertension. Stroke. 1993;24(1):49–51.
65. Challa VR, Moody DM, Bell MA. The Charcot-Bouchard aneurysm controversy: impact of a new histologic technique. J Neuropathol Exp Neurol. 1992;51(3):264–71.
66. Takebayashi S, Kaneko M. Electron microscopic studies of ruptured arteries in hypertensive intracerebral hemorrhage. Stroke. 1983;14(1):28–36.
67. Bahemuka M. Primary intracerebral hemorrhage and heart weight: a clinicopathologic case-control review of 218 patients. Stroke. 1987;18(2):531–6.
68. Brott T, Thalinger K, Hertzberg V. Hypertension as a risk factor for spontaneous intracerebral hemorrhage. Stroke. 1986;17(6):1078–83.
69. Ogasawara K, Sakai N, Kuroiwa T, Hosoda K, Iihara K, Toyoda K, et al. Intracranial hemorrhage associated with cerebral hyperperfusion syndrome following carotid endarterectomy and carotid artery stenting: retrospective review of 4494 patients. J Neurosurg. 2007;107(6):1130–6.
70. Abou-Chebl A, Reginelli J, Bajzer CT, Yadav JS. Intensive treatment of hypertension decreases the risk of hyperperfusion and intracerebral hemorrhage following carotid artery stenting. Catheter Cardiovasc Interv. 2007;69(5):690–6.
71. Nolte KB, Brass LM, Fletterick CF. Intracranial hemorrhage associated with cocaine abuse: a prospective autopsy study. Neurology. 1996;46(5):1291–6.
72. McEvoy AW, Kitchen ND, Thomas DG. Intracerebral haemorrhage and drug abuse in young adults. Br J Neurosurg. 2000;14(5):449–54.
73. Manning L, Hirakawa Y, Arima H, Wang X, Chalmers J, Wang J, et al. Blood pressure variability and outcome after acute intracerebral haemorrhage: a post-hoc analysis of INTERACT2, a randomised controlled trial. Lancet Neurol. 2014;13(4):364–73.
74. Sekhar LN, Heros RC. Origin, growth, and rupture of saccular aneurysms: a review. Neurosurgery. 1981;8(2):248–60.
75. de Paepe A, van Landegem W, de Keyser F, de Reuck J. Association of multiple intracranial aneurysms and collagen type III deficiency. Clin Neurol Neurosurg. 1988;90(1):53–6.

76. van Gijn J, Rinkel GJ. Subarachnoid haemorrhage: diagnosis, causes and management. Brain. 2001;124(Pt 2):249–78.
77. Chyatte D, Reilly J, Tilson MD. Morphometric analysis of reticular and elastin fibers in the cerebral arteries of patients with intracranial aneurysms. Neurosurgery. 1990;26(6):939–43.
78. International Study of Unruptured Intracranial Aneurysms Investigators. Unruptured intracranial aneurysms—risk of rupture and risks of surgical intervention. International Study of Unruptured Intracranial Aneurysms Investigators. N Engl J Med. 1998;339(24):1725–33.
79. Vermeer SE, Hollander M, van Dijk EJ, Hofman A, Koudstaal PJ, Breteler MM, et al. Silent brain infarcts and white matter lesions increase stroke risk in the general population: the Rotterdam Scan Study. Stroke. 2003;34(5):1126–9.
80. de Leeuw FE, de Groot JC, Oudkerk M, Witteman JC, Hofman A, van Gijn J, et al. Hypertension and cerebral white matter lesions in a prospective cohort study. Brain. 2002;125(Pt 4):765–72.
81. Fu JH, Lu CZ, Hong Z, Dong Q, Luo Y, Wong KS. Extent of white matter lesions is related to acute subcortical infarcts and predicts further stroke risk in patients with first ever ischaemic stroke. J Neurol Neurosurg Psychiatr. 2005;76(6):793–6.
82. Fazekas F, Kleinert R, Offenbacher H, Schmidt R, Kleinert G, Payer F, et al. Pathologic correlates of incidental MRI white matter signal hyperintensities. Neurology. 1993;43(9):1683–9.
83. van Swieten JC, van den Hout JH, van Ketel BA, Hijdra A, Wokke JH, van Gijn J. Periventricular lesions in the white matter on magnetic resonance imaging in the elderly. A morphometric correlation with arteriolosclerosis and dilated perivascular spaces. Brain. 1991;114(Pt 2):761–74.
84. Vermeer SE, Koudstaal PJ, Oudkerk M, Hofman A, Breteler MM. Prevalence and risk factors of silent brain infarcts in the population-based Rotterdam Scan Study. Stroke. 2002;33(1):21–5.
85. Yamauchi H, Fukuda H, Oyanagi C. Significance of white matter high intensity lesions as a predictor of stroke from arteriolosclerosis. J Neurol Neurosurg Psychiatr. 2002;72(5):576–82.
86. Arvanitakis Z, Leurgans SE, Barnes LL, Bennett DA, Schneider JA. Microinfarct pathology, dementia, and cognitive systems. Stroke. 2011;42(3):722–7.
87. Smith EE, Schneider JA, Wardlaw JM, Greenberg SM. Cerebral microinfarcts: the invisible lesions. Lancet Neurol. 2012;11(3):272–82.
88. Longstreth Jr WT, Sonnen JA, Koepsell TD, Kukull WA, Larson EB, Montine TJ. Associations between microinfarcts and other macroscopic vascular findings on neuropathologic examination in 2 databases. Alzheimer Dis Assoc Disord. 2009;23(3):291–4.
89. Neuropathology Group Medical Research Council Cognitive Function and Aging Study. Pathological correlates of late-onset dementia in a multicentre, community-based population in England and Wales. Neuropathology Group of the Medical Research Council Cognitive Function and Ageing Study (MRC CFAS). Lancet. 2001;357(9251):169–75.
90. Fan YH, Mok VC, Lam WW, Hui AC, Wong KS. Cerebral microbleeds and white matter changes in patients hospitalized with lacunar infarcts. J Neurol. 2004;251(5):537–41.
91. Wong KS, Chan YL, Liu JY, Gao S, Lam WW. Asymptomatic microbleeds as a risk factor for aspirin-associated intracerebral hemorrhages. Neurology. 2003;60(3):511–3.
92. Greenberg SM, Eng JA, Ning M, Smith EE, Rosand J. Hemorrhage burden predicts recurrent intracerebral hemorrhage after lobar hemorrhage. Stroke. 2004;35(6):1415–20.
93. Kidwell CS, Saver JL, Villablanca JP, Duckwiler G, Fredieu A, Gough K, et al. Magnetic resonance imaging detection of microbleeds before thrombolysis: an emerging application. Stroke. 2002;33(1):95–8.
94. Kakuda W, Thijs VN, Lansberg MG, Bammer R, Wechsler L, Kemp S, et al. Clinical importance of microbleeds in patients receiving IV thrombolysis. Neurology. 2005;65(8):1175–8.
95. Roob G, Lechner A, Schmidt R, Flooh E, Hartung HP, Fazekas F. Frequency and location of microbleeds in patients with primary intracerebral hemorrhage. Stroke. 2000;31(11):2665–9.
96. Kinoshita T, Okudera T, Tamura H, Ogawa T, Hatazawa J. Assessment of lacunar hemorrhage associated with hypertensive stroke by echo-planar gradient-echo T2*-weighted MRI. Stroke. 2000;31(7):1646–50.

Part III
Management of Blood Pressure for First Stroke Prevention, Immediately After Acute Stroke, and for Recurrent Stroke Prevention

Chapter 7
Cardiovascular Risk Assessment, Summary of Guidelines for the Management of Hypertension and a Critical Appraisal of the 2014 Expert Panel of the National Institutes of Health Report

Luke J. Laffin and George L. Bakris

Hypertension is one of the most prevalent health problems worldwide and the third largest cause of the global burden of disease [1]. While the prevalence of hypertension in developed countries is expected to increase by 24 %, it is projected that there will be an 80 % increase in developing nations [2]. Worldwide, 54 % of ischemic heart disease and 47 % of strokes are attributable to high blood pressure [3]. The rise in hypertension prevalence is attributed to several factors, including the overall aging of the population, a dramatic increase in obesity, and a decrease in physical activity. Untreated hypertension is associated with significant cardiovascular (CV) morbidity and mortality. It is an independent risk factor for the development of all of the clinical manifestations of cardiovascular disease (CVD), including coronary artery disease (CAD), peripheral artery disease (PAD), congestive heart failure (CHF), and stroke. In the United States, 69 % of patients who experience their first myocardial infarction (MI), 77 % with their first stroke, and 74 % with CHF have a blood pressure >140/90 mmHg [4].

It is estimated that 1/3 of individuals greater than 20 years of age has hypertension in the United States, and this number is projected to be 41 % by 2030 [4]. There is significant variation in its prevalence based on age, sex, and ethnicity. Data from the National Health and Nutrition Examination Survey (NHANES) 2011–2012 demonstrate a stepwise increase in hypertension with advancing age [5]. Among men and women ages 45–59 approximately 32 % have hypertension, compared to 65 % of individuals ages >60 years of age. From ages 20 to 64 the prevalence among men, compared to women, is higher; beyond age 65 significantly more women have hypertension than men.

L.J. Laffin, M.D. (✉) • G.L. Bakris, M.D. (✉)
ASH Comprehensive Hypertension Center, University of Chicago Medical Center, Chicago, IL, USA
e-mail: luke.laffin@uchospitals.com; gbakris@gmail.com

© Springer International Publishing Switzerland 2016
V. Aiyagari, P.B. Gorelick (eds.), *Hypertension and Stroke*, Clinical Hypertension and Vascular Diseases, DOI 10.1007/978-3-319-29152-9_7

The prevalence of hypertension in black men and women in the United States is among the highest in the world (45 % for men and 46 % for women.) This is compared to non-Hispanic white men and women with a prevalence of 33 % and 30 %, respectively, and a 30 % prevalence among Hispanic males and females [4]. Despite the considerable health consequences, the majority of people with hypertension are still not at recommended guideline goals. The data from NHANES 2009–2012 demonstrate that while 83 % of individuals with hypertension were aware of their condition, and 77 % were undergoing treatment, only 54 % had their blood pressure controlled to <140/90 mmHg. This is an improvement from 45 % in 2005–2006 [6]. Similar reports from other countries reveal a poor record of BP control, regardless of the populations studied, the accessibility to/cost of medical care, or the treatment settings [2].

In the majority of patients, the risk attributed to hypertension is driven primarily by the systolic blood pressure (SBP). As age increases both SBP and diastolic blood pressure (DBP) rise in parallel. However, after the age of 50 the DBP tends to fall or plateau, while the systolic pressure continues to increase. Consequently, SBP is the major determinant of events, particularly in patients over the age of 50 [7, 8].

The importance of pulse pressure—the difference between systolic and diastolic pressures—is controversial in predicting future events. Initial studies suggested that pulse pressure was a powerful predictor [9]. More recent analyses suggest that the significance of the pulse pressure is lessened after adjusting for the systolic pressure [10–12].

Hypertension and Cardiovascular Disease

Hypertension is a predictor of CV events in a continuous and graded manner. A meta-analysis of 61 prospective studies, including one million adults, illustrated that for each 20/10 mmHg increase in BP starting from 115/75 mmHg, the CV risk is doubled [12]. Data from the Framingham Heart Study also indicate that, compared with individuals who have normal blood pressure, the relative risk of a CV event increases as the blood pressure rises, within each age group [3]. By age 50, the overall lifetime risk of a CV event for a man with stage 1 or 2 hypertension is 62–65 %, compared to 47 % for men with normal blood pressure. The risk is 52 vs. 29 % for women [13]. For hypertensive men and women at age 50, this results in a life expectancy that is 5 years shorter than normotensive patients [14].

Studies with more than 3 years of follow-up demonstrate an independent effect of hypertension on the development of cardiovascular events in younger people as well. In a prospective study of more than 11,000 men ages 18–39 with a baseline SBP >160 mmHg, the risk of coronary heart disease increased two- to fourfold over 25 years [15]. If an individual develops left ventricular hypertrophy, his or her risk of future cardiovascular events, particularly the development of heart failure, increases even further. This accentuates the importance of recognizing and controlling hypertension early in at-risk patients.

Epidemiologic data suggest that even patients with mildly elevated blood pressure experience an increase in cardiovascular mortality. In more recent follow-up of the above cohort of men, now ages 18–49, the relative risk of CAD mortality, stroke mortality, and overall CVD mortality was increased among all hypertension subgroups. This includes men with combined systolic and diastolic hypertension, isolated systolic or diastolic hypertension, and, interestingly, men with what is termed "high-normal" BP (SBP of 130–139 mmHg or DBP 85–89) [16]. This corroborates prior work demonstrating that both men and women with high-normal BP have been shown to have more than a 50 % higher risk of cardiovascular events over 10 years than patients with normal blood pressure [17].

In the majority of patients with hypertension, their diagnosis does not occur in isolation, but rather is found in association with other CV risk factors. Investigation of risk factor clustering demonstrates that fewer than 20 % of individuals have hypertension in the absence of additional risk factors. Specifically, more than half of patients have one or two additional risk factors [18]. Unsurprisingly, the risk of CV events increases as the number of risk factors increases, even at the same level of BP [19].

Traditional CV risk factors for CAD include DM, hypertension, family history (CVD before the age of 55 in men and 65 in women), tobacco use, and age (>55 for men and >65 for women). One of the more widely used techniques to evaluate the risk of hypertension in the context of additional risk factors is the Framingham General CV risk Score (FRS). It was initially published in 1998 and updated most recently in 2008. It provides estimates of the 10-year risk of a coronary event based on a person's total cholesterol (C), HDL-C, hypertension, DM, tobacco use, and age [20].

More recently the American College of Cardiology (ACC) and the American Heart Association (AHA) jointly released an updated CV risk calculator. This model includes similar parameters to the FRS, but now includes larger numbers of African-American patients (in addition to Caucasian), includes only hard CV endpoints including fatal and nonfatal myocardial infarction and stroke, and does not include family history as a parameter [21]. This risk calculator has not been universally adopted due to concerns that it may overestimate overall CV risk [22].

Another important collection of CV risk factors, of which hypertension is one, is the metabolic syndrome. It is not truly a syndrome, but rather a compilation of risk factors combined to denote substantial increase in risk of CVD. The National Cholesterol Education Program (NCEP) Adult Treatment Panel III (ATP III) defines the metabolic syndrome as the presence of three or more of the following: (a) blood pressure elevation ($\geq$130/85 mmHg), (b) impaired fasting glucose (>100 mg/dL or drug treatment for elevated glucose), (c) increased waist circumference (>102 cm for men and 88 cm for women), (d) low HDL-C (<40 mg/dL), and (e) hypertriglyceridemia (>150 mg/dL or drug treatment for elevated triglycerides) [23]. Data from the Framingham Offspring Study demonstrated that of patients who did not have metabolic syndrome, 10 % had elevated blood pressure, compared to 32 % of the people with metabolic syndrome [24]. Subjects were followed over 8 years for the development of CV events and the development of DM. The presence of metabolic syndrome conferred a relative risk of 4–6 and 24–30 for the development of CV events and DM, respectively.

Table 7.1 Cardiovascular
risk factors

Hypertension
Diabetes mellitus
Tobacco use
Age (>55 years for men, >65 years for women)
Family history of premature cardiovascular disease (<55 years for men, <65 years for women)
CKD
Obesity
Dyslipidemia
Physical inactivity
Target organ damage
Heart
Left ventricular hypertrophy
Angina pectoris or myocardial infarction
Coronary revascularization
Heart failure
Brain
Stroke or transient ischemic attack
Chronic kidney disease
Peripheral arterial disease
Retinopathy

Much of the increased risk associated with metabolic syndrome occurs from obesity, particularly visceral adiposity. Obesity is one of the most common causes of hypertension, the prevalence of which is rising at an alarming rate. It is now estimated that 69 % of the United States population is either overweight or obese, with the latter defined as a body mass index (BMI) >30 kg/m^2 [4]. Obesity leads to several physiologic changes, including hyperinsulinemia and insulin resistance, endothelial dysfunction, increased activation of the sympathetic nervous system, sodium retention, and increased oxidative stress. Obesity is one of the major cardiovascular risk factors highlighted in Table 7.1. Population studies indicate that being obese promotes a clustering of risk factors and greatly influences their impact. Patients who are obese are more than twice as likely as lean patients to have more than three CV risk factors, a 40–60 % increased risk of a cardiac event, and up to a 100 % increase in cardiovascular death [25–27]. Data from the CRUSADE registry of national outcomes in the setting of a non-ST elevation myocardial infarction (NSTEMI) showed that among obese patients, the mean age of a first NSTEMI was 3–12 years younger than lean patients, depending on the degree of obesity [28]. Given that high BMI went from tenth to sixth in the ranking of global burden of disease between 1990 and 2010, the cardiovascular impact of obesity cannot be ignored [29].

Concurrent with the rise in obesity, hypertension, and DM is an increased risk of sequelae from these conditions, including chronic kidney disease (CKD) [30]. CKD, defined as an estimated glomerular filtration rate (eGFR) <60 mL/min, is known to be an independent risk factor for incident CVD events including all-cause mortality [31–33].

Hypertension and DM are the most common causes of CKD and patients with CKD are more likely to die of CV causes than to develop renal failure [34]. A reduced eGFR poses an increased cardiovascular risk, in part because it represents a higher prevalence of associated risk factors, such as uncontrolled hypertension and dyslipidemia. Several large studies have shown that patients with a reduced eGFR have higher blood pressure and total cholesterol, lower HDL-C, and are more likely to have ischemic heart disease, left ventricular hypertrophy, diabetes, and heart failure [35–37]. As a result, it has been postulated that reduced eGFR may be a marker for more severe vascular disease [38] and multiple cohorts demonstrate an association between reduced eGFR and risk of CVD [39]. Reduced kidney function is also associated with several abnormalities, including increased levels of inflammatory markers, enhanced coagulability, increased arterial stiffness, and endothelial dysfunction, all of which may contribute to its role in cardiovascular morbidity and mortality.

An example illustrating CKD and increased risk of CVD is provided in data from the Kaiser Permanente Renal Registry of more than one million adults. It demonstrates a graded, independent association between eGFR and CV events. Patients with an eGFR of 40–59 mL/min experienced a 40 % increase in events compared to those with normal renal function. Furthermore, there was a 100 % increase for an eGFR of 30–44 mL/min and a 340 % increase for an eGFR of less than 15 mL/min [39]. In the Valsartan in Acute Myocardial Infarction Trial (VALIANT)—a study in which patients who had a myocardial infarction complicated by heart failure were randomized to valsartan, captopril, or both—each reduction in the eGFR by 10 mL/min, starting at 80 mL/min, was associated with a hazard ratio for death and nonfatal cardiovascular events of 1.10 [40]. More specifically, high albuminuria (formerly microalbuminuria) is more often found in patients with DM and is an early marker of abnormal vascular responsiveness. As with a reduced eGFR, high albuminuria is associated with generalized endothelial dysfunction, vascular permeability, increased inflammatory markers, and abnormalities in the coagulation system (Fig. 7.1) [39]. High albuminuria is an inflammatory marker itself associated with increased CV risk and does not indicate presence of CKD. Only increases in high albuminuria to levels above 300 mg/day indicate CKD development [41] As part of the National Kidney Foundation's Kidney Early Evaluation Program (KEEP), a community-based screening program for CKD, patients with normal renal function were compared to those with a combination of moderately increased albuminuria, reduced eGFR, and anemia. The latter group had the lowest survival—93 % over 30 months vs. 98 % in the patients without kidney disease [34].

The relationship between hypertension and CVD has several important implications from diagnostic and therapeutic perspectives. First, a diagnosis of hypertension should always prompt an investigation for other CV risk factors noted in Table 7.1. Second, the presence of certain comorbidities may influence what is considered an appropriate treatment regimen, which will be discussed below. Third, previously patients with several additional risk factors had different treatment goals compared to a patient with isolated hypertension; current guidelines have moved away from different goals, but consensus for these goals is not universal.

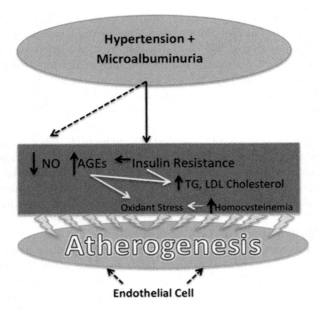

Fig. 7.1 Interaction of microalbuminuria with other factors that affect atherosclerosis development. *NO* nitric oxide, *AGEs* advanced glycation end products, *TC* triglycerides, *LDL* low density lipoproteins

Guidelines for the Management of Hypertension

The association between hypertension and other CVD risk factors, such as DM, dyslipidemia, CKD, and obesity, is the underpinning of recommendations by all national and international blood pressure guidelines written by the 2014 Expert Panel of the National Institutes of Health [42], the European Society of Hypertension–European Society of Cardiology (ESH–ESC) [43], the American and International Societies of Hypertension (ASH/ISH) [44], and the British National Institute of Clinical Excellence (NICE) guidelines [45].

The classification of hypertension was adjusted in the 2014 Expert Panel of the National Institutes of Health from the prior JNC 7 report [46]. The most significant change was increasing the target BP goals in adults of less than 60 years of age to <140/90 mmHg and for adults greater than 60 years of age to <150/90 mmHg. The other significant change was aligning the BP goals in patients with CKD or DM to those patients with only primary hypertension to <140/90 mmHg. These updated strategies for the classification and the goal treatment of hypertension in adults are shown in Table 7.2.

Pharmacotherapy of hypertension is initiated only after initial evaluation of the patient is completed, and the diagnosis of hypertension is confirmed. Additionally, if hypertension is uncomplicated, the patient must fail a trial of lifestyle modification in the presence of blood pressure elevation between 140–159 mmHg SBP and 90–100 DBP. Patients presenting with blood pressure greater than 160/100 mmHg

Table 7.2 Goal blood pressure by Guideline Committees (all expressed in mmHg)

	Year of publication	<60 yo no additional risk factors	60–79 yo no additional risk factors	>80 yo no additional risk factors	DM (any age)	CKD (any age)
014 Expert Panel (JNC 8) [38]	2014	<140/90	**<150/90**[a]	<150/90	<140/90	<140/90
ESH-ESC [39]	2013	<140/90	<140/90	<150/90	<140/90	<140/90
ISH/ASH [40]	2014	<140/90	<140/90	<150/90	<140/90	<140/90
BHS/NICE [41]	2011	<140/90	<140/90	<150/90	<140/90	<140/90

DM diabetes mellitus, *CKD* chronic kidney disease, *YO* years old
[a]If treatment leads to a blood pressure <140/<90 and is well tolerated, then treatment does not need to be adjusted

should be started on medications initially. It is important to note that lifestyle changes *must* accompany all pharmacotherapy.

Several BP measurements performed according to accepted procedural guidelines are necessary for the diagnosis of hypertension. The initial assessment should include focused medical history, particularly personal and family history of hypertension and antihypertensive medication use. Additionally, the presence of risk factors for CVD or overt CVD/target organ damage is evaluated by clinical history, physical examination as well as limited laboratory evaluation. Secondary forms of hypertension need to be excluded, with special attention to rule out commonly acquired causes of BP elevation such as sleep disorders, including, but not limited to, sleep apnea, and drug-induced hypertension. More recently in a draft statement, the United States Preventive Task Force (USPTF) recommends that 24-h ambulatory blood pressure monitoring (ABPM) be performed to confirm high blood pressure before the diagnosis of hypertension. This has not yet been formally published by the USPTF, but will likely follow the lead of 2011 published NICE guidelines that contained a similar recommendation [47]. Of note, ABPM is a better predict of mortality than office/clinic BP measurement [48].

Guideline Treatment Goals

Current guidelines highlight that a patient's overall cardiovascular risk is the basis for deciding treatment goals and when to initiate pharmacotherapy. However, there are differences among guideline writing groups with respect to which patient groups warrant more aggressive treatment goals.

For patients less than 60 years of age, the 2014 Expert Panel of the National Institutes of Health recommends starting pharmacotherapy if lifestyle intervention fails for stage 1 hypertension, with a goal blood pressure of <140/90 mmHg, but <150/90 mmHg for patients greater than 60 years of age. Aside from the more lenient BP goals in older individuals, the most significant change in current BP guidelines presented by this panel is the elimination of lower BP targets in patients with DM or CKD. Previously both patient populations had a treatment goal of ≤130/80 mmHg; however, given the paucity of evidence for these lower targets, recommendations were revised. They now align with goals in patients less than 60 years of age and are <140/90 mmHg [42].

Consensus from the AHA, ACC, and ASH is seen in recently released guidelines for individuals with CAD [49]. This updates recommendations made in 2007 by the AHA, which noted lower goals in patients with established CAD. Current recommendations again suggest that most patients with CAD should target a BP of <140/90 mmHg, but with the caveat that it may be appropriate to attempt to reach a level of 130/80 mmHg in patients with multiple CAD risk equivalents (peripheral artery disease, carotid artery disease, abdominal aortic aneurysm), or prior TIA, stroke, or MI. There are many modifiable risk factors for stroke prevention and one of the most important is BP control [50]. The most recent updated stroke guidelines review all risk factors in detail and highlight the following about BP: The committee is in agreement with the JNC 7 report, that regular BP screening and appropriate treatment, including both lifestyle modification and pharmacological therapy, are recommended. Systolic BP should be treated to a goal of <140/90 mmHg because these levels are associated with a lower risk of stroke and cardiovascular events [50]. For patients who have had a stroke, the updated guidelines report that initiation of BP lowering therapy is indicated, if previously untreated with ischemic stroke or TIA who, after the first several days, has an established BP ≥140/90 mmHg. If BP is <140/90 mmHg BP therapy is not indicated as the benefit is uncertain. Resumption of BP lowering therapy is indicated for previously treated patients with known hypertension for both prevention of recurrent stroke and prevention of other vascular events in those who have had an ischemic stroke or TIA and are beyond the first several days. In general, the goal BP to achieve with BP lowering therapy is <140/90 mmHg, however, for those with a recent lacunar stroke, it might be reasonable to target a systolic BP of <130 mmHg [51]

Historically, there has been concern that a significant lowering of blood pressure, especially DBP, could be harmful—the so-called J-curve hypothesis. One possible reason why a lower DBP could cause harm is that coronary perfusion occurs primarily during diastole. A significantly reduced diastolic pressure may, therefore, result in myocardial ischemia. Recent data suggest that in the older people, i.e., >65 years of age, those with diabetes, and those with CAD, the reduction of DBP <60 mmHg is associated with increased CVD risk [52, 53]. This was accounted for in the recent CAD and HTN guidelines and keeping DBP >60 mmHg is a Class IIA, Level of evidence C recommendation in these most recent CAD and hypertension guidelines. Note that low diastolic pressures below 60 mmHg are also associated with a higher risk for ESRD and mortality in CKD patients [54].

Overall, the preponderance of prospective randomized clinical trial data supports that BPs <140/90 mmHg reduces cardiovascular events. Levels below that threshold do not clearly improve overall cardiovascular outcomes and this drove the significant guidelines changes. The prior lower blood pressure goal recommendations or targets were not based on data from randomized prospective trials since few studies actually attained a mean BP of <130/80 mmHg (Fig. 7.2). Among ten major trials,

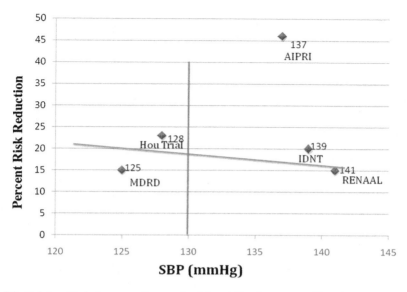

Fig. 7.2 Relationship between cardiovascular risk and blood pressure achieved

the mean SBP ranged from 132 to 151 mmHg [55–64] (Fig. 7.2). As a result, much of the data to previously support the goal of <130/80 mmHg came from epidemiologic studies and post hoc analyses of randomized clinical trials.

In patients with diabetes, the Action to Control Cardiovascular Risk in Diabetes blood pressure trial (ACCORD) was designed to answer the question of whether a lower level of blood pressure is needed to reduce cardiovascular risk [65]. Its findings were a clear driver of the more lenient BP goals in a high-risk patient population. Published in 2010, this randomized study of 4733 subjects with type 2 DM and baseline BP of 139/76 mmHg, targeted SBP of <120 mmHg in the intensive control group and <140 mmHg in the standard therapy group. The primary end-point was a composite of nonfatal MI, nonfatal stroke, or death from cardiovascular causes with mean follow-up of 4.7 years. Both groups achieved the desired BP (119 and 133 mmHg, respectively). There was no significant difference in the annual rate of the primary end-point and no difference in all-cause mortality. The lower BP goal was associated with significant reductions in total and nonfatal strokes, however significantly more serious events occurred in the intensive therapy group.

A more recent meta-analysis [66] of 40 trials (including more than 100,000 participants) demonstrated similar findings to ACCORD, i.e., the vast majority of adverse cardiovascular outcomes were not significantly different when comparing an achieved BP of 130 and 140 mmHg. However, the incidence of stroke was significantly different in patients with a goal of <130 mmHg. This clearly begs the question of what to make of the attenuated stroke risk at lower BPs as seen in ACCORD.

This is not a new finding, it is also seen in ADVANCE [67], INVEST [68], and the Ongoing Telmisartan Alone and in Combination with Ramipril Global Endpoint Trial (ONTARGET) [67]. INVEST and ONTARGET were both large international clinical trials of blood pressure lowering therapies of greater than 20,000 patients, with diabetes comprising 37% and 28% of the study subjects, respectively. Moreover, 100% of the INVEST cohort had documented CAD. Both demonstrated a systolic below 130 mmHg is associated with stroke reduction but no other CV risk benefit below that level of BP. This was also observed in the ACCOMPLISH trial of over 11,000 mostly older people, mean age of 68 year and over 65% with diabetes [69]. In ACCORD it is important to take note that the risk of serious adverse events (defined as hypotension, syncope, arrhythmia, hyperkalemia, angioedema, and renal failure) was associated with more aggressive BP control (3.3% intensive vs. 1.3% in the standard arm.). When coupled with the small absolute benefit in stroke reduction (1 in 89 patients at 5 years) the finding did not compel recent guidelines to recommend a lower BP goal. However, the new systematic analysis [66] supports that is reasonable in younger patients with prior ischemic stroke or early microvascular complications to consider a SBP of <130 mmHg if lower BPs are well tolerated with minimal side effects. Figure 7.3 provides a management algorithm for hypertension in diabetics.

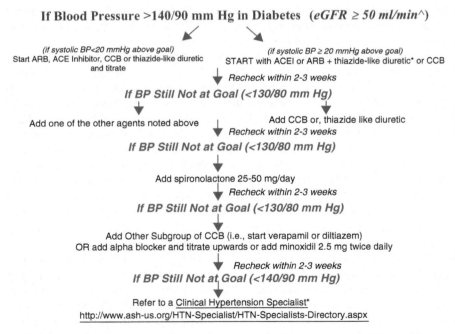

Fig. 7.3 Management algorithm for hypertension in diabetics. *Asterisk* Chlorthalidone or indapamide; # represents a physician who qualified and passed the hypertension certification examination

For kidney disease outcomes, all trials that randomized to different blood pressure levels failed to show an additional risk reduction of the lower blood pressure goal in relation to slowing the progression of kidney disease [70]. In patients with CKD, the most recent 2014 guidelines and position statements recommend starting with an inhibitor of the renin-angiotensin system. Prior guidelines have suggested that the second medication added for BP control should be a calcium channel blocker (CCB), based on outcomes of the Avoiding Cardiovascular Events through Combination Therapy in Patients Living with Systolic Hypertension (ACCOMPLISH) trial [71], however more recent data suggests addition of a diuretic or CCB as a second agent is appropriate. An exception is advanced proteinuric kidney disease, i.e., eGFR <40 mL/min with >1 g/day proteinuria [72].

Pharmacological Therapy

Multiple relatively recent trials have compared the traditional diuretic- or beta-blocker-based treatment strategies to those based on ACE inhibitors (ACEI), CCB, or angiotensin receptor blockers (ARB). In general, all major groups of antihypertensive agents have similar capacity to lower BP. A meta-analysis of 29 clinical trials that encompass 162,341 participants by the Blood Pressure Lowering Treatment Trialist's Collaboration group supports the concept that all agents that lower BP will reduce CVD risk [73]. However, some differences in the specific outcomes such as strokes (favoring diuretics and CCBs) and coronary events (favoring ACEIs and beta-blockers) exist between certain groups (Fig. 7.4). One must keep in mind that most of the trials included in the meta-analysis were secondary prevention studies.

Regardless of the choice of medication, most patients (>70 %) will eventually require more than one medication to achieve adequate BP control. For those who are greater than 20/10 mmHg above their treatment goal, i.e., stage 2 hypertension, all major guidelines recommend initiating two-drug therapy.

Diuretic therapy, in the form of thiazide diuretics, is no longer the main first-line agent for uncomplicated primary hypertension, as it was in JNC 7. Guidelines now suggest decreasing the blood pressure to <140/90 mmHg using either CCB, blockers of the renin–angiotensin system, or diuretics. Beta-blockers are not first-line therapy in most patients according to the 2014 Expert Panel of the National Institutes of Health and other recent guidelines. Although beta-blockers are well-established therapy for patients who also have ischemic heart disease, heart failure, and arrhythmias, recent data suggest that they play a more limited role in other patients. For example, in the LIFE study the ARB losartan was more effective than the beta-blocker atenolol in CV protection (particularly stroke) in hypertensive patients with electrocardiographic left ventricular hypertrophy [59]. Furthermore, in the ASCOT study hypertensive subjects randomized to amlodipine (and if needed perindopril) had fewer CV events than those randomized to atenolol (and if needed bendrofluazide), although the difference in CV protection in the ASCOT study is largely attributed

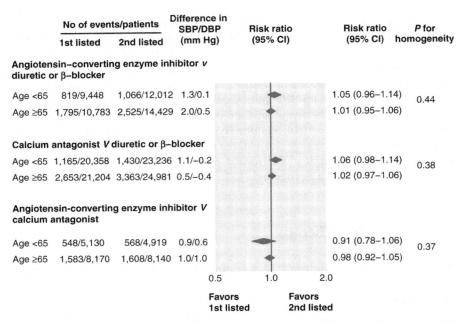

Fig. 7.4 Blood pressure-lowering regimens based on different drug classes for the outcome total major cardiovascular events and age groups <65 vs. ≥65. Negative blood pressure values indicate lower mean follow-up blood pressure in first-listed than in second-listed groups. (From Blood Pressure Lowering Treatment Trialists C, Turnbull F, Neal B, Ninomiya T, Algert C, Arima H, et al. Effects of different regimens to lower blood pressure on major cardiovascular events in older and younger adults: meta-analysis of randomised trials. BMJ. 2008;336(7653):1121, with permission)

to the greater BP reduction in the amlodipine group [60]. A meta-analysis of outcome studies of beta-blocker-based therapy (almost exclusively atenolol) in hypertension demonstrates limited stroke protection compared to that achieved by other drugs [74].

Because of these data and consistent evidence showing increased risk of new onset diabetes with beta-blockers, particularly when combined with diuretics [59, 60, 75–78], beta-blockers should not be first-line therapy in the majority of patients. The impact of various agents on glycemic control has also gained increasing attention. Multiple trials demonstrate that beta-blockers (primarily atenolol) and thiazide diuretics lead to both a worsening of glycemic control among diabetic patients and an increased incidence of new-onset diabetes with impaired fasting glucose [76, 77, 79–81]. However, retrospective analysis of outcome trials does not support the assertion that increases in diabetes translate into a higher CV event rate [81, 82]. This may relate to improvement in blood pressure, providing relatively greater CVD risk reduction trumping the risk associated with metabolic derangement. In addition, the risk of diabetes is not decreased when a thiazide is combined with an ACEI or ARB in obese patients with impaired fasting glucose [78]. Given that the primary determinant of CV risk reduction is the lowering of blood pressure and not the class of medication [73], one would ideally use medicines that do not worsen preexisting metabolic conditions. Exceptions to this rule are newer beta-blockers such as carvedilol, which also has alpha-adrenergic blocking properties, and nebivolol, which vasodilates by potentiating nitric oxide. Both agents have a neutral effect on glycemic control and enhance insulin sensitivity [83, 84].

With respect to two-drug therapy, newer data from outcome trials, such as the ACCOMPLISH, support earlier use of calcium antagonists in concert with RAS blockers. In the ACCOMPLISH trial, patients who were at high risk for CV events were randomized to benazepril plus amlodipine or hydrochlorothiazide (HCTZ) [71]. Despite comparable BPs (131.6/73.3 with amlodipine vs. 132.5/74.4 with HCTZ), the patients randomized to amlodipine experienced a 19.6 % reduction in CV events. Moreover, these similar levels of BP were borne out in a sub-study using ABPM in over 800 of the 11,506 participants. This cohort demonstrated slightly lower blood pressure in the diuretic combination group, with a CVD benefit still observed in the CCB-based therapy group. ACCOMPLISH highlights the benefit of fixed combination medicines for effective blood pressure management and risk reduction, and suggests that amlodipine should be considered as a first-line agent.

A second study examining fixed combination medications at a much earlier state of diabetes is the ADVANCE trial, which added perindopril/indapamide vs. placebo to patients with diabetes and a usual regimen, regardless of baseline blood pressure [85]. Those patients randomized to perindopril/indapamide experienced an 18 % reduction in death from cardiovascular cause, regardless of initial blood pressure.

The ONTARGET study addressed use of two renin–angiotensin system blockers [67]. Patients at high risk for CV events were randomized to either telmisartan, ramipril, or both. Telmisartan was found to be noninferior to ramipril in the prevention of CV events and has an FDA indication to be the ARB of choice in ACE inhibitor intolerant patients. Despite a superior decrease in blood pressure, the combination of both an ACEI and an ARB increased the risk of renal complications and hypotension, without any benefit in CVD outcome. Although there is data to suggest that the combination of an ACEI/ARB may be more effective in reducing death or hospitalization in patients with heart failure [86], ONTARGET suggests that there is no indication for this combination in patients with preserved ventricular function.

Consensus or Confusion?

The recent release of guidelines from various writing groups clarifies certain aspects of hypertension management among clinicians, but also confuses others. The most significant clarification is the elimination of lower BP goals in patients with CKD and DM. Prior recommendations were based on a low level of evidence and recent trials influenced this change. The most important trials contributing evidence to address this question are discussed earlier and include ACCORD trial for patients with DM. Also, encouraging was the consensus reached by the AHA, ACC, and ASH with respect to the same BP treatment goals in patients with CAD [49].

The streamlining or alignment of BP treatment goals to less than 140/90 mmHg clearly makes application easier for clinicians in a primary care setting, especially given the increasing complexity of patients with multiple comorbid conditions and the changing reimbursement structure directed toward performance-based incentives. Yet, the general application of this BP goal to patients with hypertension that are between 60 and 80 years of age, with none of the above comorbidities, remains unclear.

By far the most controversial inclusion from the 2014 Expert Panel of the National Institutes of Health is new BP goal leniency in patients greater than 60 years of age (<150/90 mmHg) without DM or CKD. In fact, it was so controversial that, within a month after guideline publication, a subset of the Expert Panel authors wrote a widely read article objecting to this BP leniency and recommending a goal of <140/90 mmHg in persons 60–80 years of age [87]. The rationale behind the "majority opinion" of the 2014 Expert Panel was a lack of definitive randomized control trial evidence to determine the optimal SBP. However, the "minority opinion" authors suggest that, although there is no definitive evidence in the form of RCTs differing between 140 and 150 mmHg in patients between 60 and 80 years of age, that the burden of evidence for increasing a BP target should be at least as strong as the evidence required to decrease recommended targets. Concurrently, their statement echoed the above sentiment that similar targets amongst the majority of patients would simplify implementation for clinicians. Guidelines from other major societies such as ASH/ISH and ESC agree with the "minority opinion" authors and recommend more stringent BP control in all patients between the ages of 60 and 80 years of age.

There is general consensus among guideline writing groups that more lenient goals are applicable in patients greater than 80 years of age. Driving this recommendation is the Hypertension in the Very Elderly Trial (HYVET), which addressed BP management in a vastly underrepresented group in clinical trials [88]. Older patients have the highest prevalence of hypertension and experience a large proportion of CV events secondary to hypertension. However, patients older than 80 years are underrepresented in clinical trials, and as such the benefits of treatment were unclear. In HYVET, patients over 80 years were randomized to indapamide, plus perindopril if needed, or placebo, for a SBP goal of 150 mmHg. Active treatment was associated with a 30 % reduction in stroke, 21 % reduction in death from any cause, and a 23 % reduction in death from cardiovascular cause. HYVET suggests that older patients do gain significant benefit from treatment of their hypertension, albeit with slightly less aggressive treatment goals (target BP 150/80 mmHg).

As a final note, guidelines are not meant to be the "holy grail" of management but merely an intellectual attempt at critical review of data from clinical trials. Their goal is to provide recommendations that can help clinicians understand how to properly apply the available data to individual patients.

References

1. Mensah GA, Bakris G. The United Nations high level meeting addresses noncommunicable diseases, but where is hypertension? J Clin Hypertens (Greenwich). 2011;13(11):787–90.
2. Mosley II WJ, Greenland P, Garside DB, Lloyd-Jones DM. Predictive utility of pulse pressure and other blood pressure measures for cardiovascular outcomes. Hypertension. 2007;49(6):1256–64.
3. Lawes CM, Vander Hoorn S, Rodgers A, International Society of Hypertension. Global burden of blood-pressure-related disease, 2001. Lancet. 2008;371(9623):1513–8.
4. Mozaffarian D, Benjamin EJ, Go AS, Arnett DK, Blaha MJ, Cushman M, et al. Heart disease and stroke statistics—2015 update: a report from the American Heart Association. Circulation. 2015;131(4):e29–322.
5. Nwankwo T, Yoon SS, Burt V, Gu Q. Hypertension among adults in the United States: National Health and Nutrition Examination Survey, 2011-2012. NCHS Data Brief. 2013;(133):1–8.
6. Lloyd-Jones D, Adams R, Carnethon M, De Simone G, Ferguson TB, Flegal K, et al. Heart disease and stroke statistics—2009 update: a report from the American Heart Association Statistics Committee and Stroke Statistics Subcommittee. Circulation. 2009;119(3):e21–181.
7. Rutan GH, Kuller LH, Neaton JD, Wentworth DN, McDonald RH, Smith WM. Mortality associated with diastolic hypertension and isolated systolic hypertension among men screened for the Multiple Risk Factor Intervention Trial. Circulation. 1988;77(3):504–14.
8. Kannel WB. Cardiovascular hazards of components of blood pressure. J Hypertens. 2002;20(3):395–7.
9. Franklin SS, Khan SA, Wong ND, Larson MG, Levy D. Is pulse pressure useful in predicting risk for coronary heart Disease? The Framingham heart study. Circulation. 1999;100(4):354–60.
10. Franklin SS, Larson MG, Khan SA, Wong ND, Leip EP, Kannel WB, et al. Does the relation of blood pressure to coronary heart disease risk change with aging? The Framingham Heart Study. Circulation. 2001;103(9):1245–9.
11. Antikainen RL, Jousilahti P, Vanhanen H, Tuomilehto J. Excess mortality associated with increased pulse pressure among middle-aged men and women is explained by high systolic blood pressure. J Hypertens. 2000;18(4):417–23.
12. Lewington S, Clarke R, Qizilbash N, Peto R, Collins R, Prospective Studies Collaboration. Age-specific relevance of usual blood pressure to vascular mortality: a meta-analysis of individual data for one million adults in 61 prospective studies. Lancet. 2002;360(9349):1903–13.
13. Lloyd-Jones DM, Leip EP, Larson MG, D'Agostino RB, Beiser A, Wilson PW, et al. Prediction of lifetime risk for cardiovascular disease by risk factor burden at 50 years of age. Circulation. 2006;113(6):791–8.
14. Franco OH, Peeters A, Bonneux L, de Laet C. Blood pressure in adulthood and life expectancy with cardiovascular disease in men and women: life course analysis. Hypertension. 2005;46(2):280–6.
15. Miura K, Daviglus ML, Dyer AR, Liu K, Garside DB, Stamler J, et al. Relationship of blood pressure to 25-year mortality due to coronary heart disease, cardiovascular diseases, and all causes in young adult men: the Chicago Heart Association Detection Project in Industry. Arch Intern Med. 2001;161(12):1501–8.
16. Yano Y, Stamler J, Garside DB, Daviglus ML, Franklin SS, Carnethon MR, et al. Isolated systolic hypertension in young and middle-aged adults and 31-year risk for cardiovascular mortality: the Chicago Heart Association Detection Project in Industry study. J Am Coll Cardiol. 2015;65(4):327–35.
17. Vasan RS, Larson MG, Leip EP, Evans JC, O'Donnell CJ, Kannel WB, et al. Impact of high-normal blood pressure on the risk of cardiovascular disease. N Engl J Med. 2001;345(18):1291–7.
18. Kannel WB. Risk stratification in hypertension: new insights from the Framingham Study. Am J Hypertens. 2000;13(1 Pt 2):3S–10.

19. Jackson R, Lawes CM, Bennett DA, Milne RJ, Rodgers A. Treatment with drugs to lower blood pressure and blood cholesterol based on an individual's absolute cardiovascular risk. Lancet. 2005;365(9457):434–41.
20. D'Agostino Sr RB, Vasan RS, Pencina MJ, Wolf PA, Cobain M, Massaro JM, et al. General cardiovascular risk profile for use in primary care: the Framingham Heart Study. Circulation. 2008;117(6):743–53.
21. Goff Jr DC, Lloyd-Jones DM, Bennett G, Coady S, D'Agostino RB, Gibbons R, et al. 2013 ACC/AHA guideline on the assessment of cardiovascular risk: a report of the American College of Cardiology/American Heart Association Task Force on Practice Guidelines. Circulation. 2014;129(25 Suppl 2):S49–73.
22. DeFilippis AP, Young R, Carrubba CJ, McEvoy JW, Budoff MJ, Blumenthal RS, et al. An analysis of calibration and discrimination among multiple cardiovascular risk scores in a modern multiethnic cohort. Ann Intern Med. 2015;162(4):266–75.
23. Alberti KG, Eckel RH, Grundy SM, Zimmet PZ, Cleeman JI, Donato KA, et al. Harmonizing the metabolic syndrome: a joint interim statement of the International Diabetes Federation Task Force on Epidemiology and Prevention; National Heart, Lung, and Blood Institute; American Heart Association; World Heart Federation; International Atherosclerosis Society; and International Association for the Study of Obesity. Circulation. 2009;120(16):1640–5.
24. Wilson PW, D'Agostino RB, Parise H, Sullivan L, Meigs JB. Metabolic syndrome as a precursor of cardiovascular disease and type 2 diabetes mellitus. Circulation. 2005;112(20):3066–72.
25. Kannel WB, Wilson PW, Nam BH, D'Agostino RB. Risk stratification of obesity as a coronary risk factor. Am J Cardiol. 2002;90(7):697–701.
26. Wilson PW, D'Agostino RB, Sullivan L, Parise H, Kannel WB. Overweight and obesity as determinants of cardiovascular risk: the Framingham experience. Arch Intern Med. 2002;162(16):1867–72.
27. Zhang C, Rexrode KM, van Dam RM, Li TY, Hu FB. Abdominal obesity and the risk of all-cause, cardiovascular, and cancer mortality: sixteen years of follow-up in US women. Circulation. 2008;117(13):1658–67.
28. Madala MC, Franklin BA, Chen AY, Berman AD, Roe MT, Peterson ED, et al. Obesity and age of first non-ST-segment elevation myocardial infarction. J Am Coll Cardiol. 2008;52(12):979–85.
29. Lim SS, Vos T, Flaxman AD, Danaei G, Shibuya K, Adair-Rohani H, et al. A comparative risk assessment of burden of disease and injury attributable to 67 risk factors and risk factor clusters in 21 regions, 1990-2010: a systematic analysis for the Global Burden of Disease Study 2010. Lancet. 2012;380(9859):2224–60.
30. Bakris GL, Ritz E, World Kidney Day Steering Committee. The message for World Kidney Day 2009: hypertension and kidney disease: a marriage that should be prevented. Am J Nephrol. 2009;30(1):95–8.
31. Tonelli M, Muntner P, Lloyd A, Manns BJ, Klarenbach S, Pannu N, et al. Risk of coronary events in people with chronic kidney disease compared with those with diabetes: a population-level cohort study. Lancet. 2012;380(9844):807–14.
32. Fox CS, Matsushita K, Woodward M, Bilo HJ, Chalmers J, Heerspink HJ, et al. Associations of kidney disease measures with mortality and end-stage renal disease in individuals with and without diabetes: a meta-analysis. Lancet. 2012;380(9854):1662–73.
33. Matsushita K, Coresh J, Sang Y, Chalmers J, Fox C, Guallar E, et al. Estimated glomerular filtration rate and albuminuria for prediction of cardiovascular outcomes: a collaborative meta-analysis of individual participant data. Lancet Diabetes Endocrinol. 2015;3(7):514–25.
34. McCullough PA, Jurkovitz CT, Pergola PE, McGill JB, Brown WW, Collins AJ, et al. Independent components of chronic kidney disease as a cardiovascular risk state: results from the Kidney Early Evaluation Program (KEEP). Arch Intern Med. 2007;167(11):1122–9.
35. Culleton BF, Larson MG, Wilson PW, Evans JC, Parfrey PS, Levy D. Cardiovascular disease and mortality in a community-based cohort with mild renal insufficiency. Kidney Int. 1999;56(6):2214–9.

36. Manjunath G, Tighiouart H, Ibrahim H, MacLeod B, Salem DN, Griffith JL, et al. Level of kidney function as a risk factor for atherosclerotic cardiovascular outcomes in the community. J Am Coll Cardiol. 2003;41(1):47–55.
37. Mann JF, Gerstein HC, Pogue J, Bosch J, Yusuf S. Renal insufficiency as a predictor of cardiovascular outcomes and the impact of ramipril: the HOPE randomized trial. Ann Intern Med. 2001;134(8):629–36.
38. Sarnak MJ, Levey AS, Schoolwerth AC, Coresh J, Culleton B, Hamm LL, et al. Kidney disease as a risk factor for development of cardiovascular disease: a statement from the American Heart Association Councils on Kidney in Cardiovascular Disease, High Blood Pressure Research, Clinical Cardiology, and Epidemiology and Prevention. Circulation. 2003;108(17):2154–69.
39. Go AS, Chertow GM, Fan D, McCulloch CE, Hsu CY. Chronic kidney disease and the risks of death, cardiovascular events, and hospitalization. N Engl J Med. 2004;351(13):1296–305.
40. Anavekar NS, McMurray JJ, Velazquez EJ, Solomon SD, Kober L, Rouleau JL, et al. Relation between renal dysfunction and cardiovascular outcomes after myocardial infarction. N Engl J Med. 2004;351(13):1285–95.
41. Bakris GL, Molitch M. Microalbuminuria as a risk predictor in diabetes: the continuing saga. Diabetes Care. 2014;37(3):867–75.
42. James PA, Oparil S, Carter BL, Cushman WC, Dennison-Himmelfarb C, Handler J, et al. 2014 evidence-based guideline for the management of high blood pressure in adults: report from the panel members appointed to the Eighth Joint National Committee (JNC 8). JAMA. 2014;311(5):507–20.
43. Mancia G, Fagard R, Narkiewicz K, Redon J, Zanchetti A, Bohm M, et al. 2013 ESH/ESC Guidelines for the management of arterial hypertension: the Task Force for the management of arterial hypertension of the European Society of Hypertension (ESH) and of the European Society of Cardiology (ESC). J Hypertens. 2013;31(7):1281–357.
44. Weber MA, Schiffrin EL, White WB, Mann S, Lindholm LH, Kenerson JG, et al. Clinical practice guidelines for the management of hypertension in the community: a statement by the American Society of Hypertension and the International Society of Hypertension. J Clin Hypertens (Greenwich). 2014;16(1):14–26.
45. Hypertension: the clinical management of primary hypertension in adults: update of clinical guidelines 18 and 34. National Institute for Health and Clinical Excellence: Guidance. London; 2011.
46. Chobanian AV, Bakris GL, Black HR, Cushman WC, Green LA, Izzo Jr JL, et al. The Seventh Report of the Joint National Committee on Prevention, Detection, Evaluation, and Treatment of High Blood Pressure: the JNC 7 report. JAMA. 2003;289(19):2560–72.
47. Krause T, Lovibond K, Caulfield M, McCormack T, Williams B, Guideline Development Group. Management of hypertension: summary of NICE guidance. BMJ. 2011;343:d4891.
48. Dolan E, Stanton A, Thijs L, Hinedi K, Atkins N, McClory S, et al. Superiority of ambulatory over clinic blood pressure measurement in predicting mortality: the Dublin outcome study. Hypertension. 2005;46(1):156–61.
49. Rosendorff C, Lackland DT, Allison M, Aronow WS, Black HR, Blumenthal RS, et al. Treatment of hypertension in patients with coronary artery disease: A scientific statement from the American Heart Association, American College of Cardiology, and American Society of Hypertension. J Am Soc Hypertens. 2015;9(6):453–498.
50. Goldstein LB, Bushnell CD, Adams RJ, Appel LJ, Braun LT, Chaturvedi S, et al. Guidelines for the primary prevention of stroke: a guideline for healthcare professionals from the American Heart Association/American Stroke Association. Stroke. 2011;42(2):517–84.
51. Kernan WN, Ovbiagele B, Black HR, Bravata DM, Chimowitz MI, Ezekowitz MD, et al. Guidelines for the prevention of stroke in patients with stroke and transient ischemic attack: a guideline for healthcare professionals from the American Heart Association/American Stroke Association. Stroke. 2014;45(7):2160–236.
52. Messerli FH, Mancia G, Conti CR, Hewkin AC, Kupfer S, Champion A, et al. Dogma disputed: can aggressively lowering blood pressure in hypertensive patients with coronary artery disease be dangerous? Ann Intern Med. 2006;144(12):884–93.

53. Protogerou AD, Safar ME, Iaria P, Safar H, Le Dudal K, Filipovsky J, et al. Diastolic blood pressure and mortality in the elderly with cardiovascular disease. Hypertension. 2007;50(1):172–80.
54. Peralta CA, Norris KC, Li S, Chang TI, Tamura MK, Jolly SE, et al. Blood pressure components and end-stage renal disease in persons with chronic kidney disease: the Kidney Early Evaluation Program (KEEP). Arch Intern Med. 2012;172(1):41–7.
55. Hansson L, Zanchetti A, Carruthers SG, Dahlof B, Elmfeldt D, Julius S, et al. Effects of intensive blood-pressure lowering and low-dose aspirin in patients with hypertension: principal results of the Hypertension Optimal Treatment (HOT) randomised trial. HOT Study Group. Lancet. 1998;351(9118):1755–62.
56. Prevention of stroke by antihypertensive drug treatment in older persons with isolated systolic hypertension. Final results of the Systolic Hypertension in the Elderly Program (SHEP). SHEP Cooperative Research Group. JAMA. 1991;265(24):3255–64.
57. Tight blood pressure control and risk of macrovascular and microvascular complications in type 2 diabetes: UKPDS 38. UK Prospective Diabetes Study Group. BMJ. 1998;317(7160):703–13.
58. Brown MJ, Palmer CR, Castaigne A, de Leeuw PW, Mancia G, Rosenthal T, et al. Morbidity and mortality in patients randomised to double-blind treatment with a long-acting calcium-channel blocker or diuretic in the International Nifedipine GITS study: Intervention as a Goal in Hypertension Treatment (INSIGHT). Lancet. 2000;356(9227):366–72.
59. Dahlof B, Devereux RB, Kjeldsen SE, Julius S, Beevers G, de Faire U, et al. Cardiovascular morbidity and mortality in the Losartan Intervention For Endpoint reduction in hypertension study (LIFE): a randomised trial against atenolol. Lancet. 2002;359(9311):995–1003.
60. Dahlof B, Sever PS, Poulter NR, Wedel H, Beevers DG, Caulfield M, et al. Prevention of cardiovascular events with an antihypertensive regimen of amlodipine adding perindopril as required versus atenolol adding bendroflumethiazide as required, in the Anglo-Scandinavian Cardiac Outcomes Trial-Blood Pressure Lowering Arm (ASCOT-BPLA): a multicentre randomised controlled trial. Lancet. 2005;366(9489):895–906.
61. Estacio RO, Jeffers BW, Gifford N, Schrier RW. Effect of blood pressure control on diabetic microvascular complications in patients with hypertension and type 2 diabetes. Diabetes Care. 2000;23 Suppl 2:B54–64.
62. Hansson L, Lindholm LH, Ekbom T, Dahlof B, Lanke J, Schersten B, et al. Randomised trial of old and new antihypertensive drugs in elderly patients: cardiovascular mortality and morbidity the Swedish Trial in Old Patients with Hypertension-2 study. Lancet. 1999;354(9192):1751–6.
63. Hansson L, Hedner T, Lund-Johansen P, Kjeldsen SE, Lindholm LH, Syvertsen JO, et al. Randomised trial of effects of calcium antagonists compared with diuretics and beta-blockers on cardiovascular morbidity and mortality in hypertension: the Nordic Diltiazem (NORDIL) study. Lancet. 2000;356(9227):359–65.
64. Staessen JA, Fagard R, Thijs L, Celis H, Arabidze GG, Birkenhager WH, et al. Randomised double-blind comparison of placebo and active treatment for older patients with isolated systolic hypertension. The Systolic Hypertension in Europe (Syst-Eur) Trial Investigators. Lancet. 1997;350(9080):757–64.
65. Group AS, Cushman WC, Evans GW, Byington RP, Goff Jr DC, Grimm Jr RH, et al. Effects of intensive blood-pressure control in type 2 diabetes mellitus. N Engl J Med. 2010;362(17):1575–85.
66. Emdin CA, Rahimi K, Neal B, Callender T, Perkovic V, Patel A. Blood pressure lowering in type 2 diabetes: a systematic review and meta-analysis. JAMA. 2015;313(6):603–15.
67. Investigators O, Yusuf S, Teo KK, Pogue J, Dyal L, Copland I, et al. Telmisartan, ramipril, or both in patients at high risk for vascular events. N Engl J Med. 2008;358(15):1547–59.
68. Cooper-DeHoff RM, Gong Y, Handberg EM, Bavry AA, Denardo SJ, Bakris GL, et al. Tight blood pressure control and cardiovascular outcomes among hypertensive patients with diabetes and coronary artery disease. JAMA. 2010;304(1):61–8.

69. Weber MA, Bakris GL, Jamerson K, Weir M, Kjeldsen SE, Devereux RB, et al. Cardiovascular events during differing hypertension therapies in patients with diabetes. J Am Coll Cardiol. 2010;56(1):77–85.
70. Upadhyay A, Earley A, Haynes SM, Uhlig K. Systematic review: blood pressure target in chronic kidney disease and proteinuria as an effect modifier. Ann Intern Med. 2011;154(8):541–8.
71. Jamerson K, Weber MA, Bakris GL, Dahlof B, Pitt B, Shi V, et al. Benazepril plus amlodipine or hydrochlorothiazide for hypertension in high-risk patients. N Engl J Med. 2008;359(23):2417–28.
72. Khosla N, Kalaitzidis R, Bakris GL. The kidney, hypertension, and remaining challenges. Med Clin North Am. 2009;93(3):697–715.
73. Blood Pressure Lowering Treatment Trialists' Collaboration, Turnbull F, Neal B, Ninomiya T, Algert C, Arima H, et al. Effects of different regimens to lower blood pressure on major cardiovascular events in older and younger adults: meta-analysis of randomised trials. BMJ. 2008;336(7653):1121–3.
74. Lindholm LH, Carlberg B, Samuelsson O. Should beta blockers remain first choice in the treatment of primary hypertension? A meta-analysis. Lancet. 2005;366(9496):1545–53.
75. Julius S, Kjeldsen SE, Weber M, Brunner HR, Ekman S, Hansson L, et al. Outcomes in hypertensive patients at high cardiovascular risk treated with regimens based on valsartan or amlodipine: the VALUE randomised trial. Lancet. 2004;363(9426):2022–31.
76. Mancia G, Grassi G, Zanchetti A. New-onset diabetes and antihypertensive drugs. J Hypertens. 2006;24(1):3–10.
77. Sarafidis PA, McFarlane SI, Bakris GL. Antihypertensive agents, insulin sensitivity, and new-onset diabetes. Curr Diab Rep. 2007;7(3):191–9.
78. Bakris G, Molitch M, Hewkin A, Kipnes M, Sarafidis P, Fakouhi K, et al. Differences in glucose tolerance between fixed-dose antihypertensive drug combinations in people with metabolic syndrome. Diabetes Care. 2006;29(12):2592–7.
79. Officers A, Coordinators for the ACRGTA, Lipid-Lowering Treatment to Prevent Heart Attack Trial. Major outcomes in high-risk hypertensive patients randomized to angiotensin-converting enzyme inhibitor or calcium channel blocker vs diuretic: The Antihypertensive and Lipid-Lowering Treatment to Prevent Heart Attack Trial (ALLHAT). JAMA. 2002;288(23):2981–97.
80. Elliott WJ, Meyer PM. Incident diabetes in clinical trials of antihypertensive drugs: a network meta-analysis. Lancet. 2007;369(9557):201–7.
81. Whelton PK, Barzilay J, Cushman WC, Davis BR, Iiamathi E, Kostis JB, et al. Clinical outcomes in antihypertensive treatment of type 2 diabetes, impaired fasting glucose concentration, and normoglycemia: Antihypertensive and Lipid-Lowering Treatment to Prevent Heart Attack Trial (ALLHAT). Arch Intern Med. 2005;165(12):1401–9.
82. Kostis JB, Wilson AC, Freudenberger RS, Cosgrove NM, Pressel SL, Davis BR, et al. Long-term effect of diuretic-based therapy on fatal outcomes in subjects with isolated systolic hypertension with and without diabetes. Am J Cardiol. 2005;95(1):29–35.
83. Bakris GL, Fonseca V, Katholi RE, McGill JB, Messerli FH, Phillips RA, et al. Metabolic effects of carvedilol vs metoprolol in patients with type 2 diabetes mellitus and hypertension: a randomized controlled trial. JAMA. 2004;292(18):2227–36.
84. Kaiser T, Heise T, Nosek L, Eckers U, Sawicki PT. Influence of nebivolol and enalapril on metabolic parameters and arterial stiffness in hypertensive type 2 diabetic patients. J Hypertens. 2006;24(7):1397–403.
85. Patel A, Group AC, MacMahon S, Chalmers J, Neal B, Woodward M, et al. Effects of a fixed combination of perindopril and indapamide on macrovascular and microvascular outcomes in patients with type 2 diabetes mellitus (the ADVANCE trial): a randomised controlled trial. Lancet. 2007;370(9590):829–40.

86. McMurray JJ, Ostergren J, Swedberg K, Granger CB, Held P, Michelson EL, et al. Effects of candesartan in patients with chronic heart failure and reduced left-ventricular systolic function taking angiotensin-converting-enzyme inhibitors: the CHARM-Added trial. Lancet. 2003;362(9386):767–71.
87. Wright Jr JT, Fine LJ, Lackland DT, Ogedegbe G, Dennison Himmelfarb CR. Evidence supporting a systolic blood pressure goal of less than 150 mm Hg in patients aged 60 years or older: the minority view. Ann Intern Med. 2014;160(7):499–503.
88. Beckett NS, Peters R, Fletcher AE, Staessen JA, Liu L, Dumitrascu D, et al. Treatment of hypertension in patients 80 years of age or older. N Engl J Med. 2008;358(18):1887–98.

Chapter 8
Acute Blood Pressure Management After Ischemic Stroke

J. Dedrick Jordan and William J. Powers

Elevation in blood pressure (BP) is common with an acute ischemic stroke; however, the acute management of the BP is a major unresolved issue. While there are clear benefits for BP reduction in the long-term for secondary stroke prevention, controversy exists in the period immediately following ischemic stroke. The main concern for the acute lowering of BP is the risk of worsening cerebral ischemia due to cerebral hypoperfusion surrounding the infarct core. Allowing the BP to be permissively elevated however may lead to an increase in the risk of hemorrhagic conversion and systemic complications. This chapter will review the current evidence that addresses the management of BP in the setting of acute ischemic stroke and how this affects neurological outcome.

Hypertension with Acute Ischemic Stroke

Incidence and Natural History

Many patients with acute ischemic stroke will present to the emergency department with BP elevation; however, it is unclear whether this represents a compensation for cerebral hypoperfusion or is related to systemic causes [1, 2]. Several studies have helped elucidate the natural history of BP changes following acute ischemic stroke.

J.D. Jordan, M.D., Ph.D. (✉) • W.J. Powers, M.D.
Departments of Neurology and Neurosurgery, University of North Carolina School of Medicine, 170 Manning Drive, POB 2118, CB #7025, Chapel Hill, NC 27599-7025, USA
e-mail: dedrick@unc.edu; powersw@neurology.unc.edu

© Springer International Publishing Switzerland 2016
V. Aiyagari, P.B. Gorelick (eds.), *Hypertension and Stroke*, Clinical Hypertension and Vascular Diseases, DOI 10.1007/978-3-319-29152-9_8

The incidence of an elevated BP has been reported to be 76.5 % in a large retrospective analysis of 276,734 patients presenting to the emergency room with acute ischemic stroke [3]. This is further supported by two large multicenter acute ischemic stroke trials, the Chinese Acute Stroke Trial (CAST) with 21,106 patients and the International Stroke Trial (IST) with 19,435 patients, that reported a systolic blood pressure (SBP) > 140 mmHg in 75 % and 80 % of patients, respectively. Furthermore, severe BP elevation, as defined as SBP > 180 mmHg, was reported in 25 % of patients in CAST and 28 % of patients in IST [4, 5].

Commonly this elevation in BP however is followed by a reduction over the next several days [1, 2, 6, 7]. A large stroke registry found that an early decrease of SBP by 20–30 % was associated with a complete neurological recovery [8]. Furthermore, an early decrease in SBP after acute ischemic stroke has been associated with recanalization of the affected vessel [9].

Effect of Hypertension on Outcome After Acute Ischemic Stroke

The optimal target for BP after acute ischemic stroke remains unclear, as several studies have demonstrated a U-shaped correlation between BP and poor outcome. Either an elevated or very low BP on admission has been associated with worse outcome.

A large observational study demonstrated early as well as late mortality in a U-shaped distribution in relation to the admission SBP. The relative risk of mortality at 1 month and 1 year increased with every 10 mmHg change in SBP above or below 130 mmHg [10]. Data from IST demonstrated that both high BP and low BP were independent prognostic indicators for poor outcome. A baseline SBP of 140–179 mmHg resulted in the lowest frequency of poor outcome [11].

Additional studies have demonstrated associations between elevated or low SBP and patient outcomes. One such study found that patients with a SBP less than 155 mmHg were more likely to die within 90 days compared to patients presenting with a SBP between 155 and 220 mmHg [12]. The Intravenous Nimodipine West European Stroke Trial found that a high initial BP, SBP greater than 160 mmHg, was a predictor for death or dependency at 21 days compared to patients who had a normal initial BP (SBP 120–160 mmHg and diastolic BP 60–90 mmHg) [13]. An analysis of the VISTA (Virtual Stroke International Stroke Trial Archive) collaboration examined the relationship between hemodynamic measures, variability in BP, and change in BP over the first 24 h after acute ischemic stroke. This study demonstrated that a persistently elevated SBP for up to 24 h was significantly associated with increased neurological impairment and poor functional outcome. Additionally, the magnitude of change in BP over this first 24 h was significantly related to poor outcome in which patients having large decreases (>75 mmHg) or increases (>25 mmHg) in BP had the highest risk of poor outcome [14]. Analysis of the Fukuoka stroke registry demonstrated that a SBP (averaged over first 48 h) range of 144–153 mmHg and above was associated with a lower probability of good neurological recovery. SBP elevation was also associated with an elevated risk of neurological deterioration and poor functional outcome [15]. These studies suggest that hypertension on admission may be a marker of other factors, such as a higher severity of stroke or a sign of premorbid hypertension, rather than an independent prognostic sign [16].

Cerebrovascular Pathophysiology and Ischemic Stroke

Under normal physiological conditions, regional cerebral blood flow (CBF) is tightly regulated through cerebral autoregulation despite variations in regional cerebral perfusion pressure (CPP) [17]. Regional CPP is equal to the local mean arterial pressure (MAP) minus local intracranial pressure (ICP). In the absence of local arterial occlusion or stenosis or local increased ICP, regional CPP is equal to systemic MAP. The cerebral vasculature will either constrict or dilate maintaining stable CBF within a mean regional CPP range of 50–150 mmHg [18, 19]. When the regional CPP falls below the lower limit of autoregulation, regional CBF is reduced resulting in cerebral ischemia. Conversely, when the regional CPP increases above the upper-limit of autoregulation regional CBF is increased, which can lead to cerebral edema or hemorrhage. The autoregulation of CBF can be affected by chronic systemic hypertension with a resultant shift to the right in the autoregulatory curve. This shift may lead to cerebral hypoperfusion even when the MAP is within the normal physiologic range of 50–150 mmHg, but below the lower limit for the right-shifted curve. Prior to the advent of modern tomographic brain imaging modalities such as CT, PET, and MRI, CBF studies in humans using the technique of radiotracer injection into the carotid artery with radioactivity detection by scintillation crystals on the scalp showed abnormalities during the initial days following ischemic stroke. These abnormalities included non-focal hemispheric decreases in CBF in response to rapid reductions in MAP; however, it was not possible to determine whether these changes were in infarcted tissue, the peri-infarct region, or non-ischemic tissue [20–22]. These studies led to the widespread view that autoregulation of CBF in response to changes in systemic blood pressure is impaired in acute ischemic stroke. More recent data using tomographic imaging techniques for CBF measurement that have better spatial resolution have produced different results from the earlier studies. In the three studies that used intravenous agents to produce rapid reduction then stabilization of BP, there was no selective impairment of autoregulation in the peri-infarct region to reduced MAP in patients studied within 6 h or 1–11 days after onset of stroke [23–25]. Two additional studies using oral agents to produce blood pressure reduction over 6–8 h also failed to demonstrate impaired autoregulation in patients 2–8 days from onset of stroke. These studies did not address patients with large edematous infarcts causing increases in ICP or those with persistent large artery occlusion causing local reduction in MAP. In these situations, when local CPP is lower than systemic MAP, a reduction in systemic MAP within the 50–150 mmHg range could cause a reduction in local CPP below the autoregulatory limit with a consequent reduction in CBF even though the autoregulatory capacity of the cerebral blood vessels is normal.

Acute Management of Blood Pressure After Ischemic Stroke

Controversy

While the long-term treatment of hypertension clearly reduces the risk of recurrent stroke, controversy exists as to the management of BP elevation in the setting of acute ischemic stroke. An elevated BP may increase the risk of secondary complications of stroke such as hemorrhagic transformation and cerebral edema [26, 27]. Additionally, if the blood pressure is aggressively lowered then cerebral perfusion may decrease to a level that leads to further cerebral ischemia [19]. Several large prospective trials have been completed within the past several years aimed at addressing these questions.

Effect on Neurological or Functional Outcome

In 2008, a Cochrane review assessed the effect of altering BP in patients with acute ischemic stroke. Twelve small randomized studies, including a total of 1153 patients, were included in the review; however, the authors felt that there was insufficient evidence to determine an effect of lowering BP on clinical outcomes [28]. Since that publication however, several large prospective trials have been completed providing more definitive data (Table 8.1).

Controlling hypertension and hypotension immediately post-stroke (CHHIPS) was a randomized, placebo-controlled, double-blind trial that compared labetalol, lisinopril, and placebo for lowering BP in 179 patients with either acute ischemic or hemorrhagic stroke and a SBP greater than 160 mmHg. While BP was reduced by 21 mmHg in the active treatment and 11 mmHg in the placebo group, there was no significant difference in primary outcome of death or dependency at 2 weeks. While there was no difference in serious adverse events between the groups, the 3 month mortality was from 20.3 to 9.7 % in the treatment group (nominal $p=0.05$, uncorrected for multiple comparisons) [29].

Angiotensin-receptor blocker candesartan for treatment of acute stroke (SCAST) was another randomized, placebo-controlled, double-blind trial conducted to determine if BP reduction with candesartan after acute ischemic or hemorrhagic stroke was beneficial. This trial included 2029 patients with acute stroke, 85 % of which were ischemic stroke, randomized to receive either candesartan or placebo for 7 days. Only a minimal SBP lowering effect was observed in the treatment arm, 5 mmHg lower in the candesartan group at day 7 compared to the placebo group. The trial did not demonstrate any significant difference in death, myocardial infarction, or recurrent stroke at 6 months between the groups while there was a slightly increased risk of poor functional outcome observed in the candesartan group at 6 months [30].

Recently, He and colleagues evaluated the impact of moderate BP reduction within 48 h of acute ischemic stroke onset on death and major disability at 14 days or hospital discharge in The Chinese Antihypertensive Trial in Acute Ischemic Stroke (CATIS) trial. CATIS randomized 4061 patients to receive either

Table 8.1 Studies evaluating the effect of blood pressure control after acute ischemic stroke

Trial	Design	Study arms/cohort	Number of patients	Time from onset to presentation (h)	Results
CHHIPS [29]	Randomized, double-blinded, prospective	Labetalol vs. lisinopril vs. placebo	179	<36	No difference in death or dependency at 2 weeks Reduced 3 month mortality in treatment arm
SCAST [30]	Randomized, double-blinded, prospective	Candesartan vs. placebo	2004	<30	Trend toward increased risk of poor functional outcome at 6 months in treatment group
CATIS [31]	Randomized, single-blind, blinded endpoint, prospective	Antihypertensive treatment vs. discontinue all antihypertensive medications	4071	<48	No difference in death or major disability at hospital discharge or at 2 weeks or 3 months
COSSACS [32]	Open, blinded-endpoint, prospective	Continue vs. discontinue preexisting antihypertensive drug	763	<48	No difference in death or dependency at 2 weeks
ENOS [33]	Randomized, single-blinded, blinded-outcome, prospective	Glyceryl trinitrate vs. no treatment; subset of patients taking antihypertensive agents on admission randomized to continue or stop these medications	4011	<48	No difference in modified Rankin Score at 90 days in either treatment comparison Patients continued on antihypertensive agents had increased risk of hospital death or have been discharged to an institution, and be dead or disabled
VENTURE [34]	Randomized, blinded-end-point, open-label, prospective	Valsartan vs. no treatment	393	<24	No reduction in death or dependency and major vascular events at 90 days Increased risk of early neurological deterioration

antihypertensive agents with a goal to lower SBP by 10–25 % within 24 h and a BP less than 140/90 mmHg within 7 days versus stopping all antihypertensive medications on admission. The primary endpoint was mortality and major disability at 14 days or at hospital discharge. While there was a significant reduction in BP in the intervention group of approximately 9 mmHg systolic from day 1–14, there was no difference in death or major disability at 2 weeks or 3 months [31].

Debate also exists whether to continue or stop antihypertensive medications that patients were receiving prior to admission with an acute ischemic stroke. The Continue Or Stop post-Stroke Antihypertensives Collaborative Study (COSSACS) assessed the efficacy and safety of continuing or stopping preexisting antihypertensive medications in patients who had an acute stroke. Patients were randomized to continue ($n = 379$; 67 % ischemic stroke) or stop ($n = 384$; 58 % ischemic stroke) their preexisting antihypertensive medications within 48 h of onset. The BP in the continue medication group was significantly lower at 2 weeks by 13/8 mmHg; however there was no difference in the primary outcome of death of dependency at 2 weeks. This trial provides data that indicates that continuing prior antihypertensive medications is safe; however, the results of this study should be taken with caution since the trial was underpowered due to the early termination of the trial and furthermore, patients with dysphagia were excluded, resulting in enrollment of a majority of patients with mild strokes (median NIHSS of 4) [32].

The Efficacy of Nitric Oxide in Stroke (ENOS) trial randomized patients with acute stroke, approximately 85 % ischemic and 15 % hemorrhagic, and elevated SBP to transdermal glyceryl trinitrate or no glyceryl trinitrate within 48 h of stroke onset. Also, a subset of patients taking antihypertensive medications prior to their stroke was also randomly assigned to stop or continue taking those previously prescribed medications. The primary outcome of this study was functional outcome as assessed via the modified Rankin Scale at 90 days. While there was a significant reduction in BP at 24 h in those receiving glyceryl trinitrate as well as those assigned to continue their previously prescribed antihypertensive agents, there was no difference in functional outcome in either group. However, patients that continued their prescribed antihypertensive medications were more likely to have died in the hospital or been discharged to an institution, and be dead or disabled by day 90 compared to those that stopped taking their antihypertensive medications on admission. Furthermore, those that continued their medications had lower cognition scores at follow-up as well as an increase in the risk for the development of pneumonia [33].

Valsartan Efficacy on Modest Blood Pressure Reduction in Acute Ischemic Stroke (VENTURE) was a randomized, open-label, blinded-end-point trial that assigned 393 subjects with acute ischemic stroke and elevated BP to either valsartan or no treatment for BP. The primary outcome was death or dependency at 90 days. Additionally, early neurological deterioration within 7 days and 90-day major vascular events were assessed. While the SBP did not differ between the two groups, the diastolic BP (DBP) was significantly lower during 7 days by approximately 2 mmHg in the treatment arm. The valsartan group did not have a reduced risk of death or dependency nor a reduction in major vascular events at 90 days, however there was a significantly increased risk of early neurological decline [34].

Based on the limited treatment data and the natural history of BP after ischemic stroke, we continue antihypertensive medications after admission either by mouth or by nasogastric tube. We often initially decrease the dose of a single medication or reduce the number of medications to guard against rapid drops in BP in the event of outpatient noncompliance. After 3 or 4 days we will begin to add medications back. For the patient with newly diagnosed hypertension or with previously known but untreated hypertension, we begin a single antihypertensive medication after 3–4 days following the Joint National Committee 8 guidelines [35]. Our practice is to avoid the use of intravenous antihypertensive medications for BP control unless there is a clear indication for rapid blood reduction, such as heart failure or myocardial ischemia. After discharge close follow-up is imperative to ensure the adequate long-term treatment of hypertension for secondary stroke prevention.

Blood Pressure Management in Patients Eligible for Thrombolytic Therapy

While the management of BP elevation in patients with acute ischemic stroke has been debated, BP lowering for patients with a BP > 185/110 mmHg is recommended for patients eligible for thrombolytic therapy.

A pilot study evaluating factors associated with intracerebral hemorrhage (ICH) following the use of thrombolytic therapy found that an increased risk of ICH was associated with elevated DBP [36]. Therefore, in the National Institute of Neurological Disorders and Stroke study, a strict BP of <185/110 mmHg was required for enrollment into the study and tight BP control was maintained for 24 h with a BP goal of <180/105 mmHg [37].

While subsequent observational studies evaluating the association of elevated BP and ICH formation have been variable [38], a study examining associations between protocol violations and outcomes in community-based recombinant tissue plasminogen activator (rt-PA) use found that when the NINDS protocol is strictly followed, hemorrhage rates are similar to those in the NINDS trial [39]. Additionally, results from the Safe Implementation of Thrombolysis in Stroke (SITS) registry demonstrated that an increased SBP 2–24 h after thrombolytic therapy was associated with worse outcome (symptomatic hemorrhage, mortality, functional dependence) at 3 months. The best outcomes were observed in patients with SBP values between 141 and 150 mmHg up to 24 h post-thrombolysis [40].

It is also important to note that thrombolytic therapy may be associated with improvement in systolic BP following successful recanalization. Mattle and colleagues reported that patients who underwent intra-arterial thrombolysis and had unsuccessful vessel recanalization had higher and sustained elevations in SBP compared to those patients with successful recanalization [9].

Guidelines for BP Management in Acute Ischemic Stroke

The current American Heart Association (AHA) and American Stroke Association (ASA) Guidelines recommend a cautious approach to lowering of BP after acute ischemic stroke. For those patients that receive thrombolysis, the BP should be reduced to less than 185/110 mmHg prior to initiation of treatment and should be maintained at less than 180/105 mmHg for 24 h after treatment. The use of intravenous labetalol and nicardipine are recommended as the first line agents although there is limited data to support this recommendation. For patients not receiving thrombolysis the guidelines recommend withholding medications unless the SBP is greater than 220 mmHg or DBP is greater than 120 mmHg. This recommendation is a consensus opinion however and not based on randomized studies [26].

The European Stroke Organization recommend similar guidelines for those treated with thrombolysis. For other patients, they do not recommend routine lowering of BP unless above 220/120 mmHg on repeated measurements, or if there is evidence of severe end-organ dysfunction [41]. The 2013 European Society of Hypertension/European Society of Cardiology Guidelines for the management of arterial hypertension recommend against BP lowering therapy in the first week after acute stroke "irrespective of BP level, although clinical judgment should be used in the face of very high SBP values" [42].

Choice of Antihypertensive Agents in Acute Ischemic Stroke

When BP reduction is required there are limited data that demonstrate the optimal antihypertensive for use in the setting of acute ischemic stroke. No large prospective comparison studies have been performed to date; however there are a few small retrospective and prospective studies evaluating efficacy and tolerability. Two comparative studies evaluated the therapeutic response and tolerability of labetalol and nicardipine following acute stroke [43, 44]. Both of these trials evaluated patients according to AHA and ASA guidelines regarding BP treatment after acute ischemic or hemorrhagic stroke and assessed patients for the first 24 h. The first study was a retrospective and non-randomized study that assessed BP reduction and BP variability between labetalol and nicardipine. Patients whom received nicardipine were more likely to achieve their BP goal at 1 h than patients whom received labetalol. Furthermore, patients treated with nicardipine required fewer dosage adjustments or need for rescue therapy with additional antihypertensive medications than those who received labetalol.

A follow-up study prospectively enrolled 54 acute ischemic or hemorrhagic stroke patients with elevated BP. The patients received either labetalol or nicardipine during the first 24 h after admission. Patients treated with nicardipine achieved a higher rate of meeting the goal BP within 60 min of drug initiation, had better maintenance of BP, and a greater percentage of time spent within the goal BP range. None of the patients randomized to nicardipine required rescue medication while 72.7 % of those randomized to labetalol required an additional agent to achieve BP goals [44]. Table 8.2 summarizes the preferred antihypertensive agents for use in the treatment of acute ischemic stroke-related hypertension.

Table 8.2 Rapidly acting antihypertensive agents for the treatment of hypertension immediately after acute ischemic stroke

Agent	Mechanism of action	Intravenous dose	Time to onset (min)	Considerations
Nicardipine	Dihydropyridine calcium channel blocker	Infusion at 5–15 mg/h	5–10	Titratable
				Invasive BP monitoring not required
				First line agent
Labetalol	Mixed α- and β-receptor antagonist	10–40 mg bolus every 15 min; max of 300 mg	5–10	May cause bradycardia
				No effect on cerebral blood flow
		Infusion at 0.5–2 mg/min		Second line agent
Hydralazine	Vasodilator	5–10 mg bolus	5–10	May increase intracranial pressure
Enalaprilat	ACE inhibitor	0.625–1.25 mg bolus every 6 h	15	Adjust dose based on renal function
				Duration of action 4–6 h

Data from [26, 40, 42]
ACE angiotensin converting enzyme

Conclusions

Blood pressure elevation after acute ischemic stroke is common and the management of this BP elevation is dependent on the clinical context. For patients that are candidates for thrombolysis, reduction and maintenance of the BP within the current guidelines is indicated as it likely reduces the risk of hemorrhagic complications. For all other patients, there is no clear benefit and potentially harm for acute blood pressure reduction.

References

1. Wallace JD, Levy LL. Blood pressure after stroke. JAMA. 1981;246:2177–80.
2. Britton M, Carlsson A, de Faire U. Blood pressure course in patients with acute stroke and matched controls. Stroke. 1986;17:861–4.
3. Qureshi AI, Ezzeddine MA, Nasar A, Suri MFK, Kirmani JF, Hussein HM, Divani AA, Reddi AS. Prevalence of elevated blood pressure in 563,704 adult patients with stroke presenting to the ED in the United States. Am J Emerg Med. 2007;25:32–8.
4. CAST: randomised placebo-controlled trial of early aspirin use in 20,000 patients with acute ischaemic stroke. CAST (Chinese Acute Stroke Trial) Collaborative Group. Lancet 1997;349:1641–49.
5. The International Stroke Trial (IST): a randomised trial of aspirin, subcutaneous heparin, both, or neither among 19435 patients with acute ischaemic stroke. International Stroke Trial Collaborative Group. Lancet 1997;349:1569–81.

6. Harper G, Castleden CM, Potter JF. Factors affecting changes in blood pressure after acute stroke. Stroke. 1994;25:1726–9.
7. Broderick J, Brott T, Barsan W, Haley EC, Levy D, Marler J, Sheppard G, Blum C. Blood pressure during the first minutes of focal cerebral ischemia. Ann Emerg Med. 1993;22:1438–43.
8. Chamorro A, Vila N, Ascaso C, Elices E, Schonewille W, Blanc R. Blood pressure and functional recovery in acute ischemic stroke. Stroke. 1998;29:1850–3.
9. Mattle HP, Kappeler L, Arnold M, Fischer U, Nedeltchev K, Remonda L, Jakob SM, Schroth G. Blood pressure and vessel recanalization in the first hours after ischemic stroke. Stroke. 2005;36:264–8.
10. Vemmos KN, Tsivgoulis G, Spengos K, Zakopoulos N, Synetos A, Manios E, Konstantopoulou P, Mavrikakis M. U-shaped relationship between mortality and admission blood pressure in patients with acute stroke. J Intern Med. 2004;255:257–65.
11. Leonardi-Bee J, Bath PMW, Phillips SJ, Sandercock PAG, IST Collaborative Group. Blood pressure and clinical outcomes in the International Stroke Trial. Stroke. 2002;33:1315–20.
12. Stead LG, Gilmore RM, Vedula KC, Weaver AL, Decker WW, Brown RD. Impact of acute blood pressure variability on ischemic stroke outcome. Neurology. 2006;66:1878–81.
13. Ahmed N, Wahlgren G. High initial blood pressure after acute stroke is associated with poor functional outcome. J Intern Med. 2001;249:467–73.
14. Sare GM, Ali M, Shuaib A, Bath PMW, for the VISTA Collaboration. Relationship between hyperacute blood pressure and outcome after ischemic stroke: data from the VISTA collaboration. Stroke. 2009;40:2098–103.
15. Ishitsuka K, Kamouchi M, Hata J, Fukuda K, Matsuo R, Kuroda J, Ago T, Kuwashiro T, Sugimori H, Nakane H, Kitazono T, Investigators FSR. High blood pressure after acute ischemic stroke is associated with poor clinical outcomes: Fukuoka Stroke Registry. Hypertension. 2014;63:54–60.
16. Jensen MB, Yoo B, Clarke WR, Davis PH, Adams HR. Blood pressure as an independent prognostic factor in acute ischemic stroke. Can J Neurol Sci. 2006;33:34–8.
17. Strandgaard S, Paulson OB. Cerebral autoregulation. Stroke. 1984;15:413–6.
18. Paulson OB, Strandgaard S, Edvinsson L. Cerebral autoregulation. Cerebrovasc Brain Metab Rev. 1990;2:161–92.
19. Lang EW, Lagopoulos J, Griffith J, Yip K, Yam A, Mudaliar Y, Mehdorn HM, Dorsch NWC. Cerebral vasomotor reactivity testing in head injury: the link between pressure and flow. J Neurol Neurosurg Psychiatr. 2003;74:1053–9.
20. Agnoli A, Fieschi C, Bozzao L, Battistini N, Prencipe M. Autoregulation of cerebral blood flow. Studies during drug-induced hypertension in normal subjects and in patients with cerebral vascular diseases. Circulation. 1968;38:800–12.
21. Paulson OB, Lassen NA, Skinhoj E. Regional cerebral blood flow in apoplexy without arterial occlusion. Neurology. 1970;20:125–38.
22. Paulson OB. Regional cerebral blood flow in apoplexy due to occlusion of the middle cerebral artery. Neurology. 1970;20:63–77.
23. Pozzilli C, Di Piero V, Pantano P, Rasura M, Lenzi GL. Influence of nimodipine on cerebral blood flow in human cerebral ischaemia. J Neurol. 1989;236:199–202.
24. Vorstrup S, Andersen A, Blegvad N, Paulson OB. Calcium antagonist (PY 108-068) treatment may further decrease flow in ischemic areas in acute stroke. J Cereb Blood Flow Metab. 1986;6:222–9.
25. Powers WJ, Videen TO, Diringer MN, Aiyagari V, Zazulia AR. Autoregulation after ischaemic stroke. J Hypertens. 2009;27:2218–22.
26. Jauch EC, Saver JL, Adams HP, Bruno A, Connors JJB, Demaerschalk BM, Khatri P, McMullan PW, Qureshi AI, Rosenfield K, Scott PA, Summers DR, Wang DZ, Wintermark M, Yonas H, Council AHAS, Council on Cardiovascular Nursing, Council on Peripheral Vascular Disease, Council on Clinical Cardiology. Guidelines for the early management of patients with acute ischemic stroke: a guideline for healthcare professionals from the American Heart Association/American Stroke Association. Stroke. 2013;44:870–947.
27. Hornig CR, Dorndorf W, Agnoli AL. Hemorrhagic cerebral infarction—a prospective study. Stroke. 1986;17:179–85.

28. Geeganage C, Bath PMW (2008) Interventions for deliberately altering blood pressure in acute stroke. Cochrane Database Syst Rev. CD000039
29. Potter JF, Robinson TG, Ford GA, Mistri A, James M, Chernova J, Jagger C. Controlling hypertension and hypotension immediately post-stroke (CHHIPS): a randomised, placebo-controlled, double-blind pilot trial. Lancet Neurol. 2009;8:48–56.
30. Sandset EC, Bath PMW, Boysen G, Jatuzis D, Kõrv J, Lüders S, Murray GD, Richter PS, Roine RO, Terént A, Thijs V, Berge E, SCAST Study Group. The angiotensin-receptor blocker candesartan for treatment of acute stroke (SCAST): a randomised, placebo-controlled, double-blind trial. Lancet. 2011;377:741–50.
31. He J, Zhang Y, Xu T, Zhao Q, Wang D, Chen C-S, Tong W, Liu C, Xu T, Ju Z, Peng Y, Peng H, Li Q, Geng D, Zhang J, Li D, Zhang F, Guo L, Sun Y, Wang X, Cui Y, Li Y, Ma D, Yang G, Gao Y, Yuan X, Bazzano LA, Chen J. Effects of immediate blood pressure reduction on death and major disability in patients with acute ischemic stroke. JAMA. 2014;311:479–89.
32. Robinson TG, Potter JF, Ford GA, Bulpitt CJ, Chernova J, Jagger C, James MA, Knight J, Markus HS, Mistri AK, Poulter NR, Investigators OBOTC. Effects of antihypertensive treatment after acute stroke in the Continue or Stop Post-Stroke Antihypertensives Collaborative Study (COSSACS): a prospective, randomised, open, blinded-endpoint trial. Lancet Neurol. 2010;9:767–75.
33. Investigators TET. Efficacy of nitric oxide, with or without continuing antihypertensive treatment, for management of high blood pressure in acute stroke (ENOS): a partial-factorial randomised controlled trial. Lancet. 2015;385:617–28.
34. Oh MS, Yu K-H, Hong K-S, Kang D-W, Park J-M, Bae H-J, Koo J, Lee J, Lee B-C. Valsartan efficacy oN modesT blood pressUre REduction in acute ischemic stroke (VENTURE) study group. Modest blood pressure reduction with valsartan in acute ischemic stroke: a prospective, randomized, open-label, blinded-end-point trial. Int J Stroke. 2015;10(5):745–51. doi:10.1111/ijs.12446.
35. James PA, Oparil S, Carter BL, Cushman WC, Dennison-Himmelfarb C, Handler J, Lackland DT, LeFevre ML, MacKenzie TD, Ogedegbe O, Smith Jr SC, Svetkey LP, Taler SJ, Townsend RR, Wright Jr JT, Narva AS, Ortiz E. 2014 evidence-based guideline for the management of high blood pressure in adults. JAMA. 2014;311:507–14.
36. Levy DE, Brott TG, Haley EC, Marler JR, Sheppard GL, Barsan W, Broderick JP. Factors related to intracranial hematoma formation in patients receiving tissue-type plasminogen activator for acute ischemic stroke. Stroke. 1994;25:291–7.
37. Tissue plasminogen activator for acute ischemic stroke. The National Institute of Neurological Disorders and Stroke rt-PA Stroke Study Group. N Engl J Med. 1995;333:1581–87.
38. Wityk RJ, Lewin JJ. Blood pressure management during acute ischaemic stroke. Expert Opin Pharmacother. 2006;7:247–58.
39. Lopez-Yunez AM, Bruno A, Williams LS, Yilmaz E, Zurru C, Biller J. Protocol violations in community-based rTPA stroke treatment are associated with symptomatic intracerebral hemorrhage. Stroke. 2001;32:12–6.
40. Ahmed N, Wahlgren N, Brainin M, Castillo J, Ford GA, Kaste M, Lees KR, Toni D, Investigators SITS. Relationship of blood pressure, antihypertensive therapy, and outcome in ischemic stroke treated with intravenous thrombolysis: retrospective analysis from Safe Implementation of Thrombolysis in Stroke-International Stroke Thrombolysis Register (SITS-ISTR). Stroke. 2009;40:2442–9.
41. European Stroke Organisation (ESO) Executive Committee, ESO Writing Committee. Guidelines for management of ischaemic stroke and transient ischaemic attack 2008. Cerebrovasc Dis. 2008;25:457–507.
42. Authors/Task Force M, Mancia G, Fagard R, Narkiewicz K, Redon J, Zanchetti A, Bohm M, Christiaens T, Cifkova R, De Backer G, Dominiczak A, Galderisi M, Grobbee DE, Jaarsma T, Kirchhof P, Kjeldsen SE, Laurent S, Manolis AJ, Nilsson PM, Ruilope LM, Schmieder RE, Sirnes PA, Sleight P, Viigimaa M, Waeber B, Zannad F, Scientific Council ESH, Redon J, Dominiczak A, Narkiewicz K, Nilsson PM, Burnier M, Viigimaa M, Ambrosioni E, Caufield M, Coca A, Olsen MH, Schmieder RE, Tsioufis C, van de Borne P, ESC Committee for Practice Guidelines (CPG), Zamorano JL, Achenbach S, Baumgartner H, Bax JJ, Bueno H, Dean V,

Deaton C, Erol C, Fagard R, Ferrari R, Hasdai D, Hoes AW, Kirchhof P, Knuuti J, Kolh P, Lancellotti P, Linhart A, Nihoyannopoulos P, Piepoli MF, Ponikowski P, Sirnes PA, Tamargo JL, Tendera M, Torbicki A, Wijns W, Windecker S, Document R, Clement DL, Coca A, Gillebert TC, Tendera M, Rosei EA, Ambrosioni E, Anker SD, Bauersachs J, Hitij JB, Caulfield M, De Buyzere M, De Geest S, Derumeaux GA, Erdine S, Farsang C, Funck-Brentano C, Gerc V, Germano G, Gielen S, Haller H, Hoes AW, Jordan JD, Kahan T, Komajda M, Lovic D, Mahrholdt H, Olsen MH, Ostergren J, Parati G, Perk J, Polonia J, Popescu BA, Reiner Z, Ryden L, Sirenko Y, Stanton A, Struijker-Boudier H, Tsioufis C, van de Borne P, Vlachopoulos C, Volpe M, Wood DA. 2013 ESH/ESC Guidelines for the management of arterial hypertension: The Task Force for the management of arterial hypertension of the European Society of Hypertension (ESH) and of the European Society of Cardiology (ESC). Eur Heart J. 2013;34:2159–219.
43. Liu-DeRyke X, Janisse J, Coplin WM, Parker Jr D, Norris G, Rhoney DH. A comparison of nicardipine and labetalol for acute hypertension management following stroke. Neurocrit Care. 2008;9:167–76.
44. Liu-DeRyke X, Levy PD, Parker D, Coplin W, Rhoney DH. A prospective evaluation of labetalol versus nicardipine for blood pressure management in patients with acute stroke. Neurocrit Care. 2013;19:41–7.

Chapter 9
Hypertensive Encephalopathy, Posterior Reversible Encephalopathy Syndrome, and Eclampsia

Karen Orjuela and Sean D. Ruland

Hypertension affects approximately a third of US adults. From 2007 to 2010, an estimated 78 million people greater than 20 years old were affected. Up to 6 % of US adults have undiagnosed hypertension [1]. This population is at risk of developing myocardial infarction, stroke, renal injury, congestive heart failure, peripheral vascular disease, and hypertensive emergencies [2].

Chronic uncontrolled blood pressure (BP) can have devastating acute neurologic complications. According to the National Health and Nutrition Evaluation Survey (NHANES) 2007–2010 report, just over half of patients with previously diagnosed hypertension were under control [3]. Uncontrolled hypertension is a major risk factor for developing stroke and present in 72 % of stroke patients [1]. End-organ dysfunction including the brain, kidneys, and heart can result from abrupt BP rises in undertreated individuals. Hypertensive encephalopathy (HE) is one of the most serious conditions acutely affecting the brain. Eclampsia, a related condition associated with pregnancy-induced hypertension, can have life-threatening consequences to both mother and fetus. This chapter will discuss the diagnosis, management, and treatment of hypertensive encephalopathy, the posterior reversible encephalopathy syndrome (PRES), and eclampsia.

K. Orjuela, M.D.
Department of Neurology, Loyola University Medical Center, Maywood, IL, USA
e-mail: korjuela@lumc.edu

S.D. Ruland, D.O. (✉)
Department of Neurology, Stritch School of Medicine, Loyola University Chicago, 2160 S. First Ave., Maywood, IL 60153, USA
e-mail: sruland@lumc.edu

© Springer International Publishing Switzerland 2016
V. Aiyagari, P.B. Gorelick (eds.), *Hypertension and Stroke*, Clinical
Hypertension and Vascular Diseases, DOI 10.1007/978-3-319-29152-9_9

Hypertensive Encephalopathy

Historical Overview

Several terms have been historically used to describe and classify acute BP elevation. The term malignant hypertension was first used by Volhard and Farh in 1914 [4, 5] after noting that many patients with severe hypertension had fundoscopic changes such as retinopathy and papilledema in addition to renal insufficiency. They defined malignant hypertension as an elevated BP with signs of acute end-organ damage [5]. Keith and Wagener subsequently broadened this definition by noting that renal dysfunction was not an obligatory requirement for acute hypertensive damage. They also used the term "accelerated hypertension" and defined it as severe BP elevation with retinal hemorrhages and exudates in the absence of papilledema [6]. Oppenheimer and Fishberg coined the term "hypertensive encephalopathy" in 1928 when they described a 19-year-old student with malignant hypertension associated with headache, convulsions, and neurologic deficits [7].

Malignant hypertension and accelerated hypertension are terms that can still be found in the medical literature. Hypertensive crisis is a term which includes hypertensive emergencies and urgencies. A hypertensive emergency is characterized by an elevation in systolic blood pressure (SBP) >180 mmHg or diastolic blood pressure (DBP) >120 mmHg associated with progressive or impending end-organ dysfunction such as HE, intracerebral hemorrhage, unstable angina pectoris, dissecting aortic aneurysm, acute kidney injury, or eclampsia. A hypertensive emergency is an acute severe rise in BP without progressive end-organ damage [8].

Epidemiology

Chronic hypertension affects approximately 1 billion adults worldwide and it is estimated that by 2025, 1.56 billion will be affected [8]. One percent of patients with chronic hypertension will experience a hypertensive crisis. In the USA, approximately 20 million emergency department visits annually are related to hypertension. Among patients at 114 US hospitals from 2005 to 2007, the incidence of SBP>180 mmHg was 14%. An independent correlation between mortality and a primary neurological reason for initial blood pressure elevation was detected [8, 9].

An Italian study reported that hypertensive crisis represented 25% of 1634 medical presentations to the emergency department during 2009. Nearly a fourth had end-organ dysfunction of which neurologic deficits accounted for 21% [10]. Undiagnosed hypertension and noncompliance with prescribed medications were found to be risk factors for presentation. The Studying the Treatment of Acute hyperTension (STAT) Registry reported younger age, African American race and history of hypertension as risk factors for hypertensive crisis [11]. More than a quarter of patients enrolled in the STAT Registry were readmitted at least once for acute severe hypertension within 90 days [12]. A retrospective study of 200 patients with malignant hypertension identified during the 1960s–1980s reported a 2-year survival rate of 50–80 % [13]. More recent studies have reported 5-year survival rates of 74 % approaching 70 % at 10 years [14, 15].

Clinical

HE accounts for nearly 16 % of all hypertensive emergencies. This phenomenon occurs when mean arterial pressure (MAP) is beyond the upper limit of cerebrovascular autoregulation, resulting in resistance vessel failure [16]. Neurological signs and symptoms occur suddenly [17]. The most common neurological manifestations are headache and visual disturbances. Others include alteration of consciousness, nausea, vomiting, seizures, and focal sensorimotor deficits [18]. It is the rate of increase rather than the absolute BP value that is thought to induce end-organ dysfunction [17].

The fundoscopic examination of individuals with HE frequently, but not always, reveals retinal exudates and hemorrhages (Keith-Wagener-Barker grade 3), and papilledema (Keith-Wagener-Barker grade 4) [19]. The presence of grade 3–4 retinopathy is associated with microvascular renal damage [20]. Even though the majority of patients with hypertensive emergency present with symptoms due to only one type of end-organ damage, evidence of other organ dysfunction is commonly seen [21]. HE can result in cerebral hemorrhage, coma, and death [16]. However, with proper treatment, it can be reversible [21].

Pathophysiology

Although the pathophysiology of HE is not completely understood, the effects of elevated BP on cerebrovascular autoregulation have been well studied. Cerebral perfusion pressure (CPP) is the difference between MAP and intracranial pressure or central venous pressure if the latter is higher [22]. Autoregulation is the intrinsic capacity of the cerebral vasculature to maintain constant cerebral blood flow (CBF) within a wide range of CPP by altering resistance in precapillary arterioles [22, 23].

The cerebrovascular resistance adapts to varying perfusion pressures, in part by activating the sympathetic nervous system and activating or suppressing the renin–angiotensin–aldosterone system (RAAS) [24]. Local mediators such as nitric oxide (NO), a vasodilator released in response to shear stress, and endothelin-1, a vasoconstrictor which activates the RAAS, are released by the endothelium and contribute to the maintenance of CBF [25]. Under normal conditions, the cerebral autoregulatory system maintains a constant CBF in the capillary bed within a MAP of 60–150 mmHg. If BP increases beyond that limit, the blood brain barrier can be damaged causing cerebral edema [16]. This limit is higher in chronic hypertensive patients.

During a hypertensive emergency, the endothelium responds to an abrupt BP increase by releasing NO. When hypertension is sustained or severe, the endothelial vasodilator response becomes overwhelmed, eventually leading to a state of increased resistance. Ongoing endothelial damage from persistent hypertension leads to production of inflammatory cytokines and increases endothelin-1. These events increase endothelial permeability, inhibit fibrinolysis, and activate coagulation [26]. An aggrandizement of the RAAS also plays a prominent role in vascular injury and tissue ischemia. These changes result in a breakdown of the blood–brain barrier, cerebral edema, and microhemorrhages [27].

Normotensive individuals can develop end-organ damage with an acute increase of DBP above as low as 100 mmHg, whereas chronically hypertensive individuals usually do not develop acute end-organ damage until DBP reaches 130 mmHg [16, 28].

Functional and structural adaptive responses in individuals with chronic hypertension protect the capillary bed from acute rises in BP due to chronic luminal narrowing and arterial hypertrophy from sustained smooth muscle contraction and increase cerebrovascular resistance [24, 29]. However, the brain is left vulnerable to ischemia at low CPP [30].

The pathophysiology of HE has been debated over the last century, but technological advances continue to provide insightful clues into its complicated pathogenesis. Acutely, there is cerebral autoregulatory failure at very high pressures [31]. One theory proposes that overregulation or spasm of cerebral vessels in response to acutely rising BP leads to decreased CBF, ischemia, intra-arterial thrombosis, and cytotoxic edema [32]. Another theory proposes a breakthrough phenomenon whereby forced vessel dilation leads to hydrostatic edema [33]. The preponderance of recent evidence supports the latter theory [34].

Insight regarding the pathophysiologic mechanism of HE can be gleaned when considering acute treatment. If HE was due to overregulation of the cerebral vasculature leading to ischemia and cytotoxic edema, [35] acute goal-directed treatment would allow for systemic BP increases to maintain CPP and prevent further ischemia [36]. However, treatment of perfusion breakthrough directs acute therapy toward a relative reduction of BP rather than permissive hypertension [8, 33].

Workup

While evaluating patients with HE, in addition to performing a thorough neurological examination, evidence for increased jugular venous pressure, abdominal bruits, abnormal peripheral pulses, and pulmonary edema should be sought. Laboratory studies should include a complete blood count, metabolic profile, urinalysis, cardiac enzymes, and toxicology studies. Additionally, an electrocardiogram and chest radiograph can be useful for detecting cardiac ischemia, left ventricular hypertrophy, pulmonary edema, and aortic dissection. Neuroimaging should be performed early to evaluate for evidence consistent with HE or alternative causes of neurological dysfunction.

Magnetic Resonance Imaging

In cases of HE, brain magnetic resonance imaging (MRI) typically reveals increased signal intensity on T2 and fluid-attenuated inversion recovery (FLAIR) sequences. Lesions can be iso- or hypointense on T1-weighted images [36]. Evidence for restricted diffusion is usually absent, supporting the perfusion breakthrough hypothesis [33, 37, 38]. However restricted diffusion can be present in nearly 25% of patients with HE and contrast enhancement can be seen in about 15% [39].

The lesions predominantly involve symmetric subcortical parieto-occipital white matter regions. Two-thirds of patients have frontal and temporal lobe involvement and a third of patients will have brainstem, cerebellum, or basal ganglia affected (Figs. 9.1 and 9.2) [38, 39]. The lesions can be asymmetric in up to 40%

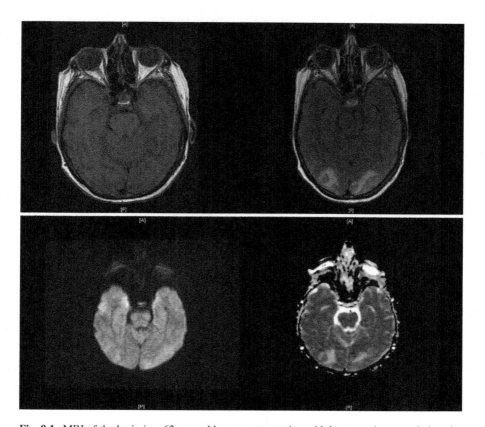

Fig. 9.1 MRI of the brain in a 62-year-old woman presenting with hypertensive encephalopathy reveals predominance of vasogenic edema in the subcortical posterior white matter. Unenhanced T1-weighted image (*upper left*) showing isointense lesion; T2-weighted FLAIR image (*upper right*) showing increased signal in posterior white matter

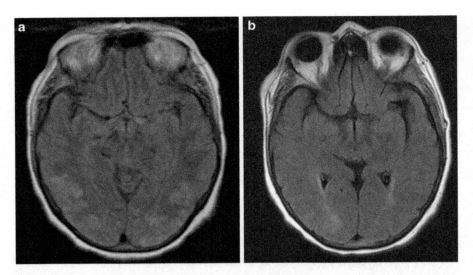

Fig. 9.2 MRI of the brain in a 21-year-old man presenting with headache, confusion, and visual scotomas. (**a**) T2-weighted FLAIR image showing increased signal in bilateral occipital and temporal lobes. (**b**) T2-weighted FLAIR image done a week later showing lesion resolution

of patients [39]. They can resolve completely with proper BP lowering [36, 38, 40]. The occipital lobe predilection is thought to be due to a paucity of sympathetic innervation in the posterior circulation, thus rendering it more susceptible to vasodilatory responses [41, 42].

Posterior Reversible Encephalopathy Syndrome

The typical neurological and imaging findings of HE are similar to the PRES. PRES has been associated with eclampsia, preeclampsia, chemotherapy regimens, immunosuppressant agents used after organ transplantation and a host of other systemic disorders and agents (Table 9.1) [43].

Two main pathophysiologic theories have been postulated with overlap to that of HE. One theory is that PRES can occur secondary to cerebral autoregulatory system impairment leading to disrupted blood brain barrier integrity. The second theory is that systemic toxicity causes endothelial dysfunction and vasogenic edema in the presence or absence of elevated BP. This has been demonstrated in animal models and supported by modern neuroimaging [30, 38, 44, 45]. In a report from the Critically Ill Posterior Reversible Encephalopathy Syndrome Study Group (CYPRESS), the most common clinical presentation was impaired consciousness,

Table 9.1 Predisposing conditions that have been associated with PRES

Medications and other agents	Systemic disorders
Aluminum toxicity	Eclampsia
Azathioprine	Hepatic encephalopathy
Bevacizumab	Hypertensive encephalopathy
Bortezomib	Infections
Caffeine	Systemic inflammatory response syndrome
Carboplatin	Multiorgan dysfunction syndrome
Cisplatin	Metabolic abnormalities
Corticosteroids	Hypomagnesemia
Cyclosporin A	Hypercalcemia
Cyclophosphamide	Hypocholesterolemia
Cytarabine	Renal disorders
Doxorubicin	Hemolytic uremic syndrome
Ephedrine	Hepatorenal syndrome
Erlotinib	Glomerulonephritis
Erythropoietin	Nephrotic syndrome
5-Fluorouracil	Rheumatologic disorders
Gemcitabine	Systemic lupus erythematosus
Granulocyte colony stimulating factor	Primary systemic sclerosis
Growth factor	Granulomatosis with polyangiitis
Interferon alfa	Polyarteritis nodosa
Intravenous immunoglobulin	Rheumatoid arthritis
Iodinated contrast	Antiphospholipid antibody syndrome
L-Asparaginase	Pheochromocytoma
Linezolid	Primary aldosteronism
Methotrexate (intravenous and intrathecal)	Tumor lysis syndrome
Midodrine	
Oxaliplatin	
Oxybutynin	
Phenylpropanolamine	
Pseudoephedrine	
Rituximab	
Sirolimus	
Sorafenib	
Sunitinib	
Tacrolimus	
Temsirolimus	
Vinblastine	
Vincristine	
Vinorelbine	

From Le EM, Loghin ME. Posterior reversible encephalopathy syndrome: a neurologic phenomenon in cancer patients. Current oncology reports. 2014;16(5):1–9, with permission followed by clinical seizures and an associated MAP more than 122 mmHg. Parieto-occipital involvement was more frequently found in CYPRESS although atypical presentations involving fronto-temporal lobes and gray matter were reported. Lesions were reversible in 43 % of patients that had follow-up imaging.

Treatment

In patients with hypertensive urgency, BP can gradually be lowered over 24–48 h with oral medications in a nonintensive care unit setting. However, all patients with hypertensive emergency should be treated with intravenous medications in an intensive care unit, commonly with invasive BP monitoring [17]. In order to prevent hypoperfusion and cerebral ischemia in patients with a right-shifted autoregulation curve, rapid BP correction should be avoided [46]. Short-acting and easily titratable continuous BP-lowering agents are preferred (Table 9.2). Intramuscular and sublingual routes are unpredictable and should be avoided [47–49]. It is reasonable to lower the DBP 10–15 % over 30–60 min or reduce MAP by 25 % over 8 h if MAP at presentation exceeds 150 mmHg [8, 22]. If neurological deterioration occurs during BP lowering, treatment should be suspended [16, 22]. Volume resuscitation with saline should be considered, as many patients presenting with hypertensive emergencies are dehydrated [47].

Recognition of simultaneous cardiac or renal involvement is important when choosing among therapeutic options. Additionally, some BP-lowering agents should be avoided during treatment of HE. Sublingual nifedipine can cause a sudden uncontrolled BP drop within 5–10 min after administration that can precipitate cerebral ischemia [47, 50]. Elderly individuals are particularly susceptible [51]. Nitroglycerine is a potent venodilator and can cause hypotension with reflex tachycardia. It also reduces preload and cardiac output which may compromise cerebral perfusion. Headache is a common side effect [47]. Hydralazine is a vasodilator that, when given parenteral, can cause an unpredictable fall in BP lasting up to 12 h [52]. Sodium nitroprusside is an arterial and venous dilator that may theoretically decrease CBF while increasing intracranial pressure although the clinical significance is contested [53]. Additionally, sodium nitroprusside contains 44 % cyanide by weight which is metabolized to thiocyanate, requiring intact liver and renal functions for adequate removal [54]. Cyanide toxicity can cause cardiac arrest, coma, encephalopathy, seizures, and irreversible focal neurological deficits. It should be avoided in patients with hereditary optic neuropathy [55, 56].

Labetalol, nicardipine, and esmolol are preferred initial agents for BP treatment in HE [22] (Table 9.2). Labetalol is a combined selective alpha 1-adrenergic and nonselective beta-adrenergic receptor blocker with sevenfold greater effect on the B receptors compared to the alpha receptors [56, 57]. Onset of action for IV labetalol is 2–5 min and peaks at 5–15 min with duration of action 2–4 h. Cardiac output and CBF are maintained while systemic vascular resistance is reduced [57]. Nicardipine is an IV dihydropyridine-derived calcium channel blocker [58]. It exhibits vascular

Table 9.2 Antihypertensive agents used in neurological emergencies

Agent	Dosing	Onset/duration of action	Advantages	Disadvantages
Esmolol	500 μg/kg IV bolus or 25–300 μg/kg/min IV infusion	60 s/10–20 min	Short acting and metabolized via red blood cells	Bradyarrhythmia, heart failure, beta blockers
Fenoldopam	0.1–0.3 mg/kg/min IV infusion	4–5 min/30–60 min	No CNS effects or toxic metabolites	Headache, tachycardia, increase intraocular pressure. Caution in intracranial hypertension and myocardial infarction. Allergic reactions when mixed with sodium met bisulfate
Hydralazine	10–20 mg IV bolus	10 min/>1 h	Safe in pregnancy	Unpredictable drop in BP, tachycardia
Labetalol	5–20 mg IV bolus every 15 min, up to 2 mg/min IV infusion	2–5 min/2–4 h	Maintains cardiac output and cerebral blood flow	Bronchospasm, bradycardia
Nicardipine	5–15 mg/h IV infusion	5–15 min/3 h	Cerebral vasodilation, reduces cerebral ischemia	Reflex tachycardia
Sodium Nitroprusside	0.25–10 μg/kg/min IV infusion	Immediate/2–3 min	Immediate onset	Possible increase in ICH, cyanide toxicity

IV intravenous, *CNS* central nervous system, *BP* blood pressure, *ICH* intracerebral hemorrhage

selectivity and has a strong cerebral vasodilator activity that has been shown to reduce cerebral ischemia. Onset of action is 5–15 min, and the duration can be up to 3 h [58]. Clevidipine is a third generation dihydropyridine-derived calcium channel blocker that has been studied in multiple trials but no specific indication exists to date for hypertensive crisis.

Esmolol is a cardioselective beta-adrenergic blocker that is extremely short acting. Onset of action is within 60 s with duration of 10–20 min. The metabolism of esmolol is via esterases in the cytosol of red blood cells and is not affected by renal or hepatic dysfunction. It may be used as both a bolus and an infusion, but is contraindicated in patients with bradyarrhythmias, heart failure, and concomitant treatment with beta blockers. Its effect can be prolonged in patients with anemia due to fewer available esterases. Lastly, IV fenoldopam, a selective dopamine-1 receptor agonist which dilates the systemic and renal arteries promoting diuresis, may be considered [59]. Its onset of action is 4–5 min, peaks within 15 min, and lasts 30–60 min [56, 59].

Fenoldopam can cause tachycardia and increased intraocular pressure. It should not be administered to patients with glaucoma and administered with caution in patients with intracranial hypertension and myocardial infarction. Allergic reactions can occur when mixed with solutions that contain sodium met bisulfate [56, 59].

Once BP is adequately controlled with initial treatment and neurological symptoms resolve, oral antihypertensive agents can be started while IV agents are slowly weaned [48]. The long-term treatment goal is blood pressure <140/90 mmHg in less than 60-year-old patients and <150/90 mmHg in patients older than 60 years. In patients with diabetes mellitus or renal disease, goal blood pressure should be <140/90 [60]. The majority of patients will require two or more agents from different drug classes to reach their goal. Specific drug classes are recommended for black Americans, diabetics, and patients with chronic kidney disease and are beyond the scope of this chapter. Adoption of lifestyle modifications should include weight loss, healthy diet, physical activity, limited alcohol intake, and smoking cessation [60]. Management strategies should focus on individual patient goals and foster adherence.

Eclampsia

Eclampsia (preeclampsia-eclampsia) is one of four hypertensive disorders of pregnancy that include chronic hypertension, chronic hypertension with superimposed preeclampsia, and gestational hypertension [61]. Its syndrome is defined by convulsive seizures in the absence of prior epilepsy in patients with established preeclampsia.

Historical Overview

Varandaeus first introduced the term eclampsia in 1619. However, its clinical presentation and pathological concepts have been recognized since ancient times. The word "eclampsia" comes from the Greek word *eklampsis*, meaning lightning, due to the striking and acute presentation reflecting the sudden onset of convulsions. Hippocrates described headaches, heaviness, and convulsions during pregnancy in the Coan Prognosis writings. During that time, the humor theory grouped all pathologies according to an imbalance between blood, phlegm, and yellow and black bile.

Hippocrates, in the fourth to fifth centuries Before Current Era (BCE), believed that the uterus traveled around the body affecting the liver, heart, brain, and kidneys to establish equilibrium. Early treatments aimed to restore balance with diet, bloodletting, and purging [62]. In 1596, during the Renaissance, a classification scheme considering a pregnant uterus an epileptic condition was proposed. Since the nineteenth century great scientific efforts have been made to understand this complex, common, and lethal disorder. The theory of vascular failure from incompetent placental spiral arteries was proposed from direct examination of tissue specimens. Aggressive management such as termination of pregnancy was considered. During the twentieth century, treatment with magnesium sulfate was introduced. Its utility in preeclampsia was first demonstrated by Horn in 1906 and, subsequently, its efficacy was established by Lazard and Dorsett in the 1920s. Since then, the knowledge about the disease has expanded although many questions remain regarding its pathogenesis. It is currently considered a form of PRES.

Epidemiology

Hypertensive disorders affect 10 % of all pregnancies worldwide. Maternal deaths related to hypertensive disorders account for 10 % of overall maternal deaths in Africa and Asia and 25 % in Latin America [61, 63]. Eclampsia occurs in 2–3 % of patients with symptoms of severe preeclampsia. Severe preeclampsia is defined as the presence of any of the following factors: two systemic BP readings >160 mmHg systolic and >110 mmHg diastolic, platelet count <100,000/µL, doubling of liver enzyme levels from baseline or right upper quadrant pain, creatinine concentration >1.1 mg/dL or twofold elevation from baseline, pulmonary edema, and visual or cerebral impairment. A third of patients with eclampsia are normotensive. In patients without severe preeclampsia, the incidence of eclampsia is 1–6 per 10,000 deliveries in developed countries and up to 157 per 10,000 deliveries in developing countries. Prior to 2013, proteinuria was considered part of the diagnostic criteria of preeclampsia but is no longer required.

Clinical Presentation

The presence of generalized tonic-clonic seizures in a patient with preeclampsia and no history of epilepsy is diagnostic of eclampsia. Other symptoms include headache, visual disturbances, and right upper quadrant pain [64, 65]. Seizures are associated with signs of fetal distress including bradycardia immediately after the seizure lasting for about 3–5 min and transient decelerations. Recurrent decelerations of fetal heart rate lasting 10–15 min should raise suspicion for occult abruptio placenta.

Approximately 90 % of patients with eclampsia present after 28 weeks of gestation. It can also occur during delivery or up to 48 h postpartum [66]. Neurological findings include brisk muscle stretch reflexes, memory deficits, and decreased visual processing and perception.

Brain imaging, preferably with MRI, should be considered in pregnant patients with neurological signs or symptoms to also assess for cerebral venous thrombosis, ischemic stroke, and intracranial hemorrhage as these may mimic eclampsia. Vascular imaging should also be considered in selected circumstances as postpartum vasculopathy, a reversible cerebral vasoconstriction syndrome, can present similarly. MRI findings in patients with eclampsia are similar to PRES.

Although twentieth century studies reported postictal abnormalities in patients with eclampsia, electroencephalography has not been proven useful.

Pathophysiology

The precise trigger for preeclampsia and eclampsia is uncertain. Complex pathogenetic theories have been proposed such as involvement of an antiangiogenic state, defective deep placentation, oxidative and endoplasmic reticulum stress, angiotensin receptor autoantibodies, platelet and thrombin activation leading to intravascular inflammation, and endothelial dysfunction disrupting angiogenesis. The antiangiogenic state involves elevated circulating levels of soluble endoglin and soluble Fms-like tyrosine kinase (sFlt1) produced predominantly by the placenta and also by circulating monocytes. sFlt-1 binds circulating and tissue-based factors such as vascular endothelial growth factor (VEGF) and placental growth factor (PlGF) inhibiting angiogenesis [67]. Maternal susceptibility factors can determine the individual clinical course of preeclamptic women.

Treatment

Magnesium sulfate remains the first line treatment for seizures in eclampsia. When compared to phenytoin and diazepam, the Eclampsia Trial Collaborative Group reported that magnesium sulfate was more effective in preventing recurrent seizures. Moreover, magnesium sulfate was shown to prevent initial seizures and reduce the risk of maternal death compared to placebo in women with preeclampsia in the Magpie Trial without any adverse impact to mother or child [68].

The loading dose of magnesium sulfate is 6 g IV over 20–30 min, with maintenance infusion of 2–3 g IV per hour. If seizures recur reload with 2 g over 5–10 min and repeat if needed. If seizures persist, treatment with benzodiazepines such as diazepam and lorazepam should be cautiously considered due to depressant effects in fetus and mother. Close monitoring of the clinical exam and serum magnesium levels is required to assess for possible toxicity. Exercise caution in patients with renal failure and infusions should be limited to less than 12 h. In cases of persistent fetal distress, prompt delivery is required. Termination of pregnancy may be considered as it is a definitive treatment for eclampsia [61, 63].

Summary

Hypertension is a prevalent disease, and nearly 1 % of hypertensive individuals will experience a hypertensive crisis in their lifetime. HE is a clinical manifestation of hypertensive crisis characterized by headache, visual disturbance, altered mental status, seizures, and focal sensorimotor deficits in the setting of an abrupt BP increase. Cerebral autoregulation can fail with an acute severe increase of BP leading to endothelial permeability, fibrin deposition, and vasogenic edema with a characteristic imaging distribution in the occipital lobes. MRI abnormalities and clinical symptoms are typically reversible with appropriate prompt treatment. Early recognition and judicious BP lowering is paramount. PRES overlaps with HE. Both have similar clinical presentation and imaging findings but PRES can be due to various medical and pharmacological etiologies. Treatment of predisposing medical conditions and removal of exacerbating medications is indicated. Eclampsia is a related neurological complication associated with pregnancy-induced hypertension characterized by headaches, seizures, and visual disturbances. Early initiation of magnesium sulfate is indicated to prevent seizures and maternal mortality.

References

1. Go AS, Mozaffarian D, Roger VL, Benjamin EJ, Berry JD, Borden WB, et al. Executive summary: heart disease and stroke statistics—2013 update: a report from the American heart association. Circulation. 2013;127(1):143–52.
2. Polgreen LA, Suneja M, Tang F, Carter BL, Polgreen PM. Increasing trend in admissions for malignant hypertension and hypertensive encephalopathy in the United States. Hypertension. 2015;65(5):1002–7.
3. Go AS, Bauman MA, Coleman King SM, Fonarow GC, Lawrence W, Williams KA, et al. An effective approach to high blood pressure control: a science advisory from the American Heart Association, the American College of Cardiology, and the Centers for Disease Control and Prevention. J Am Coll Cardiol. 2014;63(12):1230–8.
4. Rosenberg EF. The brain in malignant hypertension: a clinicopathologic study. Arch Intern Med. 1940;65(3):545–86.
5. Volhard FFTH. Die Brightsche Neirenkrankheir, KlinikPathologie Und Atlas, vol. 2. Berlin: Springer; 1914.
6. Keith Nm WHKJ. The syndrome of malignant hypertension. Arch Intern Med. 1928;41(2):141–88.
7. Oppenheimer Bs FA. Hypertensive encephalopathy. Arch Intern Med. 1928;41(2):264–78.
8. Pak KJ, Hu T, Fee C, Wang R, Smith M, Bazzano LA. Acute hypertension: a systematic review and appraisal of guidelines. Ochsner J. 2014;14(4):655–63.
9. Shorr AF, Zilberberg MD, Sun X, Johannes RS, Gupta V, Tabak YP. Severe acute hypertension among inpatients admitted from the emergency department. J Hosp Med. 2012;7(3):203–10.
10. Pinna G, Pascale C, Fornengo P, Arras S, Piras C, Panzarasa P, et al. Hospital admissions for hypertensive crisis in the emergency departments: a large multicenter Italian study. PLoS One. 2014;9(4), e93542.
11. Katz JN, Gore JM, Amin A, Anderson FA, Dasta JF, Ferguson JJ, et al. Practice patterns, outcomes, and end-organ dysfunction for patients with acute severe hypertension: the Studying the Treatment of Acute hyperTension (STAT) registry. Am Heart J. 2009;158(4):599–606.e1.
12. Gore JM, Peterson E, Amin A, Anderson Jr FA, Dasta JF, Levy PD, et al. Predictors of 90-day readmission among patients with acute severe hypertension. The cross-sectional observational Studying the Treatment of Acute hyperTension (STAT) study. Am Heart J. 2010;160(3):521–7.e1.
13. Ahmed ME, Walker JM, Beevers DG, Beevers M. Lack of difference between malignant and accelerated hypertension. Br Med J (Clin Res Ed). 1986;292(6515):235–7.
14. Lip GY, Beevers M, Beevers DG. Complications and survival of 315 patients with malignant-phase hypertension. J Hypertens. 1995;13(8):915–24.
15. Webster J, Petrie JC, Jeffers TA, Lovell HG. Accelerated hypertension—patterns of mortality and clinical factors affecting outcome in treated patients. Q J Med. 1993;86(8):485–93.

16. Manning L, Robinson TG, Anderson CS. Control of blood pressure in hypertensive neurological emergencies. Curr Hypertens Rep. 2014;16(6):436. doi:10.1007/s11906-014-0436-x.
17. Gardner CJ, Lee K. Hyperperfusion syndromes: insight into the pathophysiology and treatment of hypertensive encephalopathy. CNS Spectr. 2007;12(1):35–42.
18. Healton EB, Brust JC, Feinfeld DA, Thomson GE. Hypertensive encephalopathy and the neurologic manifestations of malignant hypertension. Neurology. 1982;32(2):127–32.
19. Elliott WJ. Clinical features in the management of selected hypertensive emergencies. Prog Cardiovasc Dis. 2006;48(5):316–25.
20. Muiesan ML, Salvetti M, Amadoro V, di Somma S, Perlini S, Semplicini A, et al. An update on hypertensive emergencies and urgencies. J Cardiovasc Med (Hagerstown). 2015;16(5):372–82.
21. Zampaglione B, Pascale C, Marchisio M, Cavallo-Perin P. Hypertensive urgencies and emergencies. Prevalence and clinical presentation. Hypertension. 1996;27(1):144–7.
22. Pancioli AM. Hypertension management in neurologic emergencies. Ann Emerg Med. 2008;51(3 Suppl):S24–7.
23. Immink RV, van den Born BJ, van Montfrans GA, Koopmans RP, Karemaker JM, van Lieshout JJ. Impaired cerebral autoregulation in patients with malignant hypertension. Circulation. 2004;110(15):2241–5.
24. Paulson OB, Waldemar G, Schmidt JF, Strandgaard S. Cerebral circulation under normal and pathologic conditions. Am J Cardiol. 1989;63(6):2C–5.
25. Cipolla MJ. Chapter 5: Control of cerebral blood flow. The Cerebral Circulation 2009. San Rafael (CA): Morgan & Claypool Life Science.
26. Verhaar MC, Beutler JJ, Gaillard CA, Koomans HA, Fijnheer R, Rabelink TJ. Progressive vascular damage in hypertension is associated with increased levels of circulating P-selectin. J Hypertens. 1998;16(1):45–50.
27. Blumenfeld JD, Laragh JH. Management of hypertensive crises: the scientific basis for treatment decisions. Am J Hypertens. 2001;14(11 Pt 1):1154–67.
28. Aggarwal M, Khan IA. Hypertensive crisis: hypertensive emergencies and urgencies. Cardiol Clin. 2006;24(1):135–46.
29. Strandgaard S, Jones JV, MacKenzie ET, Harper AM. Upper limit of cerebral blood flow autoregulation in experimental renovascular hypertension in the baboon. Circ Res. 1975;37(2):164–7.
30. Barry DI. Cerebral blood flow in hypertension. J Cardiovasc Pharmacol. 1985;7 Suppl 2:S94–8.
31. Paulson OB, Strandgaard S, Edvinsson L. Cerebral autoregulation. Cerebrovasc Brain Metab Rev. 1990;2(2):161–92.
32. Schwartz RB, Jones KM, Kalina P, Bajakian RL, Mantello MT, Garada B, et al. Hypertensive encephalopathy: findings on CT, MR imaging, and SPECT imaging in 14 cases. AJR Am J Roentgenol. 1992;159(2):379–83.
33. Schwartz RB, Mulkern RV, Gudbjartsson H, Jolesz F. Diffusion-weighted MR imaging in hypertensive encephalopathy: clues to pathogenesis. AJNR Am J Neuroradiol. 1998;19(5):859–62.
34. Hinchey JA. Reversible posterior leukoencephalopathy syndrome: what have we learned in the last 10 years? Arch Neurol. 2008;65(2):175–6.
35. Jauch EC, Saver JL, Adams HP, Bruno A, Demaerschalk BM, Khatri P, et al. Guidelines for the early management of patients with acute ischemic stroke a guideline for healthcare professionals from the American Heart Association/American Stroke Association. Stroke. 2013;44(3):870–947.
36. Bakker RC, Verburgh CA, van Buchem MA, Paul LC. Hypertension, cerebral oedema and fundoscopy. Nephrol Dial Transplant. 2003;18(11):2424–7.
37. Kinoshita T, Moritani T, Shrier DA, Hiwatashi A, Wang HZ, Numaguchi Y, et al. Diffusion-weighted MR imaging of posterior reversible leukoencephalopathy syndrome: a pictorial essay. Clin Imaging. 2003;27(5):307–15.
38. Schneider JP, Krohmer S, Gunther A, Zimmer C. Cerebral lesions in acute arterial hypertension: the characteristic MRI in hypertensive encephalopathy. Rofo. 2006;178(6):618–26.

39. Fugate JE, Claassen DO, Cloft HJ, Kallmes DF, Kozak OS, Rabinstein AA. Posterior reversible encephalopathy syndrome: associated clinical and radiologic findings. Mayo Clin Proc. 2010;85(5):427–32.
40. Price RS, Kasner SE. Hypertension and hypertensive encephalopathy. Handb Clin Neurol. 2014;119:161–7.
41. Beausang-Linder M, Bill A. Cerebral circulation in acute arterial hypertension—protective effects of sympathetic nervous activity. Acta Physiol Scand. 1981;111(2):193–9.
42. Edvinsson L, Owman C, Sjo N-O. Autonomic nerves, mast cells, and amine receptors in human brain vessels. A histochemical and pharmacological study. Brain Res. 1976;115(3):377–93.
43. Le EM, Loghin ME. Posterior reversible encephalopathy syndrome: a neurologic phenomenon in cancer patients. Curr Oncol Rep. 2014;16(5):1–9.
44. Bartynski WS. Posterior reversible encephalopathy syndrome, part 1: fundamental imaging and clinical features. AJNR Am J Neuroradiol. 2008;29(6):1036–42.
45. Porcello Marrone LC, Gadonski G, de Oliveira Laguna G, Poli-de-Figueiredo CE, da Costa BE P, Lopes MF, et al. Blood-brain barrier breakdown in reduced uterine perfusion pressure: a possible model of posterior reversible encephalopathy syndrome. J Stroke Cerebrovasc Dis. 2014;23(8):2075–9.
46. Thomas L. Managing hypertensive emergencies in the ED. Can Fam Physician. 2011;57(10):1137–97.
47. Marik PE, Varon J. Hypertensive crises: challenges and management. CHEST J. 2007;131(6):1949–62.
48. Varon J. The diagnosis and treatment of hypertensive crises. Postgrad Med. 2009;121(1):5–13.
49. Perez M, Musini V. Pharmacological interventions for hypertensive emergencies: a Cochrane systematic review. J Hum Hypertens. 2008;22(9):596–607.
50. McAllister R, Schloemer GL, Hamann SR. Kinetics and dynamics of calcium entry antagonists in systemic hypertension. Am J Cardiol. 1986;57(7):D16–21.
51. Maxwell CJ, Hogan DB, Campbell NR, Ebly EM. Nifedipine and mortality risk in the elderly: relevance of drug formulation, dose and duration. Pharmacoepidemiol Drug Saf. 2000;9(1):11–23.
52. Shepherd AM, Ludden TM, McNay JL, Lin MS. Hydralazine kinetics after single and repeated oral doses. Clin Pharmacol Ther. 1980;28(6):804–11.
53. Kondo T, Brock M, Bach H. Effect of intra-arterial sodium nitroprusside on intracranial pressure and cerebral autoregulation. Jpn Heart J. 1984;25(2):231–7.
54. Schulz V. Clinical pharmacokinetics of nitroprusside, cyanide, thiosulphate and thiocyanate. Clin Pharmacokinet. 1984;9(3):239–51.
55. Vesey C, Cole P, Simpson P. Cyanide and thiocyanate concentrations following sodium nitroprusside infusion in man. Br J Anaesth. 1976;48(7):651–60.
56. Padilla Ramos A, Varon J. Current and newer agents for hypertensive emergencies. Curr Hypertens Rep. 2014;16(7):450. doi:10.1007/s11906-014-0450-z.
57. Pearce CJ, Wallin JD. Labetalol and other agents that block both alpha-and beta-adrenergic receptors. Cleve Clin J Med. 1994;61(1):59–69.
58. Amenta F, Tomassoni D, Traini E, Mignini F, Veglio F. Nicardipine: a hypotensive dihydropyridine-type calcium antagonist with a peculiar cerebrovascular profile. Clin Exp Hypertens. 2008;30(8):808–26.
59. Wood AJ, Murphy MB, Murray C, Shorten GD. Fenoldopam—a selective peripheral dopamine-receptor agonist for the treatment of severe hypertension. N Engl J Med. 2001;345(21):1548–57.
60. James PA, Oparil S, Carter BL, Cushman WC, Dennison-Himmelfarb C, Handler J, et al. 2014 evidence-based guideline for the management of high blood pressure in adults: report from the panel members appointed to the Eighth Joint National Committee (JNC 8). JAMA. 2014;311(5):507–20.

61. American College of Obstetricians and Gynecologists, Task Force on Hypertension in Pregnancy. Hypertension in pregnancy. Report of the American College of Obstetricians and Gynecologists' Task Force on Hypertension in Pregnancy. Obstet Gynecol. 2013;122(5):1122–31.
62. Bell MJ. A historical overview of preeclampsia-eclampsia. J Obstet Gynecol Neonatal Nurs. 2010;39(5):510–8.
63. World Health Organization. WHO recommendations for prevention and treatment of pre-eclampsia and eclampsia: evidence base. 2011. http://apps.who.int/iris/bitstream/10665/44703/1/9789241548335_eng.pdf
64. Berhan Y, Berhan A. Should magnesium sulfate be administered to women with mild pre-eclampsia? A systematic review of published reports on eclampsia. J Obstet Gynaecol Res. 2015;41(6):831–42.
65. Souza JP, Gulmezoglu AM, Vogel J, Carroli G, Lumbiganon P, Qureshi Z, et al. Moving beyond essential interventions for reduction of maternal mortality (the WHO Multicountry Survey on Maternal and Newborn Health): a cross-sectional study. Lancet. 2013;381(9879):1747–55.
66. Edlow JA, Caplan LR, O'Brien K, Tibbles CD. Diagnosis of acute neurological emergencies in pregnant and post-partum women. Lancet Neurol. 2013;12(2):175–85.
67. Eiland E, Nzerue C, Faulkner M. Preeclampsia 2012. J Pregnancy. 2012;2012:1–7.
68. Altman D, Carroli G, Duley L, Farrell B, Moodley J, Neilson J, et al. Do women with pre-eclampsia, and their babies, benefit from magnesium sulphate? The Magpie Trial: a randomised placebo-controlled trial. Lancet. 2002;359(9321):1877–90.

Chapter 10
Acute Blood Pressure Management After Intracerebral Hemorrhage

Venkatesh Aiyagari

Stroke is a widely prevalent condition associated with significant morbidity and mortality. Worldwide, it is the second leading cause of death and a leading cause of disability [1]. After ischemic stroke, intracerebral hemorrhage (ICH) is the second most common stroke subtype, accounting for 10–25 % of all strokes [2]. However, the overall morbidity and mortality of ICH is significantly higher than that of ischemic stroke. Less than half of patients with ICH survive 1 year (of whom only 20–30 % live independently) and less than a third survive 5 years [2–4].

Hypertension as a Risk Factor for ICH

As discussed in detail in Chap. 2, hypertension is the most important modifiable risk factor for ICH and the risk of ICH increases linearly with an increase in the blood pressure (BP), even within the normotensive range. Hypertension is thought to lead to fibrinoid necrosis and rupture of small blood vessels leading to the formation of ICH. Long-term control of elevated BP is effective both for primary and secondary prevention of ICH. In the Perindopril Protection Against Recurrent Stroke Study (PROGRESS) of 6015 patients with a prior history of cerebrovascular disease, antihypertensive treatment lowered the absolute rates of ICH from 2 to 1 % (RRR 50 %, 95 % CI 26–67) over a mean of 3.9 years of follow-up. Among patients whose baseline stroke was an ICH, the relative risk of any stroke was reduced by 49 % (95 % CI 18–68) [5].

The impact of hypertension is not confined to hemorrhages in the "classic hypertensive locations" such as hemorrhages in the basal ganglia, thalamus, pons,

V. Aiyagari, M.B.B.S., D.M. (✉)
Departments of Neurological Surgery and Neurology and Neurotherapeutics, University of Texas Southwestern Medical Center, 5323 Harry Hines Blvd., Dallas, TX 75390, USA
e-mail: Venkatesh.aiyagari@utsouthwestern.edu

© Springer International Publishing Switzerland 2016
V. Aiyagari, P.B. Gorelick (eds.), *Hypertension and Stroke*, Clinical Hypertension and Vascular Diseases, DOI 10.1007/978-3-319-29152-9_10

or cerebellum. Inadequate BP control has been associated with a higher risk of recurrence both for lobar (hazard ratio [HR], 3.53 [95 % CI, 1.65–7.54]) and non-lobar ICH (HR, 4.23 [95 % CI, 1.02–17.52]) [6]. Active treatment of hypertension reduces the risk of amyloid angiopathy-related ICH by 77 % (95 % CI, 19–93 %), that of hypertension-related ICH by 46 % (95 % CI, 4–69 %), and that of unclassified ICH by 43 % (95 % CI, −5 to 69 %) [7].

Hypertensive Response in ICH

Elevated blood pressure is very common after an ICH. Analyzing data from the National Hospital Ambulatory Medical Care Survey, Qureshi et al. reported that of 45,330 patients with ICH presenting to hospital emergency departments in the United States, 75 % had a systolic BP≥ 140 mmHg [8]. Although many patients with ICH have preexisting hypertension, ICH itself seems to result in an elevation of the BP significantly above their usual baseline, which begins to decrease within hours or a few days after admission to the hospital [9]. A recent study also confirmed that systolic BP is substantially raised compared with usual premorbid levels after ICH, whereas acute-phase systolic BP after major ischemic stroke is much closer to the long-term premorbid level. This increase in ICH patients was due both to a rise in premorbid systolic SBP in the days and weeks before the event and to a subsequent additional increase in systolic blood pressure from the last premorbid reading. In ICH patients seen within 90 min, the highest systolic BP within 3 h of onset was 50 mmHg higher, on average, than the maximum premorbid level whereas that after ischemic stroke was 5.2 mmHg lower ($p<0.0001$) [10].

The exact cause of this acute hypertensive response is not known, but the transient nature of BP rise supports the role of stroke-specific mechanisms. These may include dysfunction of the areas of the brain involved in BP regulation, stress induced activation of neuroendocrine systems and impaired parasympathetic activity and baroreceptor sensitivity [11].

Treatment of Elevated BP in ICH

Rationale for and Against BP Reduction

While the long-term beneficial effect of lowering BP in ICH patients is widely accepted, it is not clear if elevated BP should be lowered in the acute phase of ICH. The posited advantages of acute BP lowering might include a possible reduction of hematoma expansion and cerebral edema while the disadvantages might include the risk of inducing or exacerbating cerebral ischemia with BP reduction [12].

Hematoma Expansion

Hematoma expansion is common in ICH. Among ICH patients scanned within 3 h of onset, 73 % have some hematoma expansion when scanned at 24 h, and significant hematoma expansion (>33 % increase in volume) has been seen in nearly 40 % of patients [13, 14]. Significant hematoma growth is often associated with a decline in the neurological status and is an independent predictor of mortality and functional outcome [14, 15]. Most, but not all, studies report an association between hematoma expansion and hypertension [13, 16–21]. Recently, a retrospective cohort study of the first measured BP on the scene by emergency responders in 536 ICH patients reported that elevated systolic BP (by 10 mmHg incremental: OR = 1.126, 95 % CI 1.015–1.265), diastolic BP (by 10 mmHg incremental: OR = 1.146, 95 % CI 1.019–1.303), and mean arterial pressure (MAP) (by 10 mmHg incremental: OR = 1.225, 95 % CI 1.057–1.443) were significantly associated with early neurological deterioration (defined as a ≥ 2 point decrease in the Glasgow Coma Scale (GCS) score with 24 h of arrival at the emergency department). Neurological deterioration was attributed to hematoma expansion in 83 % of cases [22]. Table 10.1 summarizes studies exploring the relationship between hematoma expansion and

Table 10.1 Relationship between hypertension and hematoma growth

Reference	Study design	Number of patients	Conclusion
Brott et al. [13]	Prospective observational	103	No association between systolic or diastolic BP and HE
Kazui et al. [19]	Retrospective	186	Systolic BP ≥ 200 mmHg at admission associated with HE
Fujii et al. [17]	Retrospective	627	Systolic BP was not a predictor of HE
Ohwaki et al. [21]	Retrospective	76	Maximum systolic BP associated with HE. Target systolic BP of ≥160 mmHg significantly associated with HE compared to ≤150 mmHg
Jauch et al. [18]	Retrospective analysis of a prospective observational study	98	No relationship between HE and systolic BP, diastolic BP, MAP or pulse pressure
Broderick et al. [16]	Retrospective analysis of a prospective study	382	No relationship between HE and baseline systolic BP or MAP
Martí-Fàbregas et al. [20]	Prospective study	60	No relationship between admission systolic BP, diastolic BP or MAP or maximum systolic, diastolic or MAP during the first 24 h and HE
Fan et al. [22]	Retrospective	536	Systolic BP, diastolic BP and MAP on-scene associated with END, which in turn was due to HE in 83 % of cases

BP blood pressure, *HE* hematoma expansion, *MAP* mean arterial blood pressure, *END* early neurological deterioration hypertension. It is important to point out that even if there is an established association between the two, it can be difficult to ascertain if hypertension led to hematoma expansion or if the expanding hematoma led to a rise in BP.

Cerebral Edema

Perihematomal edema (PHE) develops within 3 h after onset of ICH and peaks in the 2nd–4th week after onset [23]. The prognostic significance of PHE in ICH is still under investigation. Initial data from the Intensive blood pressure reduction in acute cerebral hemorrhage trial (INTERACT) suggested that the degree of, and growth in, PHE over the first 72 h are strongly related to the size of the underlying hematoma of acute ICH, and do not appear to have a major independent effect in determining the outcome from this condition [7]. Although one would expect that a higher BP would promote PHE formation by increasing the capillary hydrostatic pressure, in the INTERACT trial, lower systolic BP and baseline hematoma volume were independently associated with absolute increase in PHE volume [7]. A more recent analysis of 1138 patients enrolled in INTERACT and INTERACT2 studies found that absolute growth in PHE volume over 24 h was significantly associated with death or dependency (adjusted odds ratio, 1.17; 95 % confidence interval, 1.02–1.33 per 5 mL increase from baseline; $p = 0.025$) at 90 days, however, admission BP was not a predictor of edema growth [24]. One should note that both these studies analyzed early PHE (<72 h). Since PHE in most patients usually peaks in the 2nd–4th week, the clinical relevance of these studies of early PHE is uncertain and there is a need to study the prognostic implications of delayed PHE and its relationship with BP.

Cerebral Blood Flow and Ischemia in ICH

Cerebral blood flow (CBF) is determined by the equation: CBF = cerebral perfusion pressure (CPP)/cerebral vascular resistance (CVR) [25]. CPP is defined as MAP minus intracranial pressure (ICP). Under normal physiological conditions, as MAP fluctuates between a range of 50 and 150 mmHg, CBF is maintained at a constant state through cerebral autoregulation. This is achieved by adjustment in CVR (i.e., vasodilatation or vasoconstriction of arteriolar blood vessels occurs when MAP falls or rises). Below the lower limit of autoregulation, there may be a fall in CBF leading to cerebral ischemia, and above the upper limit there may be endothelial injury and breakdown of the blood–brain barrier leading to cerebral edema and eventually to brain hemorrhage [26]. Persons with chronic untreated hypertension have a shift of the brain autoregulatory curve to the right. Therefore, in ICH patients who have longstanding untreated hypertension, caution must be exerted when lowering BP. Abrupt lowering of the blood pressure to "normal" may lead to cerebral hypoperfusion in these patients.

Patients with large ICH or those with obstructive hydrocephalus may have increased ICP. An elevated BP in these patients may be "protective" in the sense of maintaining an adequate CPP in the face of an elevated ICP. Thus, lowering an elevated BP by a significant amount in these patients without measuring the ICP (and thus not measuring the CPP) may lead to a drop of MAP below the lower limit of autoregulation and potentially lead to cerebral hypoperfusion.

ICH itself might disrupt cerebral autoregulation, either globally or locally in the perihematomal region. Studies of CBF with single-photon emission computed tomography, positron-emission tomography (PET), CT perfusion imaging, and magnetic resonance imaging (MRI) have demonstrated that CBF is reduced in the perihematomal region [27–30]. However, the reduction in CBF does not appear to translate to cerebral ischemia. PET imaging in 19 ICH patients studied between 5 and 22 h after onset of symptoms demonstrated that both CBF and cerebral metabolic rate of oxygen (CMRO2) were reduced in the region surrounding acute ICH. In addition, the oxygen extraction fraction (OEF) was also reduced in the same region. The reduced OEF in this region, and the fact that CMRO2 was reduced to a proportionately greater degree than CBF, suggests that there is reduced metabolic demand rather than acute ischemia [30]. More recently, data from the ICH ADAPT study (see below) also suggest that the mean absolute perihematoma CBF is lower than contralateral homologous regions but above the proposed CBF threshold for ischemia [31].

Lastly, MRI observational studies have described the presence of diffusion-restricted lesions in ICH patients, suggestive of acute ischemic injury in 14–41 % of patients studied. BP lowering has been associated with the occurrence of these cerebral ischemic lesions in several of these studies [32, 33]. The authors hypothesize that BP reductions in the setting of an active vasculopathy may be a potential underlying mechanism. In a recent review of the literature, it was concluded that three studies have suggested a relationship between degree of BP lowering and DWI lesions on MRI, but two studies did not find an association, suggesting the possibility that these lesions may be an epiphenomenon resulting from underlying hypertensive cerebral microangiopathy and unrelated to BP reduction [33].

Clinical Studies of BP Reduction in ICH

In view of the reported association between hypertension and poor outcome in stroke in general, and ICH in particular, several studies of acute BP lowering in stroke have been conducted. Several of these studies studied patients with both ischemic and hemorrhagic strokes and a few studies have focused on imaging end-points. However, in the last decade, a few small and large prospective randomized studies on BP lowering in acute ICH have been conducted with the goal of determining if BP lowering is safe and effective. The studies in each section are discussed in order of publication and summarized in Table 10.2.

Table 10.2 Prospective randomized studies evaluating the effect of blood pressure reduction after intracerebral hemorrhage

Reference	Study design	Number of patients	Time from symptom onset to enrollment	BP targets	Antihypertensive agents	Conclusion
Studies enrolling patients with ischemic and hemorrhagic strokes						
CHHIPS [34]	Prospective, randomized, double-blinded	179 (25 with ICH)	<36 h	Not applicable	Labetalol, lisinopril or placebo	ICH numbers too small to draw conclusions
COSSACS [35]	Prospective, randomized, open, blinded end-point	763 (38 with ICH)	<48 h	Not applicable	Continue or discontinue previous antihypertensive agent	Data on ICH patients not presented
SCAST [36]	Prospective, randomized, double-blinded	2004 (274 with ICH)	<30 h	Not applicable	Candesartan or placebo	No association between treatment with candesartan and risk of vascular events but worse functional outcome with candesartan
ENOS [38]	Prospective, randomized, single-blinded, blinded-outcome	4000 (629 with ICH)	<48 h	Not applicable	Glyceryl trinitrate or placebo; continue or discontinue previous antihypertensive agent	No difference in functional outcome with glyceryl trinitrate
Studies enrolling patients with cerebral hemorrhage only, with imaging endpoints						
Powers et al. [39]	Prospective, randomized	14	<24 h	MAP reduction by 15%	Labetalol and nicardipine	Preserved cerebral autoregulation with BP reduction
ICH ADAPT [31]	Prospective, randomized	75	≤24 h	Systolic BP <150 or <180 mmHg	Labetalol, hydralazine, enalapril	No reduction in perihematomal cerebral blood flow with aggressive BP reduction

Studies enrolling patients with cerebral hemorrhage only, with clinical endpoints

Koch et al. [42]	Prospective, randomized	42	8 h	MAP <110 or 110–130 mmHg	Labetalol, nicardipine, sodium nitroprusside	No significant differences in early neurological deterioration, hematoma and edema growth, and clinical outcome
INTERACT [43]	Prospective, randomized, blinded end-point assessment	404	6 h	Systolic BP <140 or <180 mmHg	Variable	No significant difference in hematoma growth between the two tiers after adjustment for baseline hematoma volume and time to CT scan
ATACH [44]	Prospective, phase I dose-escalation	60	6 h	Systolic BP 170–200 or 140–170 or 110–140 mmHg	Nicardipine	Observed proportions of neurologic deterioration and serious adverse events below the pre-specified safety thresholds, and the 3-month mortality rate lower than expected in all tiers
INTERACT II [46]	Prospective, randomized, blinded end-point assessment	2839	6 h	Systolic BP <140 or <180 mmHg	Variable	No significant reduction in the rate of primary outcome of death or severe disability with intensive lowering of BP

See note added in proof for the results of the ATACH-2 trial. *BP* blood pressure, *MAP* mean arterial pressure, *ICH* intracerebral hemorrhage, *CT* computed tomography

Randomized Studies Including Ischemic Stroke and ICH

Controlling hypertension and hypotension immediately post-stroke (CHHIPS) was a pilot, randomized, double-blind, placebo-controlled trial of two blood pressure-lowering regimens within 36 h of cerebral infarction or hemorrhage. One hundred and seventy-nine patients were enrolled; however, only 25 patients had ICH (18 randomized to active treatment and 7 to placebo). While outcome data on the ICH patients was presented, the small number of patients limits the ability to draw firm conclusions about the safety or efficacy of BP reduction [34].

The Continue Or Stop post-Stroke Antihypertensives Collaborative Study (COSSACS) was a multicenter, prospective, randomized, open, blinded-endpoint trial of patients within 48 h of non-dysphagic, ischemic, or hemorrhagic stroke and within 48 h of the last dose of antihypertensive drugs. The aim was to assess the efficacy and safety of continuing or stopping preexisting antihypertensive drugs. Of 763 total enrolled patients, only 38 had ICH and subgroup analysis of the ICH patients was not presented in the published manuscript [35].

The angiotensin-receptor blocker candesartan for treatment of acute stroke (SCAST) was a randomized, placebo-controlled, double-blind trial. Patients with acute stroke (ischemic or hemorrhagic) and systolic BP of ≥ 140 mmHg were included within 30 h of symptom onset. Patients were randomly allocated to candesartan or placebo (1:1) for 7 days. There were two co-primary effect variables: the composite endpoint of vascular death, myocardial infarction, or stroke during the first 6 months; and functional outcome at 6 months, as measured by the modified Rankin Scale (mRS). Two thousand and twenty-nine patients were randomized, including 274 with ICH (144 in the candesartan and 130 in the placebo group, respectively). The main analysis of all patients showed a trend toward poorer functional outcome in the candesartan group [36]. Patients with ICH were separately studied in a pre-specified subgroup analysis [37]. There was no association between treatment with candesartan and risk of vascular events (17 of 144 [11.8 %] versus 13 of 130 [10.0 %]; hazard ratio, 1.36; 95 % confidence interval, 0.65–2.83; $p=0.41$). For functional outcome, there was evidence of a negative effect of candesartan (common odds ratio, 1.61; 95 % confidence interval, 1.03–2.50; $p=0.036$). It should be pointed out that in SCAST, treatment was started at ≈ 18 h, and the maximal difference in systolic BP of 5 mmHg was achieved on day 4. The authors concluded that the absence of benefit in SCAST might imply that treatment was started too late to limit brain injury or that angiotensin receptor blockers have unwanted properties in the acute phase of stroke [37].

In the Efficacy of Nitric Oxide in Stroke (ENOS) trial, patients admitted to hospital with an acute ischemic or hemorrhagic stroke and raised systolic blood pressure (systolic 140–220 mmHg) were randomly assigned to 7 days of transdermal glyceryl trinitrate (5 mg per day), started within 48 h of stroke onset, or to no glyceryl trinitrate (control group). A subset of patients who were taking antihypertensive drugs before their stroke was also randomly assigned to continue or stop taking these drugs. The primary outcome was function, assessed with the mRS at 90 days. Of the total 4011 patients enrolled, 629 patients presented with ICH. There was no difference in functional outcome at 90 days in ICH patients between the two groups (OR 1.03, 95 % CI: 0.78–1.36) [38].

Randomized Studies Enrolling Only ICH Patients

Studies with Imaging End-Points

Powers et al. studied 14 patients with small to moderate sized ICH (volumes 1–45 mL) imaged between 6 and 22 h after ICH. Patients were imaged using PET at baseline and after the baseline CBF measurement, randomized to receive either nicardipine or labetalol to reduce MAP by 15 %, and the CBF study was repeated. The results showed that when MAP was lowered by ~17 % from 143 ± 10 to 119 ± 11 mmHg, there was no significant change in either global CBF or perihematomal CBF, suggesting preserved autoregulation [39].

The ICH ADAPT study randomized 75 patients with ICH within 24 h of symptom onset to a systolic BP goal of <150 or <180 mmHg. The primary endpoint was perihematomal CBF measured by CT perfusion imaging. The regional CBF in the perihematomal zone was similar in both groups and aggressive BP reduction did not result in an increase in critically hypoperfused areas (CBF <18 mL/100 g/min) in the perihematomal zone or watershed areas, nor did it alter perihematomal or global CBF [31, 40]. Ipsilateral hemispheric CBF was modestly decreased in the group with the lower BP goal [31]. Additionally, the lower BP target did not lead to an increase in the volume of PHE [41].

Taken together, these two studies, albeit not very large, support the hypothesis that there is no perihematomal ischemia in CBF and lowering BP to the ranges studied does not seem to have a deleterious effect on global or perihematomal CBF.

Studies with Clinical End-Points

Koch et al. conducted a prospective randomized trial comparing two BP tiers in ICH patients to determine the safety and feasibility of aggressive BP lowering in patients with acute spontaneous ICH. Forty-two patients were enrolled and randomized to one of two MAP goals (standard BP treatment: MAP 110–130 mmHg or aggressive BP lowering: MAP< 110 mmHg) within 8 h of symptom onset. MAP was managed with antihypertensive agents during the 48 h treatment period. The primary and secondary endpoints were a clinical decline (NIHSS drop ≥ 2 points) within the first 48 h and hematoma enlargement at 24 h, respectively. Treatment was started on average 3.2 ± 2.2 h after symptom onset and target BP was achieved within 87.1 ± 59.6 min in the standard group and 163.5 ± 163.8 min in the aggressive BP treatment group. There were no significant differences in early neurological deterioration, hematoma and edema growth, and clinical outcome at 90 days. The authors concluded that aggressive BP lowering in ICH was safe and deserved further study [42].

The Intensive blood pressure reduction in acute cerebral hemorrhage trial (INTERACT) was a randomized pilot trial to assess the safety and efficiency of this treatment as a run-in phase to a larger trial. Patients with acute spontaneous ICH diagnosed by CT within 6 h of onset, elevated systolic BP (150–220 mmHg), and no definite indication or contraindication to treatment were randomly assigned to early intensive lowering of BP (target systolic BP 140 mmHg; $n = 203$) or standard guideline-based management of BP (target systolic BP 180 mmHg; $n = 201$). The primary efficacy endpoint was proportional change in hematoma volume at 24 h and secondary efficacy endpoints were absolute and substantial growth (>33 % or >12.5 mL within 24 h) of the hematoma and of the hematoma plus any intraventricular hemorrhage. Safety and clinical outcomes were assessed for up to 90 days. Mean proportional hematoma growth was 36.3 % in the guideline group and 13.7 % in the intensive group (difference 22.6 %, 95 % CI 0.6–44.5 %; $p = 0.04$) at 24 h. However, after adjustment for initial hematoma volume and time from onset to CT, median hematoma growth was no longer significantly different between the groups ($p = 0.06$). The absolute difference in volume between groups was 1.7 mL (95 % CI −0.5 to 3.9, $p = 0.13$). Intensive lowering of BP had no significant excess adverse effect on death or dependency, or on any of the clinical scales [GCS, National Institutes of Health Stroke Scale (NIHSS), mRS, Barthel index, the minimental state examination (MMSE), and the EuroQol 5D for the calculation of an overall health utility score (EQ5D)]. In a post-hoc analysis of 210 patients randomized up to 4 h from ICH onset, substantial hematoma growth was significantly less common in the intensive group (17 [15 %] of 110 patients) than the guideline group (30 [30 %] of 100 patients) (relative risk reduction 52 %, 95 % CI 30–88 %), and there was a 3.36 mL absolute difference (95 % CI 0.3–6.4 %) in hematoma volume between groups. Of note, in the intensive group, only 87 (42 %) and 133 (66 %) patients achieved the target systolic BP of 140 mmHg within 1 and 6 h after randomization, respectively [43].

The Antihypertensive Treatment of Acute Cerebral Hemorrhage (ATACH) trial was a phase I, dose-escalation, multicenter prospective study where patients with ICH with elevated BP>170 mmHg presenting within 6 h of symptom onset were studied. Patients were randomized to treatment with IV nicardipine to three systolic BP goals: 170–200 mmHg ($n = 18$), 140–170 mmHg ($n = 20$), and 110–140 mmHg ($n = 22$). Nine of 60 patients had treatment failures (all in the last tier). The observed proportions of neurologic deterioration and serious adverse events were below the pre-specified safety thresholds, and the 3-month mortality rate was lower than expected in all systolic blood pressure tiers [44]. In a subsequent post-hoc analysis, the authors were not able to find a significant relationship between the degree of SBP reduction (relative to initial SBP) and significant hematoma expansion, PHE or poor 3-month outcome [45].

Encouraged by the results of the pilot INTERACT trial, the authors conducted the subsequent INTERACT2 trial. INTERACT2 was an international, multicenter, prospective, randomized, open-treatment, blinded end-point trial. Two thousand eight hundred and thirty-nine patients with an ICH within the previous 6 h and an elevated SBP were randomized to receive intensive or guideline-recommended antihypertensive treatment (target systolic level of <140 or <180 mmHg, respectively). The primary outcome was death or major disability (defined as a score of 3–6 on the mRS) at 90 days. A pre-specified ordinal analysis was also performed to determine if there was a significant shift in the distribution of clinical outcomes on the modified Rankin score. Similar to the INTERACT study, only 33 % of patients randomized to the intensive treatment group were able to achieve the goal systolic BP of <140 mmHg within 1 h and only 53 % were able to reach it within 6 h. There was no significant difference in the primary outcome between the two groups. At 90 days, 52.0 % in the intensive-treatment group had a poor outcome, as compared with 55.6 % in the standard-treatment group (odds ratio with intensive treatment, 0.87; 95 % confidence interval [CI], 0.75–1.01; $p = 0.06$). However, the ordinal analysis showed a significant favorable shift in the distribution of scores on the mRS with intensive blood pressure-lowering treatment (pooled odds ratio for shift to higher mRS score, 0.87; 95 % CI, 0.77–1.00; $p = 0.04$). Lastly, there were no significant differences between the two groups in any of the other outcomes studied including mortality and nonfatal serious adverse events. A point worth mentioning is the fact that the difference in hematoma growth between the groups in the 24 h after baseline was not significant, suggesting that any beneficial effect of lowering BP could not be attributed to a reduction in hematoma expansion [46].

Questions have been raised about the implications and generalizability of the results of the INTERACT2 trial [47–49]. Antihypertensive treatment in INTERACT2 was not always protocol based and different agents were used based on provider preference. Post hoc analysis also seems to suggest that systolic BP variability seems to predict a poor outcome in patients with acute ICH and perhaps the benefits of early treatment to reduce systolic blood pressure to 140 mmHg might be enhanced by smooth and sustained control, and particularly by avoiding peaks in BP, which may be easier to achieve with a continuous intravenous infusion of an antihypertensive agent such as nicardipine. In addition, there was variability in other adjunct treatments. There was no difference in outcome between patients treated within 4 h or after 4 h and no effect on hematoma expansion. Patients with large hemorrhages were excluded and the majority of patients had small hemorrhages (average hematoma volume of 11 mL). The reason for use of mannitol in the majority of patients, despite small hematoma sizes, is not explained. Blood pressure control was achieved quite late, and a time when the highest risk period for hematoma expansion would have passed. The inclusion criteria allowed patients with even mild–moderate hypertension to be included. As a result, only 1873 of 2839 (66 %) subjects received any IV antihypertensive medication; 10 and 57 % of subjects randomized to intensive or standard SBP reductions, respectively, did not receive any IV antihypertensive medication. Lastly, there was a significant difference in withdrawal of life-sustaining measures between the intensive and guideline-recommended groups.

A meta-analysis of four previously discussed studies (ICH ADAPT, Koch et al., INTERACT and INTERACT2) has been recently published. Three thousand three hundred and fifteen patients were included in the meta-analysis. The results revealed that mortality was similar between patients randomized to intensive BP-lowering treatment (target systolic BP< 150 mmHg or target MAP< 110 mmHg) and those receiving guideline BP-lowering treatment (target systolic BP< 180 mmHg) (odds ratio= 1.01, 95 % confidence interval: 0.83–1.23; $p=0.914$). Intensive BP-lowering treatment tended to be associated with lower 3-month death or dependency (odds ratio= 0.87, 95 % confidence interval: 0.76–1.01; $p=0.062$) and a greater attenuation of absolute hematoma growth at 24 h (standardized mean difference ± SE: −0.110 ± 0.053; $p=0.038$) compared with guideline treatment [50].

Choice of Antihypertensive Agents

One of the main criticisms of the INTERACT and INTERACT2 is that a large percentage of patients randomized to intensive treatment were unable to be at or below the target systolic BP at 1 and even at 6 h as noted above. In both these studies, antihypertensive therapy was administered according to local protocols, alpha adrenergic antagonists like urapidil were the most commonly used agent and intravenous antihypertensive infusions were not commonly used. However, other trials have shown that faster BP control is possible. In ICH ADAPT, a strict BP lowering protocol using intravenous bolus doses of three antihypertensive agents (labetalol, hydralazine, and enalapril) allowed the target BP in the intensive group to be reached at 2 h in nearly 80 % of patients [31]. In the ATACH trial, using intravenous nicardipine infusion, the systolic BP goals were reached in 90 % of patients within 2 h [44]. In the Stroke Acute management with Urgent Risk-factor Assessment and Improvement (SAMURAI)—ICH study, intravenous nicardipine use allowed the systolic BP goal (120–160 mmHg) to be reached in a median time of 30 min (interquartile range 15–45 min). Only 7 of the enrolled 211 patients needed an additional antihypertensive agent [51]. Several small studies comparing nicardipine with labetalol for BP control in ICH seem to suggest that nicardipine is the preferred agent [52–54]. Another intravenous short-acting calcium channel blocker, clevidipine, was studied in the Evaluation of Patients with Acute Hypertension and ICH with Intravenous Clevidipine (ACCELERATE) trial. A total of 35 patients (2 of whom were later deemed ineligible) were treated in this multicenter, phase IIIb, single-arm, open-label, efficacy, and safety trial. The mean systolic BP goal of 160–140 mmHg was reached in all treated patients within the first 30 min and only one patient needed a second antihypertensive agent. Clevidipine was well tolerated and there was minimal change in the hematoma volume [55]. Commonly used antihypertensive agents with dosing guidelines are presented in Chap. 9 (Table 9.2).

Guidelines from National Societies

United States

The American Heart Association/American Stroke Association guidelines published in 2015 recommend the following:

> "1. For ICH patients presenting with systolic BP between 150 and 220 mmHg and without contraindication to acute BP treatment, acute lowering of systolic BP to 140 mmHg is safe (Class I; Level of Evidence A) and can be effective for improving functional outcome (Class IIa; Level of Evidence B).
> 2. For ICH patients presenting with systolic BP>220 mmHg, it may be reasonable to consider aggressive reduction of BP with a continuous intravenous infusion and frequent BP monitoring (Class IIb; Level of Evidence C)" [56].

Europe

The European Stroke Organization guidelines published in 2014 are:

> "In acute ICH within 6 h of onset, intensive BP reduction (systolic target < 140 mmHg in <1 h) is safe and may be superior to a systolic target < 180 mmHg. No specific agent can be recommended.
> Quality of evidence: Moderate.
> Strength of recommendation: Weak" [57].

Australia

The National Stroke Foundation (Australia) in 2010 recommended that

> "In acute primary ICH where severe hypertension is observed on several occasions within the first 24–48 h of stroke onset, antihypertensive therapy (that could include intravenous treatment) can be used to maintain a BP below 180 mmHg systolic (MAP of 130 mmHg)." This recommendation is graded GPP (Good practice point) which is defined as "Recommended best practice based on clinical experience and expert opinion" [58].

Canada

The Canadian Stroke Best Practice Recommendations published in 2015 are as follows:

> "i. BP should be assessed on initial arrival to the ED and every 15 min thereafter until it has stabilized [Evidence Level C].
> ii. BP targets in ICH patients may be challenging to achieve and require careful monitoring, and in some cases aggressive repeated dosing or intravenous infusion of antihypertensive medications [Evidence Level C].

iii. Close BP monitoring (e.g., every 30–60 min, or more frequently if above target) should continue for at least the first 24–48 h [Evidence Level B].

iv. There is presently insufficient evidence to demonstrate that lower BP targets are associated with better clinical outcomes, and research is ongoing in this area. However, there is evidence to support safety for a target systolic BP less than 140 mmHg [Evidence Level B].

v. Labetalol is recommended as a first-line treatment for acute BP management if there are no contraindications [Evidence Level B].

vi. After the first 24 h following the onset of an ICH, further BP lowering should be continued with the initiation of parenteral or oral antihypertensive medications (depending on swallowing ability), to achieve individualized BP targets that will optimize secondary stroke prevention [Evidence Level B]" [59].

Japan

The Japanese guideline recommendations published in 2011 state:

"1. The blood pressure in patients with acute ICH should be controlled to maintain the systolic BP at <180 mmHg or the MAP at <130 mmHg (Grade C1).

2. When performing surgical treatment, more aggressive lowering of BP is recommended (Grade C1).

3. There is no specially recommended hypotensive drug. Drugs that may dilate cerebral blood vessels should be administered with care because they induce brain hypertension (Grade C1)" [60].

Ongoing Research

ATACH II, the follow-up trial of ATACH, has recently halted recruitment after enrolling 1000 patients and the final results are eagerly awaited. The primary hypothesis of the trial is that intensive systolic BP reduction (Systolic BP ≤ 140 mmHg) using IV nicardipine infusion for 24-h post-randomization reduces the proportion of death and disability (mRS of 4–6) at 3 months by ≥ 10 % compared with the standard BP reduction (SBP ≤ 180 mmHg) among patients with ICH treated within 4.5 h of symptom onset [61].

Another ongoing trial of BP reduction in ICH, ICH ADAPT II, is planning to enroll 300 patients who will be randomized to two systolic BP targets (<140 or <180 mmHg). The primary endpoint is the frequency of lesions on a diffusion weighted MRI image 48 h later [62].

Conclusions

Several clinical trials of BP reduction in ICH have been conducted, however, unequivocal evidence of improved patient outcomes with intensive blood pressure reduction (e.g., a systolic BP goal <140 mmHg) has not yet been demonstrated. While awaiting the results of ATACH II, acute systolic BP reduction to a goal of <140 mmHg seemed to be safe in the majority of patients and was recommended by the American Heart Association/American Stroke Association and the European Stroke Organization guidelines. This was also supported by recent post hoc analysis of the INTERACT2 data suggesting that a target of 130–139 mmHg was associated with the lowest degree of physical dysfunction [63]. However, the recently published results of the ATACH-2 trial do not support the notion that systolic BP reduction to <140 mm Hg leads to better functional outcome compared to a systolic BP target of 140-179 mm Hg (see "Note" section below).

Hopefully, future trials will study the effect of BP reduction at even earlier time frames, when BP reduction might have a more meaningful impact on reduction of hematoma expansion. The Field Administration of Stroke Therapy–Magnesium (FAST-MAG) trial provides a model for conducting such a trial in the pre-hospital setting, perhaps facilitated by ambulances equipped with mobile CT scanners to reliably distinguish ICH from acute ischemic strokes [64].

Note

The results of the Antihypertensive Treatment of Acute Cerebral Hemorrhage II (ATACH-2) trial were published after this chapter was submitted. This multi-center, open-label trial randomized ICH patients with at least one systolic BP >180 mm Hg prior to enrollment, to two systolic BP targets: a)110–139 mm Hg (intensive treatment) and b)140–179 mm Hg (standard treatment). Treatment with IV nicardipine infusion was initiated within 4.5 hours after symptom onset and continued for the next 24 hours. Additional eligibility criteria were age $\geq$ 18 years, GCS score of $\geq$ 5 and initial ICH volume <60 cm^3. The primary outcome measure was the proportion of patients with a mRS score of 4–6 at 3 months. Enrollment was stopped for futility after a total of 1000 patients had been randomized, 500 to each systolic BP target. The primary outcome of death or disability was seen in 38.7 % in the intensive treatment group and in 37.7 % of the standard treatment group (relative risk 1.04; 95 % confidence interval 0.85–1.27), indicating no significant benefit with intensive treatment. Of note, the intensive target group also had a higher incidence of serious adverse events within 3 months of randomization. Some of the criticisms of the ATACH-2 trial are a higher proportion of treatment failure in the lower BP target group, allowing prerandomization antihypertensive treatment and a high proportion of patients with favorable characteristics at baseline [65].

References

1. Mozaffarian D, Benjamin EJ, Go AS, Arnett DK, Blaha MJ, Cushman M, et al. Heart disease and stroke statistics — 2015 update: a report from the American Heart Association. Circulation. 2015;131(4):e29–322.
2. Feigin VL, Lawes CMM, Bennett DA, Barker-Collo SI, Parag V. Worldwide stroke incidence and early case fatality reported in 56 population-based studies: a systematic review. Lancet Neurol. 2009;8(4):355–69.
3. Poon MT, Fonville AF, Al-Shahi SR. Long-term prognosis after intracerebral haemorrhage: systematic review and meta-analysis. J Neurol Neurosurg Psychiatry. 2014;85(6):660–7.

4. van Asch CJ, Luitse MJ, Rinkel GJ, van der Tweel I, Algra A, Klijn CJ. Incidence, case fatality, and functional outcome of intracerebral haemorrhage over time, according to age, sex, and ethnic origin: a systematic review and meta-analysis. Lancet Neurol. 2010;9(2):167–76.

5. Chapman N, Huxley R, Anderson C, Bousser MG, Chalmers J, Colman S, et al. Effects of a perindopril-based blood pressure-lowering regimen on the risk of recurrent stroke according to stroke subtype and medical history: the PROGRESS trial. Stroke. 2004;35(1):116–21.

6. Biffi A, Anderson CD, Battey TW, Ayres AM, Greenberg SM, Viswanathan A, et al. Association between blood pressure control and risk of recurrent intracerebral hemorrhage. JAMA. 2015;314(9):904–12.

7. Arima H, Wang JG, Huang Y, Heeley E, Skulina C, Parsons MW, et al. Significance of perihematomal edema in acute intracerebral hemorrhage: the INTERACT trial. Neurology. 2009;73(23):1963–8.

8. Qureshi AI, Ezzeddine MA, Nasar A, Suri MF, Kirmani JF, Hussein HM, et al. Prevalence of elevated blood pressure in 563,704 adult patients with stroke presenting to the ED in the United States. Am J Emerg Med. 2007;25(1):32–8.

9. Britton M, Carlsson A, de Faire U. Blood pressure course in patients with acute stroke and matched controls. Stroke. 1986;17(5):861–4.

10. Fischer U, Cooney MT, Bull LM, Silver LE, Chalmers J, Anderson CS, et al. Acute post-stroke blood pressure relative to premorbid levels in intracerebral haemorrhage versus major ischaemic stroke: a population-based study. Lancet Neurol. 2014;13(4):374–84.

11. Qureshi AI. Acute hypertensive response in patients with stroke: pathophysiology and management. Circulation. 2008;118(2):176–87.

12. Aiyagari V, Gorelick PB. Management of blood pressure for acute and recurrent stroke. Stroke. 2009;40(6):2251–6.

13. Brott T, Broderick J, Kothari R, Barsan W, Tomsick T, Sauerbeck L, et al. Early hemorrhage growth in patients with intracerebral hemorrhage. Stroke. 1997;28(1):1–5.

14. Davis SM, Broderick J, Hennerici M, Brun NC, Diringer MN, Mayer SA, et al. Hematoma growth is a determinant of mortality and poor outcome after intracerebral hemorrhage. Neurology. 2006;66(8):1175–81.

15. Lord AS, Gilmore E, Choi HA, Mayer SA, Collaboration V-I. Time course and predictors of neurological deterioration after intracerebral hemorrhage. Stroke. 2015;46(3):647–52.

16. Broderick JP, Diringer MN, Hill MD, Brun NC, Mayer SA, Steiner T, et al. Determinants of intracerebral hemorrhage growth: an exploratory analysis. Stroke. 2007;38(3):1072–5.

17. Fujii Y, Takeuchi S, Sasaki O, Minakawa T, Tanaka R. Multivariate analysis of predictors of hematoma enlargement in spontaneous intracerebral hemorrhage. Stroke. 1998;29(6):1160–6.

18. Jauch EC, Lindsell CJ, Adeoye O, Khoury J, Barsan W, Broderick J, et al. Lack of evidence for an association between hemodynamic variables and hematoma growth in spontaneous intracerebral hemorrhage. Stroke. 2006;37(8):2061–5.

19. Kazui S, Minematsu K, Yamamoto H, Sawada T, Yamaguchi T. Predisposing factors to enlargement of spontaneous intracerebral hematoma. Stroke. 1997;28(12):2370–5.

20. Marti-Fabregas J, Martinez-Ramirez S, Martinez-Corral M, Diaz-Manera J, Querol L, Suarez-Calvet M, et al. Blood pressure is not associated with haematoma enlargement in acute intracerebral haemorrhage. Eur J Neurol. 2008;15(10):1085–90.

21. Ohwaki K, Yano E, Nagashima H, Hirata M, Nakagomi T, Tamura A. Blood pressure management in acute intracerebral hemorrhage: relationship between elevated blood pressure and hematoma enlargement. Stroke. 2004;35(6):1364–7.

22. Fan JS, Chen YC, Huang HH, How CK, Yen DH, Huang MS. The association between on-scene blood pressure and early neurological deterioration in patients with spontaneous intracerebral haemorrhage. Emerg Med J. 2015;32(3):239–43.

23. Venkatasubramanian C, Mlynash M, Finley-Caulfield A, Eyngorn I, Kalimuthu R, Snider RW, et al. Natural history of perihematomal edema after intracerebral hemorrhage measured by serial magnetic resonance imaging. Stroke. 2011;42(1):73–80.

24. Yang J, Arima H, Wu G, Heeley E, Delcourt C, Zhou J, et al. Prognostic significance of perihematomal edema in acute intracerebral hemorrhage: pooled analysis from the intensive blood pressure reduction in acute cerebral hemorrhage trial studies. Stroke. 2015;46(4):1009–13.

25. Goldstein LB. Blood pressure management in patients with acute ischemic stroke. Hypertension. 2004;43(2):137–41.
26. Owens WB. Blood pressure control in acute cerebrovascular disease. J Clin Hypertens. 2011;13(3):205–11.
27. Butcher KS, Baird T, MacGregor L, Desmond P, Tress B, Davis S. Perihematomal edema in primary intracerebral hemorrhage is plasma derived. Stroke. 2004;35(8):1879–85.
28. Mayer SA, Lignelli A, Fink ME, Kessler DB, Thomas CE, Swarup R, et al. Perilesional blood flow and edema formation in acute intracerebral hemorrhage: a SPECT study. Stroke. 1998;29(9):1791–8.
29. Schellinger PD, Fiebach JB, Hoffmann K, Becker K, Orakcioglu B, Kollmar R, et al. Stroke MRI in intracerebral hemorrhage: is there a perihemorrhagic penumbra? Stroke. 2003;34(7):1674–9.
30. Zazulia AR, Diringer MN, Videen TO, Adams RE, Yundt K, Aiyagari V, et al. Hypoperfusion without ischemia surrounding acute intracerebral hemorrhage. J Cereb Blood Flow Metab. 2001;21(7):804–10.
31. Butcher KS, Jeerakathil T, Hill M, Demchuk AM, Dowlatshahi D, Coutts SB, et al. The intracerebral hemorrhage acutely decreasing arterial pressure trial. Stroke. 2013;44(3):620–6.
32. Menon RS, Burgess RE, Wing JJ, Gibbons MC, Shara NM, Fernandez S, et al. Predictors of highly prevalent brain ischemia in intracerebral hemorrhage. Ann Neurol. 2012;71(2):199–205.
33. Prabhakaran S, Naidech AM. Ischemic brain injury after intracerebral hemorrhage: a critical review. Stroke. 2012;43(8):2258–63.
34. Potter JF, Robinson TG, Ford GA, Mistri A, James M, Chernova J, et al. Controlling hypertension and hypotension immediately post-stroke (CHHIPS): a randomised, placebo-controlled, double-blind pilot trial. Lancet Neurol. 2009;8(1):48–56.
35. Robinson TG, Potter JF, Ford GA, Bulpitt CJ, Chernova J, Jagger C, et al. Effects of antihypertensive treatment after acute stroke in the Continue or Stop Post-Stroke Antihypertensives Collaborative Study (COSSACS): a prospective, randomised, open, blinded-endpoint trial. Lancet Neurol. 2010;9(8):767–75.
36. Sandset EC, Bath PM, Boysen G, Jatuzis D, Korv J, Luders S, et al. The angiotensin-receptor blocker candesartan for treatment of acute stroke (SCAST): a randomised, placebo-controlled, double-blind trial. Lancet. 2011;377(9767):741–50.
37. Jusufovic M, Sandset EC, Bath PM, Berge E, Scandinavian Candesartan Acute Stroke Trial Study Group. Blood pressure-lowering treatment with candesartan in patients with acute hemorrhagic stroke. Stroke. 2014;45(11):3440–2.
38. Bath PM, Houlton A, Woodhouse L, Sprigg N, Wardlaw J, Pocock S, et al. Statistical analysis plan for the 'Efficacy of Nitric Oxide in Stroke' (ENOS) trial. Int J Stroke. 2014;9(3):372–4.
39. Powers WJ, Zazulia AR, Videen TO, Adams RE, Yundt KD, Aiyagari V, et al. Autoregulation of cerebral blood flow surrounding acute (6 to 22 hours) intracerebral hemorrhage. Neurology. 2001;57(1):18–24.
40. Gould B, McCourt R, Gioia LC, Kate M, Hill MD, Asdaghi N, et al. Acute blood pressure reduction in patients with intracerebral hemorrhage does not result in borderzone region hypoperfusion. Stroke. 2014;45(10):2894–9.
41. McCourt R, Gould B, Gioia L, Kate M, Coutts SB, Dowlatshahi D, et al. Cerebral perfusion and blood pressure do not affect perihematoma edema growth in acute intracerebral hemorrhage. Stroke. 2014;45(5):1292–8.
42. Koch S, Romano JG, Forteza AM, Otero CM, Rabinstein AA. Rapid blood pressure reduction in acute intracerebral hemorrhage: feasibility and safety. Neurocrit Care. 2008;8(3):316–21.
43. Anderson CS, Huang Y, Wang JG, Arima H, Neal B, Peng B, et al. Intensive blood pressure reduction in acute cerebral haemorrhage trial (INTERACT): a randomised pilot trial. Lancet Neurol. 2008;7(5):391–9.
44. Antihypertensive Treatment of Acute Cerebral Hemorrhage (ATACH) Investigators. Antihypertensive treatment of acute cerebral hemorrhage. Crit Care Med. 2010;38(2):637–48.
45. Qureshi AI, Palesch YY, Martin R, Novitzke J, Cruz-Flores S, Ehtisham A, et al. Effect of systolic blood pressure reduction on hematoma expansion, perihematomal edema, and 3-month outcome among patients with intracerebral hemorrhage: results from the antihypertensive treatment of acute cerebral hemorrhage study. Arch Neurol. 2010;67(5):570–6.

46. Anderson CS, Heeley E, Huang Y, Wang J, Stapf C, Delcourt C, et al. Rapid blood-pressure lowering in patients with acute intracerebral hemorrhage. N Engl J Med. 2013;368(25):2355–65.
47. Anderson CS, Qureshi AI. Implications of INTERACT2 and other clinical trials: blood pressure management in acute intracerebral hemorrhage. Stroke. 2015;46(1):291–5.
48. Hill MD, Muir KW. INTERACT-2: should blood pressure be aggressively lowered acutely after intracerebral hemorrhage? Stroke. 2013;44(10):2951–2.
49. Qureshi AI, Palesch YY, Martin R, Toyoda K, Yamamoto H, Wang Y, et al. Interpretation and implementation of Intensive Blood Pressure Reduction in Acute Cerebral Hemorrhage Trial (INTERACT II). J Vasc Interv Neurol. 2014;7(2):34–40.
50. Tsivgoulis G, Katsanos AH, Butcher KS, Boviatsis E, Triantafyllou N, Rizos I, et al. Intensive blood pressure reduction in acute intracerebral hemorrhage: a meta-analysis. Neurology. 2014;83(17):1523–9.
51. Koga M, Toyoda K, Yamagami H, Okuda S, Okada Y, Kimura K, et al. Systolic blood pressure lowering to 160 mmHg or less using nicardipine in acute intracerebral hemorrhage: a prospective, multicenter, observational study (the Stroke Acute Management with Urgent Risk-factor Assessment and Improvement-Intracerebral Hemorrhage study). J Hypertens. 2012;30(12):2357–64.
52. Peacock 4th WF, Hilleman DE, Levy PD, Rhoney DH, Varon J. A systematic review of nicardipine vs labetalol for the management of hypertensive crises. Am J Emerg Med. 2012;30(6):981–93.
53. Liu-Deryke X, Janisse J, Coplin WM, Parker Jr D, Norris G, Rhoney DH. A comparison of nicardipine and labetalol for acute hypertension management following stroke. Neurocrit Care. 2008;9(2):167–76.
54. Liu-DeRyke X, Levy PD, Parker Jr D, Coplin W, Rhoney DH. A prospective evaluation of labetalol versus nicardipine for blood pressure management in patients with acute stroke. Neurocrit Care. 2013;19(1):41–7.
55. Graffagnino C, Bergese S, Love J, Schneider D, Lazaridis C, LaPointe M, et al. Clevidipine rapidly and safely reduces blood pressure in acute intracerebral hemorrhage: the ACCELERATE trial. Cerebrovasc Dis. 2013;36(3):173–80.
56. Hemphill 3rd JC, Greenberg SM, Anderson CS, Becker K, Bendok BR, Cushman M, et al. Guidelines for the management of spontaneous intracerebral hemorrhage: a guideline for Healthcare Professionals from the American Heart Association/American Stroke Association. Stroke. 2015;46(7):2032–60.
57. Steiner T, Al-Shahi Salman R, Beer R, Christensen H, Cordonnier C, Csiba L, et al. European Stroke Organisation (ESO) guidelines for the management of spontaneous intracerebral hemorrhage. Int J Stroke. 2014;9(7):840–55.
58. Foundation NS. Clinical guidelines for stroke management 2010 (cited 2015 11/14/2015). https://strokefoundation.com.au/~/media/strokewebsite/resources/treatment/clinical_guidelines_stroke_managment_2010_interactive.ashx?la=en
59. Casaubon LK, Boulanger JM, Blacquiere D, Boucher S, Brown K, Goddard T, et al. Canadian stroke best practice recommendations: hyperacute stroke care guidelines, update 2015. Int J Stroke. 2015;10(6):924–40.
60. Shinohara Y, Yanagihara T, Abe K, Yoshimine T, Fujinaka T, Chuma T, et al. III. Intracerebral hemorrhage. J Stroke Cerebrovasc Dis. 2011;20(4 Suppl):S74–99.
61. Qureshi AI, Palesch YY. Antihypertensive Treatment of Acute Cerebral Hemorrhage (ATACH) II: design, methods, and rationale. Neurocrit Care. 2011;15(3):559–76.
62. Butcher K. The intracerebral hemorrhage acutely decreasing arterial pressure trial II (ICH-ADAPT II). NCT02281838, 2014 (cited 2015 11/14/2015). https://clinicaltrials.gov/ct2/show/NCT02281838
63. Arima H, Heeley E, Delcourt C, Hirakawa Y, Wang X, Woodward M, et al. Optimal achieved blood pressure in acute intracerebral hemorrhage: INTERACT2. Neurology. 2015;84(5):464–71.
64. Saver JL, Kidwell C, Eckstein M, Starkman S, Investigators F-MPT. Prehospital neuroprotective therapy for acute stroke: results of the Field Administration of Stroke Therapy-Magnesium (FAST-MAG) pilot trial. Stroke. 2004;35(5):e106–8.
65. Qureshi AI, Palesch YY, Barsan WG, Hanley DF, Hsu CY, Martin RL, et al. Intensive blood-pressure lowering in patients with acute cerebral hemorrhage. N Engl J Med. 2016. [E pub ahead of print].

Chapter 11
Blood Pressure Management in Subarachnoid Hemorrhage: The Role of Blood Pressure Manipulation in Prevention of Rebleeding and the Management of Vasospasm

Zakraus K. Mahdavi, Claudia A. Perez, and Michael A. Rubin

Subarachnoid hemorrhage (SAH) is a neurological emergency that affects thousands of Americans annually. Specific guidelines have been created for the management of SAH in an effort to improve overall outcomes. For clarity, this chapter will be discussing aneurysmal SAH and not SAH associated with traumatic brain injury. The incidence of SAH varies widely within the United States, from 9.7 per 100,000 to 14.5 per 100,000 adults [1]. It has been reported that more than a quarter of patients with SAH die, and approximately half of the survivors are left with some persistent neurological deficit [1]. Patients with SAH can spend weeks in the intensive care unit. Even if their neurologic function is preserved, they may still need monitoring for development of hydrocephalus or vasospasm. In additional to open surgical and endovascular treatments to secure ruptured aneurysms, several protocols have been developed to medically manage SAH and its complications, but very few interventions have been shown in randomized controlled trials to have a significant impact. The treatment of high blood pressure and augmentation of low blood pressure is one of the main priorities with SAH and differs significantly from the approach for other types of stroke.

The clinical presentation of SAH is frequently described by a patient as the "worst headache of my life" [2]. While this phrase almost seems cliché', patients will literally use this expression to describe the intense pain that they experience

Z.K. Mahdavi, M.D.
Department of Neurological Surgery, Neurology and Neurotherapeutics, The University of Texas Southwestern Medical Center, 5323 Harry Hines Blvd., Dallas, TX 75201, USA
e-mail: zakraus.mahdavi@utsouthwestern.edu

C.A. Perez, M.D., M.S. • M.A. Rubin, M.D., M.A. (✉)
Department of Neurological Surgery, The University of Texas Southwestern Medical Center, 5323 Harry Hines Blvd., Dallas, TX 75201, USA

Department of Neurology and Neurotherapeutics, The University of Texas Southwestern Medical Center, 5323 Harry Hines Blvd., Dallas, TX 75201, USA
e-mail: claudia.perez@utsouthwestern.edu; Michael.rubin@utsouthwestern.edu

© Springer International Publishing Switzerland 2016
V. Aiyagari, P.B. Gorelick (eds.), *Hypertension and Stroke*, Clinical Hypertension and Vascular Diseases, DOI 10.1007/978-3-319-29152-9_11

from this headache. It is a severe and sudden "thunderclap" headache and may be lateralized in some patients. It can be so painful that patients will be immobilized and overwhelmed by the intensity. Patients may also have nausea, vomiting, or syncope. As the subarachnoid blood spreads, patients may develop meningismus, including photophobia and nuchal rigidity, several hours later. These symptoms may mimic the presentation of other cerebral insults, such as meningitis, spontaneous intracranial hypotension, cerebral venous sinus thrombosis, reversible cerebral vasoconstrictive syndrome, and primary thunderclap headache; consequently, these conditions ought to be considered in the differential diagnosis and a complete evaluation should include appropriate imaging and consideration of a lumbar puncture.

If the diagnosis of SAH is suspected, a prompt noncontrast head computed tomography (CT) scan should be obtained emergently, and if CT is non-confirmatory, a lumbar puncture (LP) should be considered. If the CT is performed within the first 24 h of ictus, hemorrhage will be seen in the subarachnoid spaces in 93 % of patients with SAH [3]. In the presence of SAH, an elevated RBC count would be noted in the CSF that does not diminish from tube 1 to tube 4. An LP is particularly useful in assessing for xanthochromia, which is a degradation product of hemoglobin, and indicates blood that has been present in the CSF for more than 2 h. Once the diagnosis of SAH is verified, vascular imaging should be performed with MR angiography (MRA), CT angiography (CTA), or a conventional digital subtraction angiogram (DSA) to detect an aneurysmal source. Conventional angiograms have higher sensitivity and should be performed if no aneurysm is detected on an MRA or CTA in a patient with a high suspicion for SAH (Class IIb evidence) [1]. Prompt identification of an aneurysm is a high priority so that it may be secured to reduce the risk of a rehemorrhage.

Risk Factors for Aneurysmal Subarachnoid Hemorrhage

Several risk factors for SAH exist, including hypertension, smoking, alcohol abuse, and the use of sympathomimetic drugs [1]. Data indicates a higher incidence in women [4], and African–Americans and Hispanics have a higher incidence than White-Americans [5]. The primary determinant of whether an intact aneurysm will rupture, is its size [6]; however, small aneurysms will still rupture in patients with risk factors of hypertension and smoking [7]. A patient with a first-degree family history of aneurysmal SAH has an increased risk of rupture over a patient without a family history [8]. Also, genetic disorders such as autosomal-dominant polycystic kidney disease and Type 4 Ehlers Danlos syndrome increase the risk for SAH.

According to guidelines of the American Stroke Association published in 2012, chronic hypertension should be treated as it may reduce the risk of SAH (Class 1B evidence) [1, 9]. Smoking appears to increase the risk of unruptured intracranial aneurysm formation, so smoking cessation should be advised to patients (Class IB evidence) [1]. Despite public health efforts to reduce risk factors such as hyperlipidemia, hypertension, and smoking, there has not been any significant change in the incidence of SAH over the last 30 years [10]. Interestingly enough, one study showed that the prevalence of diabetes in the aneurysmal SAH population is actually equivalent or lower than the general population [11]. In regards to hyperlipidemia, the data is unclear as to whether there is a correlation in patients with SAH, although one study in young adults aged 20–39 showed an unfavorable outcome in patients with SAH with hyperlipidemia [12].

Recently, data from the SAH international trialists (SAHIT) repository was analyzed to determine the prognostic value of premorbid hypertension in SAH. The study noted that premorbid history of hypertension was associated with a poorer outcome in SAH (OR 1.73) although when adjusted for age and neurological status (measured on the World Federation of Neurosurgical Societies (WFNS) scale), there was a decrease in the effect of premorbid hypertension, with an odds ratio of 1.37. There was also a higher chance of developing other complications including hydrocephalus, rehemorrhage, delayed cerebral ischemia (DCI), and cerebral infarctions [13].

Management of Blood Pressure Management Before the Aneurysm Is Secured

The goal of blood pressure management before an aneurysm is secured is twofold: first, to reduce the pressure enough to decrease the chance of a repeat hemorrhage, and second, to not lower it too much to cause inadequate cerebral perfusion pressure (CPP).

Blood Pressure Management and Rebleeding

A retrospective review of 273 SAH patients by Ohkuma et al. showed that a significantly higher rate of rebleeding occurs in hours 0–2 compared to hours 2–8. In addition, the risk of rebleeding for those with a systolic blood pressure of ≥ 160 mmHg was significantly higher (odds ratio 3.1, 95 % confidence interval 1.5–6.8) [14].

Another study in 1990 by Widjicks et al. retrospectively compared 134 patients with SAH for the incidence of rebleeding. The patients were divided into two groups: those that received antihypertensive treatment after hemorrhage for a systolic blood pressure goal less than 160 mmHg, and those that did not receive antihypertensive therapy [15]. While the study found a significant difference in rebleeding rates between the two groups (antihypertensive group—15 % versus untreated—33 %, $p = 0.012$), cerebral infarctions were also significantly higher in the group treated with antihypertensives (antihypertensive group 43 % versus untreated 22 %, $p = 0.03$) [16], thus illustrating the potential consequence of lowering blood pressure to reduce rebleeding risk. The current guidelines from the American Stroke Association have noted Class IIa evidence that keeping the systolic blood pressure less than 160 mmHg in an unsecured aneurysm is reasonable [1]. The Neurocritical Care Society has a similar position concluding that modest elevations in blood pressure with a MAP < 110 mmHg does not require therapy [16].

Blood Pressure Management and Intracranial Pressure

The concern over an excessive lowering of blood pressure is for related but different reasons in SAH than other forms of stroke. While perfusion of penumbra is the limiting concern of lowering blood pressure with ischemic stroke, maintaining an adequate mean arterial pressure (MAP) in the presence of raised intracranial pressure (ICP), impaired autoregulation or worsening cerebral vasospasm is the main concern with SAH. Recall that CPP is the difference between the MAP and the ICP. As subarachnoid blood interferes with the reabsorption of CSF at the arachnoid granulations, often causing increased ICPs and hydrocephalus, the ability for the brain to be perfused as a whole is in jeopardy.

Also, in the setting of brain injury, cerebral autoregulation may be altered [17]. As a result, any slight adjustment in the MAP may have a profound effect on cerebral blood flow. A clinical change associated with an intentional decrease in blood pressure may be related to exceeding the lower limit of autoregulation.

Cerebral Vasospasm and Delayed Cerebral Ischemia

After an aneurysm is secured, attention turns to the many complications that can occur with SAH. Acute hydrocephalus, cerebral edema, seizures, and hyponatremia from SIADH or cerebral salt wasting can all complicate the course after initial stabilization. Our primary focus will be what was originally termed "cerebral vasospasm" as blood pressure management in SAH is the topic of this chapter. Angiograms performed well into the course of SAH often revealed a variation in the diameter of blood vessels, i.e., vasospasm, often (but not exclusively) in the distribution of the hemorrhage, causing a deficit in local perfusion and consequent infarction (Fig. 11.1).

As the disease was studied, it became clear that patients occasionally have new deficits not attributable to any of the above complications except vasospasm, but without corresponding angiographic changes. This led to a paradigm shift that cerebral infarctions attributable to vasospasm may not be due just to variations in large vessel hemodynamics but also microscopic inflammatory changes. In addition to infarcts and clinical changes discovered in patients with normal cerebral angiograms, evidence from the Washington University in St Louis group has shown that these cerebral infarcts may be outside of the distribution of the angiographic

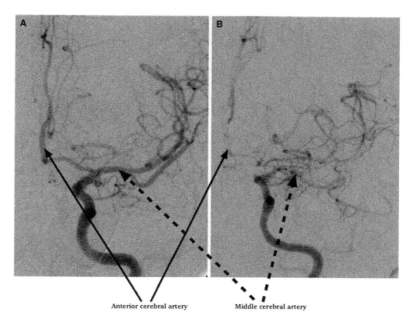

Fig. 11.1 Cerebral vasospasm: note the decrease in blood vessel diameter in both the anterior cerebral and middle cerebral arteries in panel *B* compared to panel *A* (Adapted from Fontana J, Moratin J, Ehrlich G, et al. Dynamic Autoregulatory Response After Aneurysmal Subarachnoid Hemorrhage and Its Relation to Angiographic Vasospasm and Clinical Outcome. *Neurocrit Care.* 2015;23:355–63, with permission)

vasospasm [18]. Consequently, clinical changes and angiographic vasospasm have been grouped into a condition known as DCI [18]. A proposed definition for DCI is the occurrence of a focal neurological deficit or a decrease of the Glasgow Coma Scale (GCS) by two or more points subsequent to the rupture of an aneurysm. This change should (1) last for at least 1 h, (2) not be apparent immediately after aneurysm occlusion, and (3) not be attributed to other causes by means of clinical assessment, CT or MRI scanning of the brain, and appropriate lab studies [19, 20].

The risk of developing cerebral vasospasm/DCI typically increases 3–5 days after the onset of the SAH and continues to day 14. It can present with almost any neurologic change, from a change in alertness to a focal motor deficit, depending on the arterial vascular distribution of the spasm [21]. The cause may be related to the reduced form of hemoglobin, oxyhemoglobin (OxyHb), which is present approximately 3–5 days after the blood enters the subarachnoid space and correlates with the time for red-cell lysis [22]. Although the exact mechanism is unclear, it is known that OxyHb generates activated oxygen species that can directly cause smooth muscle contraction [23]. DCI may also be related to damage that occurs to the brain in the first 72 h after the bleed onset and is termed "early brain injury." There are multiple mechanisms of early brain injury proposed, including ionic changes such as calcium influx, potassium efflux along with changes in serum magnesium levels,

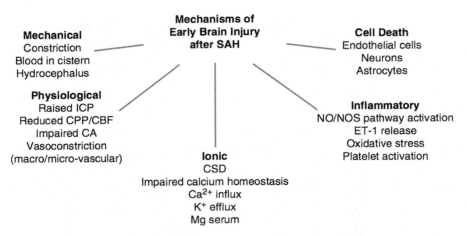

Fig. 11.2 Mechanisms of early brain injury after SAH. (From Rowland MJ, Hadjipavlou G, Kelly M, Westbrook J, Pattinson KTS. Delayed cerebral ischaemia after subarachnoid haemorrhage: looking beyond vasospasm. *British Journal of Anaesthesia.* 2012;109(3):315–329, with permission)

inflammatory pathways, and cell death (Fig. 11.2). Cortical spreading depression (CSD) has also been proposed as a mechanism behind DCI [19].

The risk of DCI is likely proportional to the amount and location of subarachnoid blood. CM Fisher developed a scale for vasospasm risk in 1980 when he noticed that, based on analysis of computerized tomography (CT) scans, the risk for vasospasm was significantly greater with subarachnoid blood clots larger than 5×3 mm and when there is 1 mm or thicker layers of blood in the fissures and cisterns. This system of grading SAHs is known as the Fisher Grade [21]. The Fisher grade ranges from 1 to 4 and grades subarachnoid blood seen on a CT scan. A grade of 1 indicates no evidence of hemorrhage. A grade of 2 indicates SAH < 1 mm thick, 3 is >1 mm thick, and 4 is for any thickness with intraventricular hemorrhage or intraparenchymal hemorrhage. A variant of this scale is the Modified Fisher Scale that reliably predicts the risk of symptomatic vasospasm [24].

Traditional Management of Blood Pressure After an Aneurysm Is Mechanically Secured

The classic teaching of patient management with vasospasm was to follow what was known as "Triple-H therapy" or "HHH." This approach includes maintaining *H*ypervolemia, elevated blood pressure (*H*ypertension), and *H*emodilution [25]. Although this practice was widely adopted, it has not been proven in a prospective, randomized controlled trial [26]. This concept was introduced in 1982 by Kassell et al., who noted that hypervolemic hypertensive therapy reversed the neurological deterioration in proven spasm in 47 of 58 patients [27]. Awad et al. in 1987 expanded on this research and noted that earlier surgical intervention along with treatment of vasospasm with hypervolemic hemodilution (defined as maintaining a hematocrit of 33–38 %, a central venous pressure of 10–12 mmHg, and a systolic blood pressure of 160–200 mmHg in patients with a secured aneurysm) resulted in improved outcomes [28]. Their study noted that after completion of the therapy, 47.6 % were neurologically normal, 24 % maintained a stable neurological status, and 16 % were noted to worsen. In 1988, Solomon et al. reported a case series with 125 patients with ruptured aneurysmal SAH, who were treated with prompt surgery along with initiation of prophylactic hypervolemic hypertensive therapy [29]. Ten patients developed DCI, which was reversible in six cases. This case series resulted in the widespread adoption of Triple-H therapy for treatment for vasospasm in patients with secured aneurysms.

The theory behind Triple-H therapy is largely based on the hemodynamics of a blood vessel with a narrowing diameter. Additionally, there is a loss of cerebral autoregulation thought to be secondary to a shift of cerebrovascular resistance from the penetrating arterioles to the major blood vessels, which occurs as the arterial narrowing increases. According to fluid dynamics described by Poiseuille's Law as noted below:

$$Q = \frac{\Delta P * \pi * r^4}{8 * L * n}$$

In this equation, Q is flow, ΔP is the pressure gradient, r is the vessel radius, L is vessel length, and n is viscosity. In the setting of a significantly smaller fixed radius due to vasospasm, the only remaining variables to adjust flow are the pressure gradient and blood viscosity [23, 30]. Figure 11.3 illustrates the normal functioning of cerebral autoregulation where the diameter changes to maintain constant flow, while Fig. 11.4 illustrates the changes that occur in cerebral vasospasm and how increasing blood pressure may overcome the deficiencies in the pathologic flow dynamics. Consequently, the first element of "Triple H" was to induce hypertension with vasopressors. Hypervolemia (the second "H") likely causes an increase in intravascular volume as well as causing hemodilution (the third "H") which is posited to reduce viscosity, which has an inverse relation with blood flow.

Systemic Complications of SAH Caused by Treatment of DCI

The treatment of SAH with "Triple H therapy" sometimes leads to systemic complications limiting the use of the traditional therapy. This has led to an approach to attempt to limit the systemic complications to preserve the benefit of intervention. The most common iatrogenic complication is pulmonary edema, which can be difficult to differentiate from its occurrence as a complication of SAH [16].

Cerebral Autoregulation

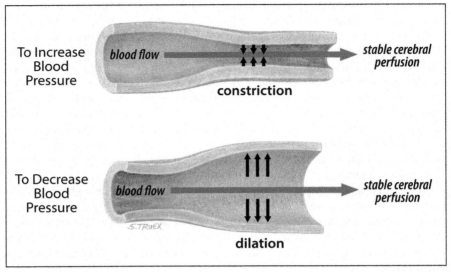

Fig. 11.3 Illustration of cerebral autoregulation with the goal of maintaining a stable cerebral perfusion pressure

This can lead to lower arterial oxygen saturation as well as decreased perfusion pressure, thus lowering delivery of oxygen to the brain. Very high crystalloid volume expansion is also associated with pulmonary edema even outside of any consistent heart failure or neurogenic pulmonary edema (discussed below) [31]. The frequent occurrence of pulmonary edema has led to a movement away from supra hypervolemic states. The most current recommendations from the Neurocritical Care Society emphasize euvolemia over hypervolemia [16]. This is corroborated by a study in 2000 by Lennihan et al., who randomized 82 patients post-clipping to hypervolemic therapy or euvolemic therapy, and CBF was measured using 133-xenon clearance. It was noted that despite the hypervolemic group receiving significantly more fluid and having higher central venous pressures as well as higher pulmonary artery diastolic pressures, there was no difference in global CBF between the two groups [32]. As a result, the study recommended avoiding hypovolemia, but also noted that hypervolemia is unlikely to provide an additional benefit.

Less common complications caused by traditional triple-H therapy include dilutional hyponatremia [31] as well as myocardial infarction (reported in about 2 % of patients). Although uncommon, hypertension induction with SAH can cause a neurologic deficit by inducing a phenomenon called reversible leukoencephalopathy syndrome (RLS), sometimes known with the word "posterior" added to the beginning. This condition was first described independent of SAH. Usually caused by an abrupt increase in blood pressure or found in patients being treated with immune suppression regiments or collagen vascular disease, the patient presents with nausea,

Vasospasm

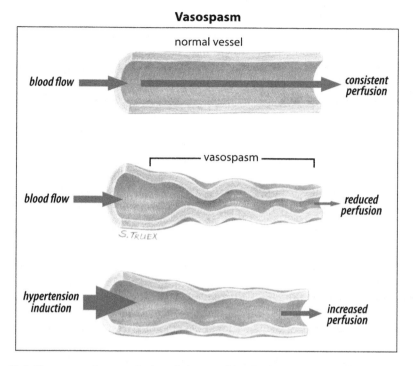

Fig. 11.4 Vasospasm alters cerebral perfusion, resulting in decreased cerebral perfusion. With hypertension induction, the goal is to increase perfusion pressure

headache, and visual disturbances and is found to have diffuse and symmetrical parietal and occipital white matter edema; however, edema has been described outside of these typical regions. Paramount to this diagnosis is its reversibility; when the offending agent is removed, the condition reverses. Multiple cases of RLS occurring during hemodynamic augmentation associated with SAH have been reported including one with CT perfusion showing increased blood volume in regions demonstrating edema and decreased mean transient time [33]. A review from the Mayo group cites three cases in the literature as well as three of their own where a neurologic deficit led to treatment for vasospasm followed by a further decline later attributed to RLS that is reversed when hemodynamic augmentation is reduced [34].

Contemporary Data and Treatment for DCI

Work has been published trying to delineate which elements of "Triple H" therapy are actually more likely to provide benefit.

Hypervolemia and Hemodilution

Hypervolemia and hemodilution studies have not shown a clear benefit. An animal stroke model showed that intravascular volume expansion can increase local blood flow to ischemic areas which appeared independent of MAP, the effect of which was limited to the extent that the animals developed heart failure. In order to assess whether the initial increase in cerebral blood flow may be related to the relative hemodilution seen in volume expansion, control animals underwent exchange transfusion with equivalent volumes of dextran-40 and whole blood. Blood volume and cardiac output were held constant and there was no alteration in local cerebral blood flow [35].

A study examining the effects of isovolemic and hypervolemic hemodilution in patients with vasospasm after SAH showed that isovolemic hemodilution caused an increase in global cerebral blood flow and also an increase in the volume of ischemic brain area with a pronounced reduction in the cerebral delivery of oxygen (CDRO2). These subjects underwent autotransfusion with previously removed blood to create a hypervolemic hemodiluted state that did not improve CBF and CDRO2 [36]. As an alternative to hemodilution, there has been some research evaluating whether maintaining higher hemoglobin levels improves outcomes. A study in 2006 evaluated hemoglobin levels in 103 patients with aneurysmal SAH. It was noted that higher levels of hemoglobin at Day 0 along with higher mean hemoglobin levels tended to predict a lower risk of cerebral infarction. In addition, higher mean hemoglobin levels were associated with lower odds of a poor outcome (odds ratio, 0.57 per g/dL; 95 % CI, 0.38–0.87; $P=0.009$) [37].

Induced Hypertension

Clinical data and animal models in SAH suggest that induced HTN, when compared with induced hypervolemia and hemodilution, is more effective in increasing regional cerebral blood flow and brain tissue oxygenation. While hypervolemic and hemodiluted states can slightly increase regional blood flow, they fail to improve brain tissue oxygenation. Triple-H therapy compared to induced hypertension alone failed to improve regional blood flow and the introduction of hypervolemic hemodilution reversed the initial effect of induced hypertension on brain tissue oxygenation [38].

Data does show that hypertension induction may reverse clinical changes associated with vasospasm/DCI. A study evaluating the efficacy of hypervolemia with either moderately induced hypertension or aggressively induced hypertension to increase brain tissue partial oxygenation (PO2), as measured by tissue oxygenation probe in angiographically verified vasospasm after SAH, found that moderate hypertension in euvolemic, hemodiluted patients can be an effective method of improving cerebral oxygenation. Moderately induced HTN was associated with lower complication rates than hypervolemia or aggressive induced HTN [39]. Clinical studies appear to support normovolemic induced HTN as an effective therapy in reducing ischemic symptoms attributed to cerebral vasospasm [40]. It has also been noted that patients with ongoing angiographic vasospasm and reduced cerebral blood flow measured by Xenon-enhanced CT had reversal of neurological deficits with dopamine induced hypertension and significant increase in regional blood flow. Similar effects were seen with phenylephrine [41, 42].

Studies citing improved cerebral blood flow with dopamine induced hypertension in ischemic territories have found a paradoxical effect on CBF in nonischemic territories and, in fact, have shown decreased cerebral blood flow [43]. Studies using serial O-positron emission tomographic (PET) imaging have shown that cerebral vasospasm is related to decreased cerebral perfusion, and there is additional regional hypoperfusion and oligemia in patients and cerebral regions without evidence of angiographic vasospasm [44]. Cerebral autoregulation is disrupted in ischemic and nonischemic areas associated with increased incidence of vasospasm and DCI after SAH [45, 46].

Cardiac Output Augmentation

As an alternative to targeting blood pressure augmentation, cardiac output augmentation with inotropic support has shown to provide benefit. Animal studies show a decrease in cerebral blood flow when cardiac output is decreased despite maintaining stable arterial blood flow [47]. This raises the question as to whether impaired cerebral autoregulation in ischemic areas as seen in SAH may create a greater dependence on perfusion pressure from cardiac function (CO). Levy et al. showed that in patients who were clinically refractory to hypervolemic therapy, dobutamine increasing cardiac output seemed to reverse neurological deficits [48]. One study examining patients with vasospasm after SAH found an independent influence on cerebral blood flow with augmentations in cardiac output independent of MAP. In this study, both phenylephrine and dobutamine were equally effective in increasing cerebral blood flow [49]. Of note, an interesting study published in 2003 used a xenon blood flow tomography-based system to quantitate CBF, and noted a direct relationship between increases in cardiac output (CO) via the use of dobutamine and CBF [49].

Others argue that the solution is neither blood pressure augmentation nor cardiac augmentation but altering the pulsatility of blood flow, as cerebral perfusion may not be completely dependent on CPP as a linear relationship (simple expedient). Local cerebral blood flow appears to be dependent on pulse pressure especially in ischemia. Studies comparing the effect of pulse pressure in ischemic and nonischemic brain showed a significant effect in cerebral blood flow when perfusion was changed from non-pulsatile to pulsatile blood flow, in ischemic brain tissue CBF increased 55 %, the effect was much less in nonischemic brain it increased 16 % [47].

Current Recommendations

Based on current NCS clinical guidelines, patients clinically suspected of DCI should undergo a trial of induced hypertension (moderate quality evidence, strong recommendation). The choice of vasopressor should be based on the pharmacologic properties of the agents (e.g., inotropy, tachycardia) (moderate quality evidence, strong recommendation). Blood pressure augmentation should progress in a stepwise fashion with assessment of neurologic function at each MAP level to determine if a higher blood pressure target is appropriate (poor quality evidence, strong recommendation). While there was no clear consensus on specific MAP or SBP ranges used, a targeted percent increase from baseline of 20 % is typically used. Blood pressure targets should be adjusted based on individual patient response to initial elevation of blood pressure. Common medications, dosing, and blood pressure parameters used in the induction of hypertension are illustrated in Table 11.1.

If patients with DCI do not improve with blood pressure augmentation, a trial of inotropic therapy may be considered (low quality evidence, strong recommendation). There is no specific blood pressure cutoff for supramaximal HTN before transition to inotropes (although most studies maintained SBP < 220), the indication for inotrope was lack of response to induced hypertension. Some centers avoid use of inotropes given concern for reduction in blood pressure. Inotropes with prominent B-2 agonist properties (e.g., dobutamine) may lower MAP and require increases in vasopressor dosage (high quality evidence, strong recommendation) [16]. In the studies reviewed there was mainly invasive pulmonary arterial (Swanz-Ganz) catheter monitoring of cardiac output with use of inotropes [48, 49]. A particular means of measuring volume and pressure augmentation is not recommended, however placement of central lines and/or pulmonary artery catheters may not provide an advantage over noninvasive technologies.

Complications of SAH That May Limit Blood Pressure and Volume Augmentation in the Treatment of DCI

Besides the cardiopulmonary complications caused by the treat of DCI, the inflammatory state induced by an aneurysmal rupture can causes several systemic complications limiting the modification of blood pressure to maximize cerebral perfusion. Cardiac dysfunction as a result of SAH is not uncommon. A review of 617 patients with SAH found that 14.1 % of them had features concerning for a cardiac evaluation with 46 % of them having a myocardial infarction, 63 % an arrhythmia, and 31 % of them having heart failure [50]. Stress cardiomyopathy (SCM) is a well-documented feature of SAH. While its pathophysiology is not completely understood, a massive cardiac response likely caused by a catecholamine surge associated with the initial hemorrhage can lead to diffuse ECG changes, cardiac ischemia, and

Table 11.1 Common medications used to induce hypertension

Drug name	Initial dose	Maintenance dose	Max doses used in refractory shock	Doses used in induced HTN to treat DCI	Targets used in induced HTN to treat DCI
Norepinephrine [38, 57]	0.1–0.15 mcg/kg/min	0.025–0.05 mcg/kg/min	0.5–0.75 mcg/kg/min; up to 3.3 mcg/kg/min		MAP>130 or SBP 200–220
Epinephrine [39]	0.014 mcg/kg/min	0.014–0.14 mcg/kg/min	0.14–0.5 mcg/kg/min	0.1–0.5 mcg/kg/min	CPP >120 mmHg (SBP >220 mmHg were avoided)
Phenylephrine [41, 49]	0.5–2 mcg/kg/min	0.25–1.1 mcg/kg/min	1.1–6 mcg/kg/min	4.8 mcg/kg/min	MAP 120–150, 112–173
Dopamine [39, 40, 42, 43, 58]	2–5 mcg/kg/min	5–20 mcg/kg/min	20 to >50 mcg/kg/min	5–20 mcg/kg/min, one study used up to 46 mcg/kg/min	MAP 95–150, CPP 80–120 mmHg, SBP 160–200

Takotsubo

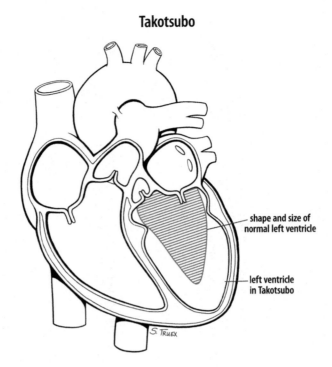

Fig. 11.5 Takotsubo cardiomyopathy: left ventricle changes in size and shape

cardiac failure. This heart failure is self-limited and will often resolve within days to weeks.

Paramount in distinguishing SCM as its own entity is that the distribution of the cardiac failure is not consistent with a single vascular territory as seen in coronary artery disease. The classic presentation includes apical left ventricular dysfunction, which led to the description of the phenomenon as "Takotsubo Cardiomyopathy" as it is similar in appearance to a trap used by Japanese fishermen to catch octopus (Fig. 11.5); however, there are also subtypes where the dysfunction is primarily in the basal segment. A series of 2276 patients found that 79.9 % of cases have apical ballooning while the remainder had apical sparing [51]. This phenomenon is likely not restricted to SAH and has been reported in acute ischemic stroke as well as peripheral nervous disease, and seizure [52, 53].

Managing heart failure in these patients is extremely challenging while balancing strategies to reduce the likelihood of DCI; the usual method of hypervolemia and hypertension with SAH are the antithesis of the approach of managing acute heart failure. Usually, afterload reduction and diuresis with lowering of blood pressure and the avoidance of peripheral alpha constriction are helpful in heart failure; however, these strategies may lead to reduced cerebral perfusion at a most delicate point in vasospasm management. The best approach is to manage the heart failure only as much as is necessary to allow for adequate forward flow and acceptable amount of pulmonary edema without decreasing alveolar to arterial oxygenation. If possible, tolerate the heart failure during the period of maximum likelihood of cerebral vasospasm and correct the failure when the risk has lessened. Often, the natural history of heart failure caused by SAH is short-lived and may improve without the need for specific interventions.

Respiratory insufficiency and failure are also common with SAH. A review of 70 patients with SAH showed that 80 % had some impairment of oxygenation with 14 % with pneumonia, 16 % with neurogenic pulmonary edema, 27 % from atelectasis and the remained without a defined etiology [54]. While this study did not show a correlation between respiratory issues and vasospasm, another found that symptomatic vasospasm (vasospasm with a clinical change) increased in frequency from 31 to 63 % for those with respiratory issues ($P < 0.001$) [55]. "Neurogenic pulmonary edema" is likely caused by the same inflammatory cascade or catecholamine surge SCM, this time causing a change in pulmonary capillary bed pressure or permeability [56]. As this condition is not necessarily caused by heart failure or volume overload, it does not always respond to diuresis in the same manner as other causes of pulmonary edema.

Summary

SAH is a neurological emergency affecting anywhere between 9.7 and 14.5 in 100,000 adults yearly within the United States. Risk factors for SAH include hypertension, smoking, alcohol use, and the use of sympathomimetic drugs. Patients will frequently describe it as being the "worst headache of my life." If there is concern for SAH, a prompt head CT should be obtained, and if negative, an LP should be performed. If a diagnosis of SAH is made, vascular imaging to identify a source of the hemorrhage should then be pursued.

Guidelines from the American Stroke Association have suggested maintaining a systolic blood pressure < 160 mmHg or MAP < 110 mmHg in the setting of an unsecured aneurysm. Once the aneurysm has been secured, the next key in management is avoidance of DCI. This was initially thought to be due to vasospasm, but data now shows that patients can have deficits without evidence of vasospasm. The risk of DCI increases around days 3–5 and continues to day 14. Several mechanisms have been proposed that contribute to DCI.

Current data suggests that Triple-H therapy, which was once widely adopted in the practice of prevention of diffuse cerebral injury, can cause systemic complications, particularly pulmonary edema, that result in higher risk than reward. The current recommendation is for induced hypertension; MAPs should be titrated in a stepwise manner with a focus on the effects on the neurological exam to determine a need for further titration. Management of SAH and diffuse cerebral injury continues to evolve as our understanding of the disease process and its associated complications are better understood.

References

1. Connolly Jr ES, Rabinstein AA, Carhuapoma JR, et al. Guidelines for the management of aneurysmal subarachnoid hemorrhage: a guideline for healthcare professionals from the American Heart Association/American Stroke Association. Stroke. 2012;43(6):1711–37.
2. Gorelick PB, Hier DB, Caplan LR, Langenberg P. Headache in acute cerebrovascular disease. Neurology. 1986;36(11):1445–50.
3. Perry JJ, Stiell IG, Sivilotti ML, et al. Sensitivity of computed tomography performed within six hours of onset of headache for diagnosis of subarachnoid haemorrhage: prospective cohort study. Br Med J. 2011;343:d4277.
4. Shea AM, Reed SD, Curtis LH, Alexander MJ, Villani JJ, Schulman KA. Characteristics of nontraumatic subarachnoid hemorrhage in the United States in 2003. Neurosurgery. 2007;61(6):1131–7; discussion 1137–8.
5. Labovitz DL, Halim AX, Brent B, Boden-Albala B, Hauser WA, Sacco RL. Subarachnoid hemorrhage incidence among Whites, Blacks and Caribbean Hispanics: the Northern Manhattan Study. Neuroepidemiology. 2006;26(3):147–50.
6. Lall RR, Eddleman CS, Bendok BR, Batjer HH. Unruptured intracranial aneurysms and the assessment of rupture risk based on anatomical and morphological factors: sifting through the sands of data. Neurosurg Focus. 2009;26(5):E2.
7. Etminan N, Beseoglu K, Steiger HJ, Hanggi D. The impact of hypertension and nicotine on the size of ruptured intracranial aneurysms. J Neurol Neurosurg Psychiatry. 2011;82(1):4–7.
8. Broderick JP, Brown Jr RD, Sauerbeck L, et al. Greater rupture risk for familial as compared to sporadic unruptured intracranial aneurysms. Stroke. 2009;40(6):1952–7.
9. Thompson BG, Brown Jr RD, Amin-Hanjani S, et al. Guidelines for the management of patients with unruptured intracranial aneurysms: a guideline for Healthcare Professionals from the American Heart Association/American Stroke Association. Stroke. 2015;46(8):2368–400.
10. Lovelock CE, Rinkel GJ, Rothwell PM. Time trends in outcome of subarachnoid hemorrhage: population-based study and systematic review. Neurology. 2010;74(19):1494–501.
11. Adams Jr HP, Putman SF, Kassell NF, Torner JC. Prevalence of diabetes mellitus among patients with subarachnoid hemorrhage. Arch Neurol. 1984;41(10):1033–5.
12. Chotai S, Ahn SY, Moon HJ, et al. Prediction of outcomes in young adults with aneurysmal subarachnoid hemorrhage. Neurol Med Chir. 2013;53(3):157–62.
13. Jaja BN, Lingsma H, Schweizer TA, et al. Prognostic value of premorbid hypertension and neurological status in aneurysmal subarachnoid hemorrhage: pooled analyses of individual patient data in the SAHIT repository. J Neurosurg. 2015;122(3):644–52.
14. Ohkuma H, Tsurutani H, Suzuki S. Incidence and significance of early aneurysmal rebleeding before neurosurgical or neurological management. Stroke. 2001;32(5):1176–80.
15. Wijdicks EF, Vermeulen M, Murray GD, Hijdra A, van Gijn J. The effects of treating hypertension following aneurysmal subarachnoid hemorrhage. Clin Neurol Neurosurg. 1990;92(2):111–7.
16. Diringer MN, Bleck TP, Claude Hemphill 3rd J, et al. Critical care management of patients following aneurysmal subarachnoid hemorrhage: recommendations from the Neurocritical Care Society's Multidisciplinary Consensus Conference. Neurocrit Care. 2011;15(2):211–40.
17. Lang EW, Diehl RR, Mehdorn HM. Cerebral autoregulation testing after aneurysmal subarachnoid hemorrhage: the phase relationship between arterial blood pressure and cerebral blood flow velocity. Crit Care Med. 2001;29(1):158–63.
18. Brown RJ, Kumar A, Dhar R, Sampson TR, Diringer MN. The relationship between delayed infarcts and angiographic vasospasm after aneurysmal subarachnoid hemorrhage. Neurosurgery. 2013;72(5):702–8.
19. Rowland MJ, Hadjipavlou G, Kelly M, Westbrook J, Pattinson KTS. Delayed cerebral ischaemia after subarachnoid haemorrhage: looking beyond vasospasm. Br J Anaesth. 2012;109(3):315–29.

20. Vergouwen MDI, Vermeulen M, van Gijn J, et al. Definition of delayed cerebral ischemia after aneurysmal subarachnoid hemorrhage as an outcome event in clinical trials and observational studies: proposal of a Multidisciplinary Research Group. Stroke. 2010;41(10):2391–5.
21. Heros RC, Zervas NT, Varsos V. Cerebral vasospasm after subarachnoid hemorrhage: an update. Ann Neurol. 1983;14(6):599–608.
22. Weir B, Macdonald RL, Stoodley M. Etiology of cerebral vasospasm. Acta Neurochir Suppl. 1999;72:27–46.
23. Lee KH, Lukovits T, Friedman JA. "Triple-H" therapy for cerebral vasospasm following subarachnoid hemorrhage. Neurocrit Care. 2006;4(1):68–76.
24. Frontera JA, Claassen J, Schmidt JM, et al. Prediction of symptomatic vasospasm after subarachnoid hemorrhage: the modified fisher scale. Neurosurgery. 2006;59(1):21–7; discussion 21–7.
25. Treggiari MM, Participants in the International Multi-Disciplinary Consensus Conference on the Critical Care Management of Subarachnoid Hemorrhage. Hemodynamic management of subarachnoid hemorrhage. Neurocrit Care. 2011;15(2):329–35.
26. Oropello JM, Weiner L, Benjamin E. Hypertensive, hypervolemic, hemodilutional therapy for aneurysmal subarachnoid hemorrhage. Is it efficacious? No. Crit Care Clin. 1996;12(3):709–30.
27. Kassell NF, Peerless SJ, Durward QJ, Beck DW, Drake CG, Adams HP. Treatment of ischemic deficits from vasospasm with intravascular volume expansion and induced arterial hypertension. Neurosurgery. 1982;11(3):337–43.
28. Awad IA, Carter LP, Spetzler RF, Medina M, Williams Jr FC. Clinical vasospasm after subarachnoid hemorrhage: response to hypervolemic hemodilution and arterial hypertension. Stroke. 1987;18(2):365–72.
29. Solomon RA, Fink ME, Lennihan L. Early aneurysm surgery and prophylactic hypervolemic hypertensive therapy for the treatment of aneurysmal subarachnoid hemorrhage. Neurosurgery. 1988;23(6):699–704.
30. Aaslid R. Hemodynamics of cerebrovascular spasm. Acta Neurochir Suppl. 1999;72:47–57.
31. Sen J, Belli A, Albon H, Morgan L, Petzold A, Kitchen N. Triple-H therapy in the management of aneurysmal subarachnoid haemorrhage. Lancet Neurol. 2003;2(10):614–21.
32. Lennihan L, Mayer SA, Fink ME, et al. Effect of hypervolemic therapy on cerebral blood flow after subarachnoid hemorrhage : a randomized controlled trial. Stroke. 2000;31(2):383–91.
33. Wartenberg KE, Parra A. CT and CT-perfusion findings of reversible leukoencephalopathy during triple-H therapy for symptomatic subarachnoid hemorrhage-related vasospasm. J Neuroimaging. 2006;16(2):170–5.
34. Giraldo EA, Fugate JE, Rabinstein AA, Lanzino G, Wijdicks EF. Posterior reversible encephalopathy syndrome associated with hemodynamic augmentation in aneurysmal subarachnoid hemorrhage. Neurocrit Care. 2011;14(3):427–32.
35. Keller TS, McGillicuddy JE, LaBond VA, Kindt GW. Volume expansion in focal cerebral ischemia: the effect of cardiac output on local cerebral blood flow. Clin Neurosurg. 1982;29:40–50.
36. Ekelund A, Reinstrup P, Ryding E, et al. Effects of iso- and hypervolemic hemodilution on regional cerebral blood flow and oxygen delivery for patients with vasospasm after aneurysmal subarachnoid hemorrhage. Acta Neurochir. 2002;144(7):703–12; discussion 703–12.
37. Naidech AM, Drescher J, Ault ML, Shaibani A, Batjer HH, Alberts MJ. Higher hemoglobin is associated with less cerebral infarction, poor outcome, and death after subarachnoid hemorrhage. Neurosurgery. 2006;59(4):775–9; discussion 779–780.
38. Muench E, Horn P, Bauhuf C, et al. Effects of hypervolemia and hypertension on regional cerebral blood flow, intracranial pressure, and brain tissue oxygenation after subarachnoid hemorrhage. Crit Care Med. 2007;35(8):1844–51; quiz 1852.
39. Raabe A, Beck J, Keller M, Vatter H, Zimmermann M, Seifert V. Relative importance of hypertension compared with hypervolemia for increasing cerebral oxygenation in patients with cerebral vasospasm after subarachnoid hemorrhage. J Neurosurg. 2005;103(6):974–81.

40. Otsubo H, Takemae T, Inoue T, Kobayashi S, Sugita K. Normovolaemic induced hypertension therapy for cerebral vasospasm after subarachnoid haemorrhage. Acta Neurochir. 1990;103(1–2):18–26.
41. Muizelaar JP, Becker DP. Induced hypertension for the treatment of cerebral ischemia after subarachnoid hemorrhage. Direct effect on cerebral blood flow. Surg Neurol. 1986;25(4):317–25.
42. Touho H, Karasawa J, Ohnishi H, Shishido H, Yamada K, Shibamoto K. Evaluation of therapeutically induced hypertension in patients with delayed cerebral vasospasm by xenon-enhanced computed tomography. Neurol Med Chir. 1992;32(9):671–8.
43. Darby JM, Yonas H, Marks EC, Durham S, Snyder RW, Nemoto EM. Acute cerebral blood flow response to dopamine-induced hypertension after subarachnoid hemorrhage. J Neurosurg. 1994;80(5):857–64.
44. Dhar R, Diringer MN. Relationship between angiographic vasospasm, cerebral blood flow, and cerebral infarction after subarachnoid hemorrhage. Acta Neurochir Suppl. 2015;120:161–5.
45. Fontana J, Moratin J, Ehrlich G, et al. Dynamic autoregulatory response after aneurysmal subarachnoid hemorrhage and its relation to angiographic vasospasm and clinical outcome. Neurocrit Care. 2015;23:355–63.
46. Otite F, Mink S, Tan CO, et al. Impaired cerebral autoregulation is associated with vasospasm and delayed cerebral ischemia in subarachnoid hemorrhage. Stroke. 2014;45(3):677–82.
47. Tranmer BI, Gross CE, Kindt GW, Adey GR. Pulsatile versus nonpulsatile blood flow in the treatment of acute cerebral ischemia. Neurosurgery. 1986;19(5):724–31.
48. Levy ML, Rabb CH, Zelman V, Giannotta SL. Cardiac performance enhancement from dobutamine in patients refractory to hypervolemic therapy for cerebral vasospasm. J Neurosurg. 1993;79(4):494–9.
49. Joseph M, Ziadi S, Nates J, Dannenbaum M, Malkoff M. Increases in cardiac output can reverse flow deficits from vasospasm independent of blood pressure: a study using xenon computed tomographic measurement of cerebral blood flow. Neurosurgery. 2003;53(5):1044–51; discussion 1042–51.
50. Ahmadian A, Mizzi A, Banasiak M, et al. Cardiac manifestations of subarachnoid hemorrhage. Heart Lung Vessel. 2013;5(3):168–78.
51. Abd TT, Hayek S, Cheng JW, Samuels OB, Wittstein IS, Lerakis S. Incidence and clinical characteristics of takotsubo cardiomyopathy post-aneurysmal subarachnoid hemorrhage. Int J Cardiol. 2014;176(3):1362–4.
52. Murthy SB, Shah S, Venkatasubba Rao CP, Suarez JI, Bershad EM. Clinical characteristics of myocardial stunning in acute stroke. J Clin Neurosci. 2014;21(8):1279–82.
53. Porto I, Della Bona R, Leo A, et al. Stress cardiomyopathy (tako-tsubo) triggered by nervous system diseases: a systematic review of the reported cases. Int J Cardiol. 2013;167(6):2441–8.
54. Vespa PM, Bleck TP. Neurogenic pulmonary edema and other mechanisms of impaired oxygenation after aneurysmal subarachnoid hemorrhage. Neurocrit Care. 2004;1(2):157–70.
55. Friedman JA, Pichelmann MA, Piepgras DG, et al. Pulmonary complications of aneurysmal subarachnoid hemorrhage. Neurosurgery. 2003;52(5):1025–32.
56. Junttila E, Ala-Kokko T, Ohtonen P, et al. Neurogenic pulmonary edema in patients with nontraumatic intracerebral hemorrhage: predictors and association with outcome. Anesth Analg. 2013;116(4):855–61.
57. De Araujo LC, Zappulla RA, Yang WC, Hollin SA. Angiographic changes to induced hypertension in cerebral vasospasm. Case report. J Neurosurg. 1978;49(2):312–5.
58. Brown FD, Hanlon K, Mullan S. Treatment of aneurysmal hemiplegia with dopamine and mannitol. J Neurosurg. 1978;49(4):525–9.

Chapter 12
Recurrent Stroke Prevention: Diuretic and Angiotensin-Converting Enzyme Inhibitors (ACEIs)—The PROGRESS Trial

Thomas K.A. Linden and Geoffrey A. Donnan

Background to the Progress Study

The rationale and design of the Perindopril Protection Against Secondary Stroke Study (PROGRESS) was published in 1996 [1], while recruitment had already commenced in 1995. The study design involved a randomized, double-blind, placebo-controlled trial approach in which the blood pressure-lowering component was the angiotensin-converting enzyme inhibiting agent perindopril with and without the addition of the thiazide-like diuretic indapamide. The primary outcome measure was recurrent stroke of all types (fatal, nonfatal, ischaemic and hemorrhagic). The total sample size was over 7000 patients from almost 200 centres in ten countries worldwide with a follow-up of a mean 4 years. The major findings were published in 2001. PROGRESS was the first study to show definitively that ACEI-based blood pressure-lowering regimens reduced the risk of recurrent stroke. This was particularly for haemorrhagic stroke and, importantly, was independent of baseline blood pressure. In other words, the benefits were not only for hypertensive patients, but for all participants.

Before PROGRESS, there was quite strong evidence that treatment of hypertension was a powerful means of primary stroke prevention (*see* Chaps. 2 and 3).

T.K.A. Linden, M.D., Ph.D. (✉)
Institute of Neuroscience and Physiology, Gothenburg University,
Box 100, Gothenburg 405 30, Sweden

The Florey Institute of Neuroscience and Mental Health,
30 Royal Parade, Melbourne, VIC 3052, Australia

Department of Neurology, Sahlgrenska University Hospital, Gothenburg, Sweden
e-mail: thomas.linden@neuro.gu.se

G.A. Donnan, M.D., F.R.C.P., F.R.A.C.P.
The Florey Institute of Neuroscience and Mental Health,
30 Royal Parade, Melbourne, VIC 3052, Australia
e-mail: geoffrey.donnan@florey.edu.au

© Springer International Publishing Switzerland 2016
V. Aiyagari, P.B. Gorelick (eds.), *Hypertension and Stroke*, Clinical
Hypertension and Vascular Diseases, DOI 10.1007/978-3-319-29152-9_12

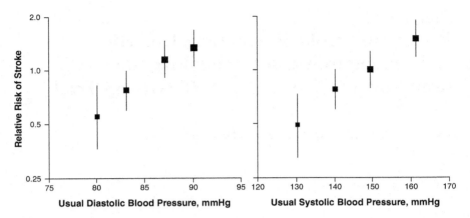

Fig. 12.1 The UKTIA study showed the association between rising blood pressure and increased risk for stroke, both for diastolic and systolic blood pressure and also in normotensive individuals (From Rodgers A, MacMahon S, Gamble G, Slattery J, Sandercock P, Warlow C. Blood pressure and risk of stroke in patients with cerebrovascular disease. The United Kingdom Transient Ischaemic Attack Collaborative Group. BMJ (Clin Res Ed). 1996;313(7050):147, with permission)

A number of meta-analyses of the existing evidence established that blood pressure reduction was associated with fewer incident stroke events [2] and there was a view, however questioned, that the introduction of blood pressure-lowering agents since the 1950s was a major contributor to the gradual reduction of mortality from stroke from about that time [3]. It was apparent that there was a linearly increasing risk between elevation of blood pressure and risk for stroke based on both epidemiological and clinical trial evidence [4]. Some suggested that there may be a J-shaped relationship between blood pressure and stroke risk [5]. However, the evidence regarding risk for recurrent stroke and its association with blood pressure was less clear. Perhaps some of the more persuasive information came from a further analysis of the United Kingdom Transient Ischemic Attack Study [6], which was published at about the time of the commencement of PROGRESS. The authors were able to demonstrate that in people with established cerebrovascular disease, blood pressure level is an important risk factor not only in the hypertensive range, but also in what in many countries still today is considered normotensive (Fig. 12.1).

An important inference from the study was that a consistent 5 mmHg lowering of blood pressure would yield a secondary stroke risk reduction by a third. Interestingly, there was no "safe" blood pressure level, thus establishing the continuous relationship between blood pressure and stroke risk and questioning the concept of the J-shaped curve.

The UKTIA study was, however, not a blood pressure-lowering treatment trial. As mentioned earlier, the effect of hypertension treatment on first-stroke incidence had been studied in a meta-analysis approach comprising almost 50,000 individuals and 5 years of follow-up from the Hypertension Detection and Follow-up Programme (HDFP), the Medical Research Council Hypertension Trial (MRC), the Systolic

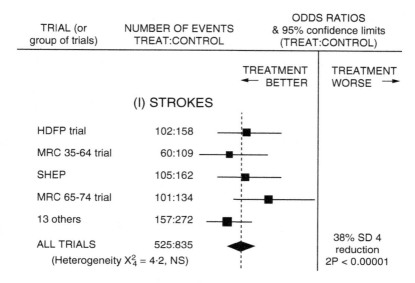

Fig. 12.2 Stroke odds ratio reduction in pooled unconfounded antihypertensive drug trials comprising almost 50,000 patients and 5 years of follow-up. *Solid squares* represent the treatment: control odds ratios. The *squares' sizes* correspond to the relative weight of the trial in the pooled measure. The *horizontal lines* denote 95 % confidence intervals for the individual or combined studies, as does the *diamond shape* for the pooled data (From Collins R, MacMahon S. Blood pressure, antihypertensive drug treatment and the risks of stroke and of coronary heart disease. Br Med Bull. 1994;50(2):272–98, with permission)

Hypertension in the Elderly Trial (SHEP) and 13 smaller trials [7]. The mean effect of the average decline in blood pressure of 6 mmHg was a relative reduction of 38 %, equally for fatal and non-fatal, strokes (Fig. 12.2).

The initial attempts to establish the effect of blood pressure lowering as a secondary stroke prevention strategy produced two studies with conflicting results (*see* Chaps. 2 and 3). Both were conducted during the 1970s and were diuretic based. One showed a significant secondary stroke risk reduction [8], but the other did not [9]. The pooled data of these two studies estimated, however, a reduced secondary stroke risk from antihypertensive treatment by 38 %, but with a large confidence interval. The uncertainty was increased by the more recently published Dutch TIA trial [10] and the Swedish TEST trial [11]. Both of these were atenolol-based studies, produced relatively small decreases in blood pressure and were negative. The efficacy of atenolol in cardiovascular disease prevention has been questioned, and its use as a first-line agent more recently has been banned by the National Institute of Clinical Excellence in the United Kingdom. The combined results from these four trials predicted only a 19 % decrease in secondary stroke risk by hypertension treatment—a figure thus much lower than that which could be inferred both from primary prevention trials and epidemiological studies. Some support for these modest possible secondary prevention effects came from some experimental studies. For example, the suggestion that chronic treatment of spontaneously hypertensive rats with ACEIs caused regression of vascular changes associated with the development of hypertension [12].

These uncertainties provided the major rationale for the PROGRESS study. At the time, antihypertensives were not considered standard treatment for stroke patients and their value was debated. The high recurrence of stroke after the initial event was already known but became even more evident after the publication of the UKTIA trial (5 % stroke recurrence in the first year and 3 % for each of the following 4 years). The introduction of ACEIs as potent antihypertensive agents into clinical practice also constituted a strong rationale for conducting the trial.

Perindopril and Indapamide

Perindopril is an inhibitor of the angiotensin-converting enzyme (ACE), a kinase that converts angiotensin I (AT1) to angiotensin II (AT2) by stripping its two terminal amino acids. This translates into lower blood pressure by decreased concentrations of the strong vasoconstrictor AT2. Perindopril exerts its action by reducing peripheral vascular resistance with resulting decreased blood pressure, increased peripheral blood flow (in particular in end organs as the brain and the kidney) with no change in heart rate. ACE also inactivates bradykinin which constitutes a proposed adjuvant blood pressure-lowering mechanism. Increasing the activity in the kallikrein–bradykinin system is believed to be the mechanism behind the cough that may occur with ACE inhibitors [13]. Perindopril is converted in the liver into its active metabolite perindoprilat, which is its only metabolite with ACE-inhibiting properties. Perindopril is eliminated via the urine with an effective half-life of just over 24 h, which allows steady state after 4 days and once-daily dosage. The decrease in blood pressure stabilizes rapidly, normally within a month. Perindopril has been shown effective in mild, moderate as well as severe hypertension [14] (Fig. 12.3).

Indapamide is a diuretic chemically related to the thiazide-class diuretics. It increases the secretion of salt and water by inhibiting the resorption of sodium and chloride in the kidneys' distal tubuli. This leads in turn to increased excretion of potassium and magnesium. Its immediate blood pressure-lowering effect is a result of the decreased plasma volume, while the long-term blood pressure lowering is to a larger extent accountable to a decrease of the total peripheral vascular resistance [15]. Indapamide is rapidly absorbed from the gastrointestinal tract and immediately active. It is mainly eliminated through metabolization and urinary excretion. It can be given once daily, and steady-state plasma concentration is reached within a week. Indapamide has been proven effective in clinical studies of mild and moderate hypertension, but is to be combined with another class of drugs in severe hypertension. Thiazides and related diuretics show a plateau effect in its antihypertensive action, while side effects are dose related.

The treatment of hypertension with perindopril and indapamide shows an additive synergistic effect from both drugs. Further, the ACEI lessens the risk for

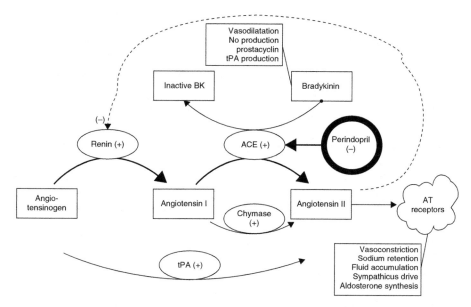

Fig. 12.3 By the action of renin, angiotensinogen (AG) is converted to angiotensin I (AT1) and then by the action of angiotensin-converting enzyme (ACE) to angiotensin II. There are however alternative metabolic routes to AT2 from AT1, and also directly from AG. AT2 exerts a blood pressure increasing effect by increasing vasoconstriction, but has also other effects. AT2 also negatively feeds back on renin, modulating its action. ACE also inactivates the cytokine bradykinin, which may be responsible for some of the ACE inhibitor specific side effects

hypokalemia, which is a common clinical problem in the treatment of hypertension with thiazide diuretics.

Design of the Progress Trial

Organization

PROGRESS was an academic initiative and conducted as an industry-independent, multicentre study. The trial was coordinated by the University of Auckland, New Zealand, but directed from seven regional centres in Australia, China, France, Italy, Japan, Sweden and the United Kingdom. An independent monitoring committee was established to oversee unblinded safety data throughout the course of the study. The aim was to determine balance of benefits and risks conferred by an ACE-inhibitor-based blood pressure-lowering regimen among patients with a history of stroke or TIA and a wide range of blood pressure at entry. The trial design was that of a secondary stroke prevention study and thus included patients with already manifest cerebrovascular disease, defined as TIA (also amaurosis fugax) or stroke (ischaemic or haemorrhagic with the exception of subarachnoid haemorrhage) within the past 5 years. Given that this was a pharmacological treatment trial, the inclusion and exclusion criteria stipulated that participants could not have a contra-indication for any of the interventional compounds or have a medical condition that could preclude full participation in the study. Importantly, patients did not need to be hypertensive (defined as blood pressure above 160 mmHg systolic or 90 mmHg diastolic) to be included. In other words, patients were treated with blood pressure-lowering agents or placebo even if they were normotensive at entry. Patients who were already on ACEI were not excluded, but it was recommended that those treated with other antihypertensives were preferred.

The sample size was calculated from the conservative (*see* the UKTIA study [6] above) assumption of a 1.5–2 % annual rate of recurrent stroke and a blood pressure difference between those on active substance and placebo of 4 mmHg. Sampling for a 90 % power of detecting a 30 % secondary stroke risk reduction over 4–5 years would require a minimum of 200 strokes in the control group and thus 3000 patients in each treatment arm.

The main outcome of the study was recurrent stroke, ischaemic or haemorrhagic, by the WHO definition [16]. Secondary outcomes in the main study included stroke, death or disability at 6–12 months, and total serious cardiovascular events including death, cognitive impairment, disability and dependency by the Barthel [17] and Lindley [18] classifications. A number of substudies were incorporated such as the investigation of genetic variations [19], impacts of age [20], sex and region [21], diabetes [22], silent brain infarcts [23], platelet volume [24], natriuretic peptide [25] and C-reactive protein [26], cerebral white-matter changes [27], blood lipids [28], inflammation and haemostasis [29, 30], atrial fibrillation [31] as well as health services-related research [32, 33].

Implementation of the Trial

Patients were selected by clinicians at participating centres in Australia, Belgium, China, France, Japan, Italy, New Zealand, Sweden and the United Kingdom. After informed consent, all participants entered an open-label run-in phase during which all were given perindopril increased up to 4 mg/day over 4 weeks. The study group chose this rather unconventional design to test in all eligible patients whether they tolerated the study drug before randomization, thus minimizing the number of drop-outs due to non-tolerance and increasing study power. At randomization, patients were allocated to active substance or placebo. If there was a contraindication to diuretics, this determined as to whether it was added to the randomized perindopril or placebo (clinician discretion). Otherwise, randomization to active substance inferred giving both perindopril and indapamide or placebo. The daily dose was 4 mg of perindopril and 2.5 mg of indapamide, except for in Japan where 2.0 mg was the standard dose, due to local regulations. The randomization procedure involved stratification for age group, sex, region and baseline blood pressure as well

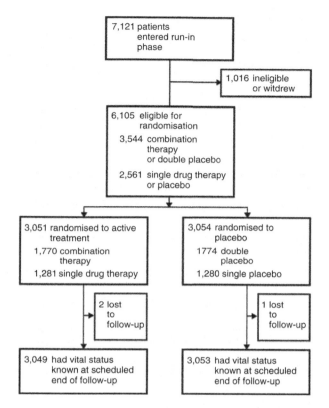

Fig. 12.4 The design and logistics of the PROGRESS trial. An eligible 7121 patients went through the run-in phase to yield the 6000+ patients tolerating the trial drug and ready to be included in the study (From PROGRESS Collaborative Group. Randomised trial of a perindopril-based blood-pressure-lowering regimen among 6105 individuals with previous stroke or transient ischaemic attack. Lancet. Sept 29 2001;358(9287):1033–41, with permission)

as stroke subtype and mono/combination therapy. The patients were then seen after 2 weeks, 1, 3, 6, 9 and 12 months and then half-yearly for the duration of the study.

Results

From the 7121 patients entering the run-in phase, 1016 withdrew during the subsequent 4 weeks. The main reasons were blood pressure-lowering related causes, including dizziness (3.4 %), the ACEI specific cough (2.7 %) and proposed intolerance (2.3 %). This left 6105 patients for randomization by the above-mentioned procedure—3051 to active treatment and 3054 to placebo. Fifty-eight percent of patients in both groups were assigned to combination therapy (Fig. 12.4). When the inclusion phase was over, baseline characteristics were presented [34, 35] showing a balanced distribution between patients on active treatment and placebo, respectively. About half of all randomized patients were classified as hypertensive from their blood pressure at the first visit. The mean initial blood pressure for all participants was 147/86 and 159/94 mmHg among those classified as hypertensive. The mean blood pressure of non-hypertensive patients was 136/79 mmHg. The assignment to single or combination therapy was, however, not randomized and was based on individual clinician preference. The patients allocated to combination treatment were younger, to a larger extent men, had higher blood pressure and more often had coronary heart disease.

The mean follow-up time for those surviving for the length of the study was 4.1 years, and a mean 3.9 years for all those patients entered, or a total of 23,782 patient-years. Twenty-two percent of the patients had discontinued their medication at the end of the study (or their death before that), equally distributed among patients on active treatment or placebo and hypertensive or normotensive. In patients receiving active treatment, 11.9 % discontinued it because of an active decision to do so, or side effects such as 2.2 % due to cough. An additional 2.2 % were diagnosed with heart failure and were actively treated with an ACEI. In the placebo group, 9.5 % discontinued medication because of an active decision to do so, or because of side effects. An additional 2.3 % discontinued because of heart failure. During the course of the trial, only three cases of angio-edema were recorded, none of them fatal.

For the whole study base, patients assigned to active treatment had a systolic blood pressure reduction of 9.0 mmHg compared to patients assigned to placebo, and a diastolic blood pressure reduction of 4 mmHg. These differences appeared shortly after the initiation of treatment and then were maintained without much change during the remainder of the study (Fig. 12.5).

The reduction of blood pressure was much greater, 12/5.0 mmHg, among the patients on combination therapy compared to 4.9/2.8 mmHg for those on ACEI monotherapy. The blood pressure reduction did not differ much between patients classified as normotensive or hypertensive at study entry.

During the course of the trial, 727 stroke events were recorded in the participants. This affected 10 % ($n = 307$) of the active-treatment group and 14 % ($n = 420$) of the patients that were given placebo, yielding a relative risk that was 28 % (95%CI: 17–38 %) lower in the perindopril/indapamide group. The distribution of ischaemic to haemorrhagic stroke was about 5:1 and similar in both groups. There were, however, more strokes in the placebo group with a fatal or disabling outcome (Fig. 12.6).

The cumulative incidence curves diverged after about 6 months and continued to separate throughout the remainder of the study. The active-treatment arm had a yearly incidence of 2.7 % compared to 3.8 % in the placebo group. This was not modified by subgrouping ischaemic/haemorrhagic stroke, time from stroke to enrollment or ethnic background. The two treatment arms showed the same picture for incidence of major vascular events with an annual incidence in the treatment group of 4.1 % compared to 5.5 % in the placebo group (Fig. 12.7).

When patients treated with the combination of perindopril and indapamide were considered separately, they were found to have had a blood pressure lowering of

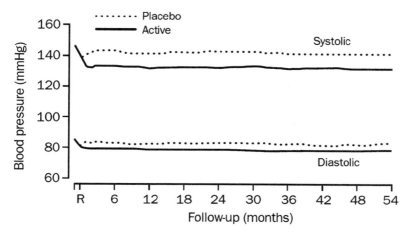

Fig. 12.5 Blood pressure change in study groups. A 9/4 mmHg drop in blood pressure in the active-treatment group was observed soon after institution of treatment that remained more or less unchanged during the course of the study (From PROGRESS Collaborative Group. Randomised trial of a perindopril-based blood-pressure-lowering regimen among 6105 individuals with previous stroke or transient ischaemic attack. Lancet. Sept 29 2001;358(9287):1033–41, with permission)

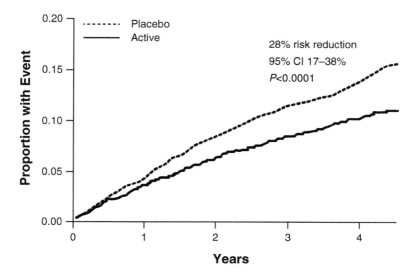

Fig. 12.6 Cumulative incidence of stroke in the two treatment arms of the PROGRESS trial. After a similar incidence for the first 6 months, there is markedly lower incidence in the active-treatment arm for the remainder of the study (From PROGRESS Collaborative Group. Randomised trial of a perindopril-based blood-pressure-lowering regimen among 6105 individuals with previous stroke or transient ischaemic attack. Lancet. Sept 29 2001;358(9287):1033–41, with permission.)

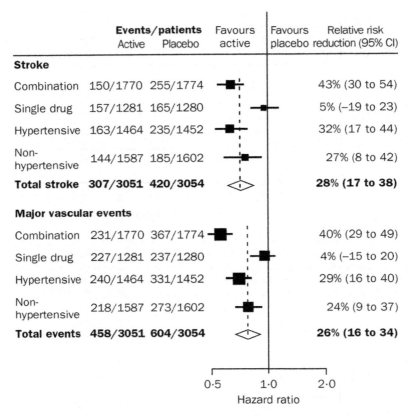

Fig. 12.7 Effects of active treatment vs. placebo on stroke and major vascular events in subgroups of patients [34]. The position of *black squares* represents the effect size and their area the underlying number of patients in subgroups with *horizontal lines* denoting 95 % confidence interval of the effect size. The *diamonds* denote the overall effect size and its confidence interval

12/5 mmHg (as mentioned earlier) and had a 43 % lower risk of recurrent stroke. This was significantly different from the effect of monotherapy, where there was an observed 5/3 mmHg lowering of blood pressure and a recurrent stroke risk indistinguishable from that of the placebo group. This absence of effect remained after subgroup stratification. The effect of the combination therapy was observed in all subgroups as well, with a risk reduction of 46 % for fatal or disabling stroke, 36 % for ischaemic stroke and 76 % for haemorrhagic stroke, but with a large (95%CI: 55–87 %) confidence interval. The same picture was observed for secondary outcome events. Combination therapy reduced the risk of major vascular events by 40 % compared to placebo, while treatment with perindopril only did not. Combination therapy was also associated with a 42 % reduction in non-fatal myocardial infarction.

During the course of the study, 1026 patients had a major vascular event of which 379 were fatal. Patients in the active-treatment group had fewer non-fatal strokes, deaths from coronary heart disease and non-fatal myocardial infarction. The rate of

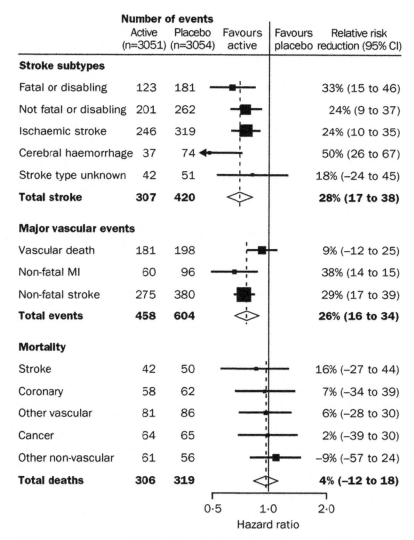

Fig. 12.8 Effects in study arms on subtypes of stroke, major vascular events and mortality. *MI* myocardial infarction. Conventions as in Fig. 12.5 (From PROGRESS Collaborative Group. Randomised trial of a perindopril-based blood-pressure-lowering regimen among 6105 individuals with previous stroke or transient ischaemic attack. Lancet. Sept 29 2001;358(9287):1033–41, with permission)

overall vascular death was, however, not discernable between groups. During the follow-up period 625 patients died, of whom 379 from vascular causes, but this was similar between treatment groups. The number of hospital admissions during the study was 9 % lower in the active-treatment group, and their median hospital stay was 2.5 days shorter (Fig. 12.8).

The PROGRESS investigators also published data on the effect of Perindopril-based therapy on cognitive decline [36]. Patients meeting DSM-IV dementia criteria were recorded in 6.3 % ($n=193$) of the actively treated participants compared to 7.1 % ($n=217$) in the placebo group, resulting in a non-significant 12 % risk reduction. However, the risk for overall cognitive decline, measured as a 3-or-more-point decline in the Mini-Mental-State-Examination [37], was 19 % (9.1 % vs. 11 %; 95 % CI: 4–32 %) less in the group receiving active treatment. In the subgroup analysis, there was a significant 34 % reduction of risk for the composite measure "dementia with recurrent stroke".

To summarize the overall PROGRESS results, blood pressure lowering with a perindopril-based regime showed a significant 28 % risk reduction on the primary outcome measure of recurrent fatal or non-fatal stroke of any type. This was the first study to definitively show that blood pressure lowering could be an effective secondary stroke prevention strategy. Importantly, the benefits were independent of the baseline blood pressure; in other words, the participants did not need to be hypertensive to benefit from active treatment and normotensive participants had similar reductions in recurrent stroke risk. While taken in the context of subgroup analyses, combination therapy was particularly efficacious, as was the effect on the likelihood of developing intracerebral haemorrhage as an outcome event.

Context and Interpretation

The same lack of evidence or conflicting study data that constituted the rationale for the PROGRESS study also inspired other researchers to investigate related research questions at around the same time. For example, data from the Heart Outcomes Prevention Evaluation (HOPE) study [38], the Losartan Intervention for Endpoint Reduction in Hypertension (LIFE) study [39] and the Study on Cognition and Prognosis in the Elderly (SCOPE) study[40] were published and provide support for as well as contrast to the PROGRESS findings. As previously mentioned, the clear message from the PROGRESS study was that blood pressure lowering significantly lowers the risk of recurrent stroke and that this is not restricted to certain stroke subtypes, age groups, gender, hypertensive or normotensive status. Further, the treatment regime was also proven feasible and safe, with only a few percent of withdrawals during the 4 years of the study and only a slight excess of minor side effects in the active-treatment group over placebo. It also showed that the J-shaped risk curve concept suggested by previous studies was most likely the result of confounding, since the effect of active treatment was the same regardless of baseline blood pressure.

The HOPE trial provides one of the most important comparisons to the PROGRESS study. Here, the investigators studied the ACEI ramipril, which in monotherapy in stroke patients yielded a 3/1 mmHg blood pressure reduction, a 32 % secondary stroke risk reduction and a 20 % myocardial infarction risk reduction compared to placebo. This was a stronger risk reduction than predicted from epidemiological data alone, consistent with the PROGRESS findings and led to the hypothesis of a secondary stroke risk lowering effect by ACEIs which is additive to the effects of lowering blood pressure alone. However, this must be balanced by the finding that when a subset of HOPE patients were studied with 24 h blood pressure monitoring, the blood pressure reduction was greater. Also, the patients with the lowest baseline blood pressure did not show benefit of ramipril in the HOPE study.

Although the LIFE study design was quite different in that asymptomatic hypertensive patients with left ventricular hypertrophy were recruited, the results were of importance in the context of PROGRESS. The effects of losartan, an angiotensin II type 1 receptor blocker (ARB), belonging to another class of agents modulating the renin–angiotensin–aldosterone system (RAAS) were investigated. When compared to a beta blocker, atenolol, there was a stroke risk reduction despite no between-groups difference in blood pressure, thus strengthening the additive-effect-hypothesis for agents interfering with the RAAS system. The LIFE investigators also found a 25 % diabetes incidence reduction in the treatment group, adding another proposed benefit to these classes of drugs. The SCOPE trial investigators studied candesartan, another ARB class drug, compared to placebo in elderly mildly hypertensive persons, finding a 28 % reduced stroke risk, seemingly independent of blood pressure lowering. In addition, other studies have shown ACEIs and ARBs may reverse functional cardiac failure [41] and promote vascular remodelling [42]. Two other studies later added to the knowledge base on RAAS modulators: The ONTARGET [43] study investigated the ARB telmisartan, the ACEI ramipril, or the combination of both for reducing vascular outcomes including stroke in people over 55 years old with vascular disease. The TRANSCEND [44] study investigated telmisartan against placebo in patients that were candidates for treatment with but showed adverse effects to ACEI. Since up to one in five patients are intolerant to ACEI, there was hope that ARB treatments would be more feasible and still give the same vascular protection. The HOPE study had already showed benefit of ramipril in a similar cohort and the intention of ONTARGET was to show, besides greater protection by the ACEI + ARB combination, that ARB was better tolerated and not inferior in effect to ramipril. It failed, however, to show any effect of the combination beyond that of either drug alone, while there were more adverse effects, and this despite 2.4/1.4 mmHg greater blood pressure lowering. The TRANSCEND study could not show any benefit of telmisartan over placebo in reducing neither primary nor secondary outcomes, maybe due to under-powering caused by a lower than expected event rate in the study or the fact that many of the subjects had received RAAS modulators already before randomization into the study. The PROFESS [45] study failed to show benefit of telmisartan over placebo for protection against recurrent stroke in 20,000 stroke patients despite a 3.8/2.0 mmHg lower blood pressure in the ARB group, thus weakening the support for effects of this drug class on recurrent stroke. However, less than half of the patients were followed for at least 2 years.

There are pragmatic implications of the results of the PROGRESS trial. For example, if there is a linear relationship between blood pressure and stroke risk, it seems reasonable that stroke sufferers be prescribed antihypertensive treatment even though they fall short of being diagnosed as hypertensive. The finding that perindopril alone did not result in as much protection against secondary stroke unless a thiazide-like diuretic (indapamide) is added has been widely debated. The difference should first be considered in the context of the subanalysis and then in the degree of blood pressure achieved. The 5/3 mmHg blood pressure lowering would be associated to an anticipated 30 % reduction in secondary stroke risk [46]. Subsequent studies have investigated whether the effects of this particular combination are unique, a class effect between any ACEI (or even ARB) and diuretic or rather attributable to the blood pressure lowering per se. The latter has in subsequent meta-analyses seemed more likely, both in general [47] and regarding specific questions as baseline blood pressure [48], body mass index [49] or cardiovascular risk [50]. The fact that individual study physicians decided on monotherapy or combination therapy may also have contributed to a confounding of the results, selecting patients that most would have benefited from perindopril. The study was not powered to answer the question of secondary stroke risk reduction by indapamide treatment alone. The Chinese PATS [51] trial however evaluated indapamide against placebo for stroke risk reduction in 5665 patients and reported a hazard ratio of 0.71 (95 % CI 0.58–0.88). A report from the Blood Pressure Lowering Treatment Trialists' Collaboration found all major classes of antihypertensives effective in preventing first strokes. So, is secondary stroke prevention different and which should be the drug of choice? We still lack final evidence on whether there are strong class effects of ACEIs [52] or whether individual drug characteristics within the class outweigh the common features. Further, genetic profiling and drug substitution studies [53, 54] suggest that antihypertensive treatment may yet need individual tailoring of pharmacotherapy for optimizing results, for instance, depending on whether individuals are high-renin, low-renin or aldosterone-sensitive. Recent developments in gene-wide association studies have suggested potential targets for further research.

Regardless, PROGRESS results have provided a milestone of specific evidence for secondary stroke prevention. The effect of the tested intervention is quite powerful with the possibility to avoid one serious vascular event in every 11 patients treated with perindopril and indapamide over 5 years, in addition to those of other preventive measures such as lifestyle adjustment and the use of antiplatelet agents or statins. The PROGRESS results have changed the way we approach blood pressure lowering in stroke patients. Its legacy is that it has manifested itself as the realms of standard poststroke management.

References

1. PROGRESS Management Committee. PROGRESS—perindopril protection against recurrent stroke study: status in July 1996. J Hypertens Suppl. 1996;14(6):S47–51.
2. MacMahon S, Rodgers A. The effects of blood pressure reduction in older patients: an overview of five randomized controlled trials in elderly hypertensives. Clin Exp Hypertens. 1993;15(6):967–78.

3. Bonita R, Beaglehole R. Does treatment of hypertension explain the decline in mortality from stroke? Br Med J (Clin Res Ed). 1986;292(6514):191–2.
4. MacMahon S, Rodgers A. Blood pressure, antihypertensive treatment and stroke risk. J Hypertens Suppl. 1994;12(10):S5–14.
5. Irie K, Yamaguchi T, Minematsu K, Omae T. The J-curve phenomenon in stroke recurrence. Stroke. 1993;24(12):1844–9.
6. Rodgers A, MacMahon S, Gamble G, Slattery J, Sandercock P, Warlow C. Blood pressure and risk of stroke in patients with cerebrovascular disease. The United Kingdom Transient Ischaemic Attack Collaborative Group. BMJ. 1996;313(7050):147.
7. Collins R, MacMahon S. Blood pressure, antihypertensive drug treatment and the risks of stroke and of coronary heart disease. Br Med Bull. 1994;50(2):272–98.
8. Carter AB. Hypotensive therapy in stroke survivors. Lancet. 1970;1(7645):485–9.
9. Hypertension-Stroke Cooperative Study Group. Effect of antihypertensive treatment on stroke recurrence. JAMA. 1974;229(4):409–18.
10. The Dutch TIA. Trial Study Group. Trial of secondary prevention with atenolol after transient ischemic attack or nondisabling ischemic stroke. Stroke. 1993;24(4):543–8.
11. Eriksson S, Olofsson BO, Wester PO. Atenolol in secondary prevention after stroke. Cerebrovasc Dis. 1995;5:21–5.
12. Lee RM, Delaney KH, Lu M. Perindopril treatment prolonged the lifespan of spontaneously hypertensive rats. J Hypertens. 1995;13(4):471–6.
13. Ferrari R, Pasanisi G, Notarstefano P, Campo G, Gardini E, Ceconi C. Specific properties and effect of perindopril in controlling the renin-angiotensin system. Am J Hypertens. 2005;18(9 Pt 2):142S–54S.
14. EMEA. Perindopril product resume. The European Medicines Agency: London, UK; 2005.
15. SMPA. Indapamide product resume. Sweden: The Swedish Medical Products Agency; 2009.
16. WHO. Cerebrovascular disorders. Geneva: World Health Organisation; 1978.
17. Mahoney FI, Barthel DW. Functional evaluation: the Barthel Index. Md State Med J. 1965;14:61–5.
18. Lindley RI, Waddell F, Livingstone M, Warlow CP, Dennis MS, Sandercock P. Can simple questions assess outcome after stroke? Cerebrovas Dis. 1994;4:314–24.
19. Harrap SB, Tzourio C, Cambien F, et al. The ACE gene I/D polymorphism is not associated with the blood pressure and cardiovascular benefits of ACE inhibition. Hypertension. 2003;42(3):297–303.
20. Ratnasabapathy Y, Lawes CM, Anderson CS. The Perindopril Protection Against Recurrent Stroke Study (PROGRESS): clinical implications for older patients with cerebrovascular disease. Drugs Aging. 2003;20(4):241–51.
21. Rodgers A, Chapman N, Woodward M, et al. Perindopril-based blood pressure lowering in individuals with cerebrovascular disease: consistency of benefits by age, sex and region. J Hypertens. 2004;22(3):653–9.
22. Berthet K, Neal BC, Chalmers JP, et al. Reductions in the risks of recurrent stroke in patients with and without diabetes: the PROGRESS Trial. Blood Press. 2004;13(1):7–13.
23. Hasegawa Y, Yamaguchi T, Omae T, Woodward M, Chalmers J. Effects of perindopril-based blood pressure lowering and of patient characteristics on the progression of silent brain infarct: the Perindopril Protection against Recurrent Stroke Study (PROGRESS) CT Substudy in Japan. Hypertens Res. 2004;27(3):147–56.
24. Bath P, Algert C, Chapman N, Neal B. Association of mean platelet volume with risk of stroke among 3134 individuals with history of cerebrovascular disease. Stroke. 2004;35(3):622–6.
25. Campbell DJ, Woodward M, Chalmers JP, et al. Perindopril-based blood pressure-lowering therapy reduces amino-terminal-pro-B-type natriuretic peptide in individuals with cerebrovascular disease. J Hypertens. 2007;25(3):699–705.
26. Campbell DJ, Woodward M, Chalmers JP, et al. Prediction of heart failure by amino terminal-pro-B-type natriuretic peptide and C-reactive protein in subjects with cerebrovascular disease. Hypertension. 2005;45(1):69–74.

27. Dufouil C, Chalmers J, Coskun O, et al. Effects of blood pressure lowering on cerebral white matter hyperintensities in patients with stroke: the PROGRESS (Perindopril Protection Against Recurrent Stroke Study) Magnetic Resonance Imaging Substudy. Circulation. 2005;112(11):1644–50.
28. Patel A, Woodward M, Campbell DJ, et al. Plasma lipids predict myocardial infarction, but not stroke, in patients with established cerebrovascular disease. Eur Heart J. 2005;26(18):1910–5.
29. Woodward M, Lowe GD, Campbell DJ, et al. Associations of inflammatory and hemostatic variables with the risk of recurrent stroke. Stroke. 2005;36(10):2143–7.
30. Campbell DJ, Woodward M, Chalmers JP, et al. Soluble vascular cell adhesion molecule 1 and N-terminal pro-B-type natriuretic peptide in predicting ischemic stroke in patients with cerebrovascular disease. Arch Neurol. 2006;63(1):60–5.
31. Arima H, Hart RG, Colman S, et al. Perindopril-based blood pressure-lowering reduces major vascular events in patients with atrial fibrillation and prior stroke or transient ischemic attack. Stroke. 2005;36(10):2164–9.
32. Chalmers J, Chapman N. Challenges for the prevention of primary and secondary stroke: the importance of lowering blood pressure and total cardiovascular risk. Blood Press. 2001;10(5–6):344–51.
33. Arima H, Chalmers J, Woodward M, et al. Lower target blood pressures are safe and effective for the prevention of recurrent stroke: the PROGRESS trial. J Hypertens. 2006;24(6):1201–8.
34. PROGRESS Collaborative Group. Randomised trial of a perindopril-based blood-pressure-lowering regimen among 6,105 individuals with previous stroke or transient ischaemic attack. Lancet. 2001;358(9287):1033–41.
35. Committee PM. PROGRESS—Perindopril Protection Against Recurrent Stroke Study: characteristics of the study population at baseline. J Hypertens. 1999;17(11):1647–55.
36. Tzourio C, Anderson C, Chapman N, et al. Effects of blood pressure lowering with perindopril and indapamide therapy on dementia and cognitive decline in patients with cerebrovascular disease. Arch Intern Med. 2003;163(9):1069–75.
37. Folstein MF, Folstein SE, McHugh PR. "Mini-mental state". A practical method for grading the cognitive state of patients for the clinician. J Psychiatr Res. 1975;12(3):189–98.
38. Yusuf S, Sleight P, Pogue J, Bosch J, Davies R, Dagenais G. Effects of an angiotensin-converting-enzyme inhibitor, ramipril, on cardiovascular events in high-risk patients. The Heart Outcomes Prevention Evaluation Study Investigators. N Engl J Med. 2000;342(3):145–53.
39. Dahlof B, Devereux RB, Kjeldsen SE, et al. Cardiovascular morbidity and mortality in the Losartan Intervention For Endpoint reduction in hypertension study (LIFE): a randomised trial against atenolol. Lancet. 2002;359(9311):995–1003.
40. Lithell H, Hansson L, Skoog I, et al. The Study on Cognition and Prognosis in the Elderly (SCOPE): principal results of a randomized double-blind intervention trial. J Hypertens. 2003;21(5):875–86.
41. Tamura T, Said S, Harris J, Lu W, Gerdes AM. Reverse remodeling of cardiac myocyte hypertrophy in hypertension and failure by targeting of the renin-angiotensin system. Circulation. 2000;102(2):253–9.
42. McVeigh GE. Effects of perindopril on cardiovascular remodeling. Am J Cardiol. 2001;88(7A):28i–35i.
43. Yusuf S, Teo KK, Pogue J, et al. Telmisartan, ramipril, or both in patients at high risk for vascular events. N Engl J Med. 2008;358(15):1547–59.
44. Yusuf S, Teo K, Anderson C, et al. Effects of the angiotensin-receptor blocker telmisartan on cardiovascular events in high-risk patients intolerant to angiotensin-converting enzyme inhibitors: a randomised controlled trial. Lancet. 2008;372(9644):1174–83.
45. Yusuf S, Diener HC, Sacco RL, et al. Telmisartan to prevent recurrent stroke and cardiovascular events. N Engl J Med. 2008;359(12):1225–37.
46. Staessen JA, Wang JG, Thijs L. Cardiovascular protection and blood pressure reduction: a meta-analysis. Lancet. 2001;358(9290):1305–15.

47. Turnbull F, Neal B, Ninomiya T, et al. Effects of different regimens to lower blood pressure on major cardiovascular events in older and younger adults: meta-analysis of randomised trials. BMJ. 2008;336(7653):1121–3.
48. McAlister FA. Renin Angiotension System Modulator Meta-Analysis Investigators. Angiotensin-converting enzyme inhibitors or angiotensin receptor blockers are beneficial in normotensive atherosclerotic patients: a collaborative meta-analysis of randomized trials. Eur Heart J. 2012;33(4):505–14.
49. Ying A, Arima H, Czernichow S, et al. Blood Pressure Lowering Treatment Trialists' Collaboration, Effects of blood pressure lowering on cardiovascular risk according to baseline body-mass index: a meta-analysis of randomised trials. Lancet. 2015;385(9971):867–74.
50. Sundström J, Arima H, Woodward M, et al. Blood Pressure Lowering Treatment Trialists' Collaboration, Blood pressure-lowering treatment based on cardiovascular risk: a meta-analysis of individual patient data. Lancet. 2014;384(9943):591–8.
51. PATS Collaborating Group. Post-stroke antihypertensive treatment study. A preliminary result. Chin Med J (Engl). 1995;108(9):710–17.
52. Teo KK, Yusuf S, Pfeffer M, et al. Effects of long-term treatment with angiotensin-converting-enzyme inhibitors in the presence or absence of aspirin: a systematic review. Lancet. 2002;360(9339):1037–43.
53. Mackenzie IS, Brown MJ. Genetic profiling versus drug rotation in the optimisation of antihypertensive treatment. Clin Med (Lond). 2002;2(5):465–73.
54. Franceschini N, Chasman DI, Cooper-DeHoff RM, Arnett DK. Genetics, ancestry, and hypertension: implications for targeted antihypertensive therapies. Curr Hypertens Rep. 2014;16(8):461.

Chapter 13
Blood Pressure Variability, Antihypertensive Therapy and Stroke Risk

Muhammad U. Farooq, Jiangyong Min, Lawrence K.S. Wong, and Philip B. Gorelick

Hypertension is considered by many experts to be the "crown jewel" of stroke prevention as it is the most important modifiable risk factor for stroke [1–3]. Blood pressure has been determined traditionally with a cuff in the office that determines systolic and diastolic measures based on appearance and disappearance of the Korotkoff sounds, respectively. Multiple blood pressure studies have led to a substantial body of scientific data recognizing raised blood pressure as a major risk factor for stroke [4–6]. Observations in the early 1990s showed that mean blood pressure lowering alone might not explain all of the benefit of antihypertensive therapy [7]. The theme was revisited by Rothwell et al. in 2010, and these investigators showed that visit-to-visit systolic blood pressure variability, independent of mean blood pressure, predicted stroke, and certain blood pressure lowering agents were more effective in reducing blood pressure variability based on clinical trial evidence [8–11]. In this chapter we review circadian patterns and types of blood pressure variability and discuss blood pressure variability as a risk for stroke, the means to measure it, its long-term consequences, and how blood pressure variability is being incorporated into stroke prevention guidelines for diagnosis and treatment of hypertension.

M.U. Farooq, M.D., F.A.C.P., F.A.H.A. (✉) • J. Min, M.D., Ph.D.
Division of Stroke and Vascular Neurology, Mercy Health Hauenstein Neurosciences,
200 Jefferson Street SE, Grand Rapids, MI 49503, USA
e-mail: farooqmu@mercyhealth.com

L.K.S. Wong, M.D.
Department of Medicine and Therapeutics, Faculty of Medicine, Prince of Wales Hospital,
Chinese University of Hong Kong, 9/F., Lui Che Woo Clinical Science Building,
Hong Kong, China

P.B. Gorelick, M.D., M.P.H., F.A.C.P.
Professor, Department of Translational Science and Molecular Medicine, College of Human
Medicine, Michigan State University, 220 Cherry Street SE Room H 3037, Grand Rapids, MI
49503, USA

Medical Director, Mercy Health Hauenstein Neurosciences, 220 Cherry Street SE
Room H 3037, Grand Rapids, MI 49503, USA

© Springer International Publishing Switzerland 2016   233
V. Aiyagari, P.B. Gorelick (eds.), *Hypertension and Stroke*, Clinical
Hypertension and Vascular Diseases, DOI 10.1007/978-3-319-29152-9_13

Circadian Blood Pressure, Blood Pressure Variability, Its Significance and Long-Term Consequences

Circadian rhythms play a crucial role in the function of cardiovascular and cerebrovascular systems. They are intrinsically regulated by the circadian system which involves hypothalamic nuclei and other components of autonomic nervous system. There are also various other neuronal and hormonal circuits involved in the circadian system. These circuits work through a complicated interaction, which connects directly or indirectly and provides output to various organs including the heart, brain, and blood vessels [12–14]. This system is responsible for diurnal variations and oscillations in our heart rate and blood pressure over 24 h periods. Normally, blood pressure displays a daily rhythm and is highest in the morning and falls progressively to reach its lowest level during sleep. Thus, one's pulse and blood pressure exhibit significant time-of-day dependent oscillations. However, dysfunction of circadian rhythms can lead to significant effects on the heart and brain [15–17].

It is well documented that cerebrovascular and cardiovascular events may occur more often at certain times during the day in relation to circadian rhythms [16]. The rise in blood pressure in the morning around the awakening time known as "morning surge," for example, is a physiological phenomenon. However, an exacerbated morning blood pressure surge is a risk factor for major vascular complications [16, 18]. It has been noted that the association between morning blood pressure surge and cardiovascular risk has a threshold rather than a linear relationship [19]. An early morning peak of acute myocardial infarction was first reported in the 1980s and persists despite advancement in medical care [17]. This association also has been observed with stroke, whereby there is a significantly higher risk in the morning [16]. Therefore, a proper understanding of the importance of circadian patterns of pulse and blood pressure may help improve management of patients with hypertension and those who are at risk of further vascular complications such as stroke.

The diurnal variation in blood pressure as mentioned above is well known and several diurnal and sleep blood pressure patterns in normotensive and hypertensive subjects have been identified, called "dipping patterns." These are characterized by following four important diurnal patterns of blood pressure variability (Table 13.1):

Increase of mean blood pressure is an important cause of arterial disease, but it does not account for all blood pressure related risk of vascular events [8]. Blood pressure variability, beyond mean blood pressure, adds important information to stroke risk [3, 7]. The investigators of the Swedish Trial in Old Patients with Hypertension (STOP) noted that antihypertensive therapy lowered stroke risk more than one would expect attributed only to mean blood pressure lowering [6]. After 2 years, follow-up data showed that blood pressure variability predicted cardiac complications including left ventricular hypertrophy [31]. Rothwell and colleagues resurrected this valuable concept and provided additional clarity and definition to previously unanswered questions including the rapid effect of some of the antihypertensive medications on the reduction of the incidence of stroke [8]. This may

Table 13.1 Blood pressure variability patterns in normal and hypertensive individuals

Type of blood pressure "dipping patterns"	Characteristics of blood pressure "dipping patterns"	Associations and significance of blood pressure "dipping patterns"
Normal dippers	Characterized by 10–20 % reduction in blood pressure from day to night	Physiological and is a normal pattern of blood pressure variability
Non-dippers	Characterized by <10 % reduction in nighttime blood pressure	– Seen in elderly, postmenopausal women and African-Americans
		– Increased risk of vascular complications
Reverse dippers	Characterized by >20 % rise in nighttime blood pressure	Increased risk of vascular complications including intracerebral hemorrhage and microbleeds
Extreme dippers	Characterized by >20 % fall in nighttime blood pressure	Increased risk of vascular complications including small vessel ischemic disease and lacunar infarcts

Data from references [20–30]

help to explain why amlodipine was more effective in reducing risk of vascular complications as compared to valsartan in Valsartan Antihypertensive Long-term Use Evaluation Trial and why there is suboptimal effect of nonselective beta-blockers in stroke prevention as compared to other antihypertensive medications [11, 32]. Therefore, we now have strong evidence that day-to-day and visit-to-visit systolic blood pressure variability is significantly associated with the risk of cerebrovascular and cardiovascular events independent of mean blood pressure [3, 7, 8]. There is an important association between variability of early morning blood pressure and vascular complications which may be driven by the morning surge in blood pressure. Morning surge of blood pressure is associated with various neurohormonal abnormalities including sympathetic nervous system, renin-angiotensin system, and changes in plasma cortisol and plasminogen. It is important to note that blood pressure surge does not occur only on awakening in the morning but also may occur after an afternoon nap. Episodic blood pressure surges may be responsible for high maximum systolic blood pressure as well as diurnal variability in blood pressure and stroke risk [16, 18, 19, 31, 33–36].

Studies have shown that nighttime blood pressure variability is a better predictor of long-term vascular outcomes than daytime variability especially in patients with hypertension [33, 37–41]. There may be a greater likelihood of brain injury during nighttime as compared to daytime due to various dipping patterns including non-dipping and extreme dipping. There is an association of blunted decline in blood pressure in non-dippers during sleep and higher incidence of vascular events including white matter lesions and silent strokes as seen on MRI brain studies. Other adverse outcomes in non-dippers included increase in both cardiac and stroke related mortality [33, 41–47]. There is also some concern about the reproducibility of daytime blood pressure associations due to interference by daytime activities.

Therefore, cardiovascular risk stratification might not be very accurate if based only on daytime blood pressure determinations. On the other hand, these various patterns of blood pressure variability provide a potential opportunity to take corrective and preventive measures in blood pressure management such as by using drugs that target the sympathetic nervous system and renin-angiotensin system [19, 48, 49].

The abovementioned dipping patterns are affected and influenced by duration and quality of sleep. Short sleep duration has been associated with silent brain infarcts in hypertensive persons. One should also consider sleep disorders in patients with excessive nighttime blood pressure variability and non-dipping sleep pattern as an increase in nighttime blood pressure may be an indicator of an underlying sleep disorder. Non-dipping pattern in hypertensive patients is associated with obstructive sleep apnea. This can also lead to an increased risk of cardiovascular and cerebrovascular complications. Therefore, proper management of sleep disorders such as obstructive sleep apnea by using continuous positive airway pressure may help to control blood pressure during nighttime and minimize excessive variability and dipping patterns [50–52].

In addition to the complications associated with significant blood pressure variability as mentioned above, there are various short- and long-term deleterious effects of instability and variability of blood pressure on the nervous system as the brain does not tolerate blood pressure variability well. Significant blood pressure fluctuations result in excessive mechanical and sheer stress on the vascular system, leading to endothelial cell damage, advancement of atherosclerosis and platelet activation resulting in thromboembolic phenomenon and consequent major vascular events such as ischemic stroke. The long-term end-organ damage to the brain results in other complications including small vessel ischemic disease, cerebral atrophy, and memory and cognitive impairment. This is summarized in Fig. 13.1.

Data about various blood pressure dipping patterns in normal and hypertensive patients using ambulatory/portable blood pressure monitoring, which will be discussed in the next section, are obtained from studies conducted by Kario, Nakamura, Klarenbeek and Aznaouridis and colleagues. These studies have

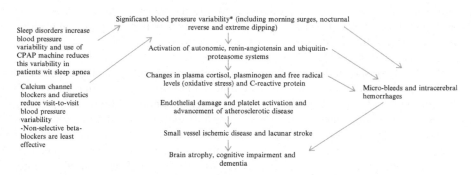

Fig. 13.1 Pathophysiology of blood pressure variability, its related complications and treatment strategies [8–11, 16–19, 31–34, 50–52]. *CPAP* continuous positive airway pressure. *Asterisk* can be measured by home blood pressure monitoring and/or by ambulatory blood pressure monitoring

shown that extreme dippers are prone to have both silent and clinical brain ischemia especially if treated with blood pressure lowering medications which further drop blood pressure during sleep. Markers of ischemic disease on magnetic resonance imaging of the brain include not only findings suggestive of small vessel ischemic disease and lacunar infarcts but also micro bleeds. Thus, there may be hypotension during sleep and an excessive rise in blood pressure in the morning hours (blood pressure surge), respectively. Moreover, in patients with reverse dipping, there is a higher risk of intracerebral hemorrhage and related complications. In addition, there is a possible role for inflammation, as high-sensitive C-reactive protein is associated with clinical strokes in addition to silent brain ischemia in these hypertensive patients. Aznaouridis et al. also studied the potential utility of an ambulatory systolic–diastolic pressure gradient index (ASDPRI) [18, 27–29, 53–60].

Calcium channel blockers may prevent these complications by minimizing blood pressure variations. There may be direct effects on neuronal circuits and central control of blood pressure, helping to explain a rapid onset of protection from cardiovascular events [3, 8, 61]. The effect of different medication groups on blood pressure will be discussed later in this chapter. We will now focus on how to accurately measure blood pressure variability.

Measurement of Blood Pressure Variability

Home blood pressure monitoring (HBPM) and ambulatory blood pressure monitoring (ABPM) are effective methods to monitor diurnal blood pressure variability. Blood pressure measurements done in a physician's office may have limitations, whereas blood measurements taken in a patient's home may be a better predictor of future vascular complications [62]. HBPM and ABPM are very important means to monitor blood pressure variability as up to 35 % of patients diagnosed with hypertension may have white coat hypertension or isolated elevation in blood pressure in the medical office setting leading to an incorrect diagnosis [63]. Other indications and advantages of HBPM or ABPM include obtaining accurate information about masked hypertension, episodic hypertension, symptomatic hypotension, and nocturnal hypertension [62].

Now, remote transmission of home blood pressure readings is available. Using this technology, blood pressure readings can be transmitted to a data collection center via a wireless technology [64]. These techniques also offer a practical method of assessing the effects of antihypertensive treatment on blood pressure variability and drug resistant hypertension. ABPM is superior to HBPM in some regards. For example, isolated nocturnal hypertension may be present in 7 % of hypertensive patients and ABPM is the only and most accurate way to make this determination. It can also monitor the effect of drug therapy on early morning fluctuations in blood pressure as well as other time windows in a 24-h period [26, 62, 64, 65].

APBM is a cost-effective way to monitor blood pressure variability in both primary and specialist care settings [62, 64]. It not only provides information to help guide adjustment of antihypertensive therapy, but also helps to detect patients with white coat hypertension. The cost of care for hypertension including medications and associated complications exceeds that of the cost of monitoring and associated testing [62, 66, 67]. Whereas ABPM has advantages over other techniques including HBPM, it also has limitations. These include requirement of special equipment, time needed to fit the device, possible discomfort related to the technology especially during nighttime, and the need for staff training, data evaluation, higher cost and limited availability [21, 62]. There are some other challenges when using this technique in children, patients with obesity, cardiac arrhythmias, renal failure and during pregnancy related to lack of formal validation protocols [62].

On the other hand, advancement in technology provides advantages in favor of ABPM use such as concomitant measurement of pulse pressure, pulse wave velocity, central blood pressure, and arterial stiffness. Moreover, accessories such as position and activity sensors have been developed to determine the patient's position and also physical activity which allows an estimation of sleep and awake periods, activity and rest, respectively [62]. Overall, ABPM is a useful technique, and it is becoming a standard practice in targeted blood pressure management in developed countries around the globe [65].

Blood Pressure Variability as a Risk for Stroke: What Guidelines Recommend for Clinical Practice

Many national and international guidelines including those of the American Society of Hypertension, American Heart Association/American Stroke Association (AHA/ASA), European Society of Hypertension, and British Society of Hypertension recommend HBPM to study intraindividual variability in pulse and blood pressure patterns [68–72]. Furthermore, it's routine use for initial diagnosis of hypertension was recommended by the UK National Clinical Guideline Center (NCGC) in 2011 [73]. The 2014 AHA/ASA primary stroke prevention guideline acknowledges that intraindividual blood pressure variability is associated with risk of stroke beyond mean blood pressure assessment and that nocturnal blood pressure determination by ABPM may provide additional useful information [74]. However, the 2014 AHA/ASA guidance statement on recurrent stroke prevention generally remains silent on the issue [57]. The European Society of Hypertension recommends the use of HBPM or ABPM in individuals with stage I hypertension in the office and who are at low or moderate total cardiovascular risk and in those who have high-normal office blood pressure or normal blood pressure with asymptomatic organ damage [62, 65].

Epidemiological observational studies and clinical trials have shown the benefit of reducing blood pressure with the use of antihypertensive medications for reduction of cardiovascular and cerebrovascular events. The class of drug used in the management of hypertension and to reduce blood pressure variability may affect stroke risk and related complications [3, 4, 75–77].

Ideally, antihypertensive medications should reduce mean blood pressure and also blood pressure variability [9, 11]. Medications such as calcium channel blockers and diuretics, which reduce blood pressure variability, may be more beneficial in reducing stroke risk than medications such as nonselective beta-blockers which do not reduce variability [3, 11]. One of the mechanisms by which calcium channel blockers and diuretics may reduce blood pressure variability is their effects on central control of blood pressure and morning blood pressure surges [61].

Calcium channel blockers and thiazide diuretics reduced maximum systolic blood pressure and systolic blood pressure variability in the Anglo-Scandinavian Cardiac Outcomes Trial-Blood Pressure Lowering Arm (ASCOT-BPLA) and Medical Research Council 2 (MRC-2) studies. The effect of calcium channel blockers and thiazide diuretics on vascular events was compared with beta-blockers and renin-angiotensin system inhibitors [78–80]. Rothwell and colleagues analyzed the ASCOT-BPLA and MRC-2 databases and emphasized the differences in effects of beta-blockers and calcium channel blockers on variability of blood pressure and the prognostic implications including risk of stroke after transient ischemic attack. In the ASCOT-BPLA arm, the patients with the highest residual intersession variability of systolic blood pressure when on treatment remained at greater risk of subsequent stroke (CI 2.32–4.54; $p < 0.0001$, hazard ratio 3.25). The stroke risk was independent of mean systolic blood pressure. Moreover, visit-to-visit variability in systolic blood pressure was greater in patients randomized to atenolol treatment than in the group who received amlodipine. Therefore, Rothwell and colleagues suggested using antihypertensive medications which reduce blood pressure variability to optimally reduce stroke risk [9, 11, 78–80].

Webb and colleagues evaluated the effect of antihypertensive treatment on interindividual variance in blood pressure and outcomes in 389 clinical trials. They found maximum reduction (19 %) in interindividual systolic blood pressure variation with calcium channel blockers (variance ratio 0.81, 95 % CI 0.76–0.86, $p < 0.0001$). The effect was less marked with non-loop diuretics where there was a 13 % reduction in interindividual systolic blood pressure variation (variance ratio 0.87, CI 0.79–0.96, $p = 0.007$). Interestingly, they reported an increase of 8 % with angiotensin-converting enzyme inhibitors (variance ratio 1.08, CI 1.02–1.15, $p = 0.008$) and 16 % with angiotensin receptor blockers (variance ratio 1.16, CI 1.07–1.25, $p = 0.0002$). The increase in interindividual systolic blood pressure variation was maximum at 17 % with beta-blockers (variance ratio 1.17, CI 1.07–1.28, $p = 0.0007$). The analysis revealed a significant relationship between interindividual systolic blood pressure variation and difference between drug classes and risk of subsequent stroke. It was noted that a lower standard deviation of systolic blood pressure with variance ratio ~≤ 0.8 was associated with a significantly reduced risk of stroke (odd ratio 0.79, 95 % CI 0.71–0.87) in spite of small reductions in mean systolic blood pressure [10].

In the abovementioned data we do not have information about the effect of time of day on blood pressure variability. Webb et al. [81] addressed this concern by using HBPM for one month in 500 consecutive transient ischemic attack or minor stroke patients and determining mean, maximum, and variability in systolic blood pressure. This is the first study showing the effect of antihypertensive medications on day-to-day home blood pressure variability. Patients were treated according to a standard protocol, and differences in systolic blood pressure variability were documented (3–10 days before and 8–15 days after starting or adjusting the doses of antihypertensive medications). They reported that there was a significant reduction ($p=0.015$) in variability in home systolic blood pressure after treatment with calcium channel blockers/ diuretics (7.8 %) as compared with renin-angiotensin system inhibitors (4 %). It was primarily due to an effect on maximum systolic blood pressure and not on mean systolic blood pressure ($p=0.001$). Moreover, there was a class difference and maximum effect on early morning systolic blood pressure variability ($p=0.002$). The drug class effect persisted with combinations of diuretics and renin-angiotensin system inhibitors [81]. These findings are consistent with the data from other randomized control trials and explain the reduction of stroke risk with an appropriate choice of antihypertensive medication. The study also emphasizes the value of using HBPM as a potential tool for monitoring of blood pressure variability in patients taking antihypertensive medications.

Conclusion

There is increased recognition of the value of the determination of blood pressure variability and deviations of daytime and nighttime circadian blood pressure patterns. Local and regional guidance statements, especially in developed countries, have now included such information and may include discussion of management strategies. Blood pressure variability, for example, may be reduced in practice by use of calcium channel blocking agents and certain types of diuretics. Further ABPM research will help to elucidate populations and subgroups most prone to blood pressure variability and best management practices. ABPM is an important diagnostic technology for the detection and diagnosis of raised blood pressure.

References

1. Gorelick PB, Farooq MU, Min J. Population-based approaches for reducing stroke risk. Expert Rev Cardiovasc Ther. 2015;13(1):49–56.
2. Gorelick PB, Goldstein LB, Ovbiagele B. New guidelines to reduce risk of atherosclerotic cardiovascular disease: implications for stroke prevention in 2014. Stroke. 2014;45(4):945–7.
3. Gorelick PB. Reducing blood pressure variability to prevent stroke? Lancet Neurol. 2010;9(5):448–9.
4. Lawes CM, Bennett DA, Feigin VL, Rodgers A. Blood pressure and stroke: an overview of published reviews. Stroke. 2004;35(4):1024.
5. Sundstrom J, Arima H, Jackson R, et al. Effects of blood pressure reduction in mild hypertension: a systematic review and meta-analysis. Ann Intern Med. 2015;162(3):184–91.
6. Blood Pressure Lowering Treatment Trialists C, Sundstrom J, Arima H, et al. Blood pressure-lowering treatment based on cardiovascular risk: a meta-analysis of individual patient data. Lancet. 2014;384(9943):591–8.

7. Carlberg B, Lindholm LH. Stroke and blood-pressure variation: new permutations on an old theme. Lancet. 2010;375(9718):867–9.
8. Rothwell PM. Limitations of the usual blood-pressure hypothesis and importance of variability, instability, and episodic hypertension. Lancet. 2010;375(9718):938–48.
9. Rothwell PM, Howard SC, Dolan E, et al. Prognostic significance of visit-to-visit variability, maximum systolic blood pressure, and episodic hypertension. Lancet. 2010;375(9718):895–905.
10. Webb AJ, Fischer U, Mehta Z, Rothwell PM. Effects of antihypertensive-drug class on inter-individual variation in blood pressure and risk of stroke: a systematic review and meta-analysis. Lancet. 2010;375(9718):906–15.
11. Rothwell PM, Howard SC, Dolan E, et al. Effects of beta blockers and calcium-channel blockers on within-individual variability in blood pressure and risk of stroke. Lancet Neurol. 2010;9(5):469–80.
12. Cooke HM, Lynch A. Biorhythms and chronotherapy in cardiovascular disease. Am J Hosp Pharm. 1994;51(20):2569–80.
13. Muller JE, Mangel B. Circadian variation and triggers of cardiovascular disease. Cardiology. 1994;85 Suppl 2:3–10.
14. Smolensky MH, D'Alonzo GE. Medical chronobiology: concepts and applications. Am Rev Respir Dis. 1993;147(6 Pt 2):S2–19.
15. White WB. Circadian variation of blood pressure: clinical relevance and implications for cardiovascular chronotherapeutics. Blood Press Monit. 1997;2(1):47–51.
16. Elliott WJ. Circadian variation in the timing of stroke onset: a meta-analysis. Stroke. 1998;29(5):992–6.
17. Cohen MC, Rohtla KM, Lavery CE, Muller JE, Mittleman MA. Meta-analysis of the morning excess of acute myocardial infarction and sudden cardiac death. Am J Cardiol. 1997;79(11):1512–6.
18. Kario K, Pickering TG, Umeda Y, et al. Morning surge in blood pressure as a predictor of silent and clinical cerebrovascular disease in elderly hypertensives: a prospective study. Circulation. 2003;107(10):1401–6.
19. Kario K. Morning surge in blood pressure and cardiovascular risk: evidence and perspectives. Hypertension. 2010;56(5):765–73.
20. Mancia G, Facchetti R, Bombelli M, Grassi G, Sega R. Long-term risk of mortality associated with selective and combined elevation in office, home, and ambulatory blood pressure. Hypertension. 2006;47(5):846–53.
21. White WB, Gulati V. Managing hypertension with ambulatory blood pressure monitoring. Curr Cardiol Rep. 2015;17(2):2.
22. Di Iorio A, Marini E, Lupinetti M, Zito M, Abate G. Blood pressure rhythm and prevalence of vascular events in hypertensive subjects. Age Ageing. 1999;28(1):23–8.
23. Harshfield GA, Hwang C, Grim CE. Circadian variation of blood pressure in blacks: influence of age, gender and activity. J Hum Hypertens. 1990;4(1):43–7.
24. Sherwood A, Thurston R, Steffen P, Blumenthal JA, Waugh RA, Hinderliter AL. Blunted nighttime blood pressure dipping in postmenopausal women. Am J Hypertens. 2001;14(8 Pt 1):749–54.
25. Cuspidi C, Giudici V, Negri F, Sala C. Nocturnal nondipping and left ventricular hypertrophy in hypertension: an updated review. Expert Rev Cardiovasc Ther. 2010;8(6):781–92.
26. Fan HQ, Li Y, Thijs L, et al. Prognostic value of isolated nocturnal hypertension on ambulatory measurement in 8711 individuals from 10 populations. J Hypertens. 2010;28(10):2036–45.
27. Kario K, Shimada K. Risers and extreme-dippers of nocturnal blood pressure in hypertension: antihypertensive strategy for nocturnal blood pressure. Clin Exp Hypertens. 2004;26(2):177–89.
28. Kario K, Matsuo T, Kobayashi H, Imiya M, Matsuo M, Shimada K. Nocturnal fall of blood pressure and silent cerebrovascular damage in elderly hypertensive patients. Advanced silent cerebrovascular damage in extreme dippers. Hypertension. 1996;27(1):130–5.
29. Kario K, Shimada K, Pickering TG. Abnormal nocturnal blood pressure falls in elderly hypertension: clinical significance and determinants. J Cardiovasc Pharmacol. 2003;41 Suppl 1:S61–6.

30. Pierdomenico SD, Bucci A, Costantini F, Lapenna D, Cuccurullo F, Mezzetti A. Circadian blood pressure changes and myocardial ischemia in hypertensive patients with coronary artery disease. J Am Coll Cardiol. 1998;31(7):1627–34.

31. Frattola A, Parati G, Cuspidi C, Albini F, Mancia G. Prognostic value of 24-hour blood pressure variability. J Hypertens. 1993;11(10):1133–7.

32. Julius S, Kjeldsen SE, Weber M, et al. Outcomes in hypertensive patients at high cardiovascular risk treated with regimens based on valsartan or amlodipine: the VALUE randomised trial. Lancet. 2004;363(9426):2022–31.

33. Fagard RH, Celis H, Thijs L, et al. Daytime and nighttime blood pressure as predictors of death and cause-specific cardiovascular events in hypertension. Hypertension. 2008;51(1):55–61.

34. Patel PV, Wong JL, Arora R. The morning blood pressure surge: therapeutic implications. J Clin Hypertens (Greenwich). 2008;10(2):140–5.

35. Bursztyn M, Ginsberg G, Hammerman-Rozenberg R, Stessman J. The siesta in the elderly: risk factor for mortality? Arch Intern Med. 1999;159(14):1582–6.

36. Bursztyn M, Mekler J, Ben-Ishay D. The siesta and ambulatory blood pressure: is waking up the same in the morning and afternoon? J Hum Hypertens. 1996;10(5):287–92.

37. Boggia J, Li Y, Thijs L, et al. Prognostic accuracy of day versus night ambulatory blood pressure: a cohort study. Lancet. 2007;370(9594):1219–29.

38. Brotman DJ, Davidson MB, Boumitri M, Vidt DG. Impaired diurnal blood pressure variation and all-cause mortality. Am J Hypertens. 2008;21(1):92–7.

39. Hermida RC, Ayala DE, Fernandez JR, Mojon A. Sleep-time blood pressure: prognostic value and relevance as a therapeutic target for cardiovascular risk reduction. Chronobiol Int. 2013;30(1–2):68–86.

40. Ohkubo T, Hozawa A, Yamaguchi J, et al. Prognostic significance of the nocturnal decline in blood pressure in individuals with and without high 24-h blood pressure: the Ohasama study. J Hypertens. 2002;20(11):2183–9.

41. White WB. The riskiest time for the brain: could the nighttime be the right time for intervention? Hypertension. 2007;49(6):1215–6.

42. Staessen JA, Thijs L, Fagard R, et al. Predicting cardiovascular risk using conventional vs ambulatory blood pressure in older patients with systolic hypertension. Systolic Hypertension in Europe Trial Investigators. JAMA. 1999;282(6):539–46.

43. Celis H, Staessen JA, Thijs L, et al. Cardiovascular risk in white-coat and sustained hypertensive patients. Blood Press. 2002;11(6):352–6.

44. Clement DL, De Buyzere ML, De Bacquer DA, et al. Prognostic value of ambulatory blood-pressure recordings in patients with treated hypertension. N Engl J Med. 2003;348(24):2407–15.

45. Fagard RH, Van Den Broeke C, De Cort P. Prognostic significance of blood pressure measured in the office, at home and during ambulatory monitoring in older patients in general practice. J Hum Hypertens. 2005;19(10):801–7.

46. Dolan E, Stanton A, Thijs L, et al. Superiority of ambulatory over clinic blood pressure measurement in predicting mortality: the Dublin outcome study. Hypertension. 2005;46(1):156–61.

47. Schwartz GL, Bailey KR, Mosley T, et al. Association of ambulatory blood pressure with ischemic brain injury. Hypertension. 2007;49(6):1228–34.

48. Kario K. Proposal of RAS-diuretic vs. RAS-calcium antagonist strategies in high-risk hypertension: insight from the 24-hour ambulatory blood pressure profile and central pressure. J Am Soc Hypertens. 2010;4(5):215–8.

49. Kario K, White WB. Early morning hypertension: what does it contribute to overall cardiovascular risk assessment? J Am Soc Hypertens. 2008;2(6):397–402.

50. Wolf J, Hering D, Narkiewicz K. Non-dipping pattern of hypertension and obstructive sleep apnea syndrome. Hypertens Res. 2010;33(9):867–71.

51. Martinez-Garcia MA, Capote F, Campos-Rodriguez F, et al. Effect of CPAP on blood pressure in patients with obstructive sleep apnea and resistant hypertension: the HIPARCO randomized clinical trial. JAMA. 2013;310(22):2407–15.

52. Eguchi K, Hoshide S, Ishikawa S, Shimada K, Kario K. Short sleep duration is an independent predictor of stroke events in elderly hypertensive patients. J Am Soc Hypertens. 2010;4(5):255–62.

53. Kario K, Pickering TG, Matsuo T, Hoshide S, Schwartz JE, Shimada K. Stroke prognosis and abnormal nocturnal blood pressure falls in older hypertensives. Hypertension. 2001;38(4):852–7.
54. Kario K, Pickering TG, Hoshide S, et al. Morning blood pressure surge and hypertensive cerebrovascular disease: role of the alpha adrenergic sympathetic nervous system. Am J Hypertens. 2004;17(8):668–75.
55. Kario K, Ishikawa J, Pickering TG, et al. Morning hypertension: the strongest independent risk factor for stroke in elderly hypertensive patients. Hypertens Res. 2006;29(8):581–7.
56. Ishikawa J, Tamura Y, Hoshide S, et al. Low-grade inflammation is a risk factor for clinical stroke events in addition to silent cerebral infarcts in Japanese older hypertensives: the Jichi Medical School ABPM Study, wave 1. Stroke. 2007;38(3):911–7.
57. Kernan WN, Ovbiagele B, Black HR, et al. Guidelines for the prevention of stroke in patients with stroke and transient ischemic attack: a guideline for healthcare professionals from the American Heart Association/American Stroke Association. Stroke. 2014;45(7):2160–236.
58. Klarenbeek P, van Oostenbrugge RJ, Rouhl RP, Knottnerus IL, Staals J. Ambulatory blood pressure in patients with lacunar stroke: association with total MRI burden of cerebral small vessel disease. Stroke. 2013;44(11):2995–9.
59. Nakamura K, Oita J, Yamaguchi T. Nocturnal blood pressure dip in stroke survivors. A pilot study. Stroke. 1995;26(8):1373–8.
60. Aznaouridis K, Vlachopoulos C, Protogerou A, Stefanadis C. Ambulatory systolic-diastolic pressure regression index as a predictor of clinical events: a meta-analysis of longitudinal studies. Stroke. 2012;43(3):733–9.
61. de Champlain J, Karas M, Toal C, Nadeau R, Larochelle P. Effects of antihypertensive therapies on the sympathetic nervous system. Can J Cardiol. 1999;15:8–14.
62. O'Brien E, Parati G, Stergiou G, et al. European Society of Hypertension position paper on ambulatory blood pressure monitoring. J Hypertens. 2013;31(9):1731–68.
63. White WB. Ambulatory blood-pressure monitoring in clinical practice. N Engl J Med. 2003;348(24):2377–8.
64. Omboni S, Gazzola T, Carabelli G, Parati G. Clinical usefulness and cost effectiveness of home blood pressure telemonitoring: meta-analysis of randomized controlled studies. J Hypertens. 2013;31(3):455–67. discussion 467-458.
65. O'Brien E, Parati G, Stergiou G. Ambulatory blood pressure measurement: what is the international consensus? Hypertension. 2013;62(6):988–94.
66. Krakoff LR. Cost-effectiveness of ambulatory blood pressure: a reanalysis. Hypertension. 2006;47(1):29–34.
67. Tamaki Y, Ohkubo T, Kobayashi M, et al. Cost effectiveness of hypertension treatment based on the measurement of ambulatory blood pressure. Yakugaku Zasshi. 2010;130(6):805–20.
68. Mancia G, Fagard R, Narkiewicz K, et al. 2013 ESH/ESC Guidelines for the management of arterial hypertension: the Task Force for the management of arterial hypertension of the European Society of Hypertension (ESH) and of the European Society of Cardiology (ESC). J Hypertens. 2013;31(7):1281–357.
69. O'Brien E, Asmar R, Beilin L, et al. Practice guidelines of the European Society of Hypertension for clinic, ambulatory and self blood pressure measurement. J Hypertens. 2005;23(4):697–701.
70. Pickering T. Recommendations for the use of home (self) and ambulatory blood pressure monitoring. American Society of Hypertension Ad Hoc Panel. Am J Hypertens. 1996;9(1):1–11.
71. Pickering TG, Hall JE, Appel LJ, et al. Recommendations for blood pressure measurement in humans and experimental animals: part 1: blood pressure measurement in humans: a statement for professionals from the Subcommittee of Professional and Public Education of the American Heart Association Council on High Blood Pressure Research. Circulation. 2005;111(5):697–716.
72. Williams B, Poulter NR, Brown MJ, et al. Guidelines for management of hypertension: report of the fourth working party of the British Hypertension Society, 2004-BHS IV. J Hum Hypertens. 2004;18(3):139–85.
73. Krause T, Lovibond K, Caulfield M, McCormack T, Williams B, Guideline DG. Management of hypertension: summary of NICE guidance. BMJ. 2011;343:d4891.

74. Meschia JF, Bushnell C, Boden-Albala B, et al. Guidelines for the primary prevention of stroke: a statement for healthcare professionals from the American Heart Association/ American Stroke Association. Stroke. 2014;45(12):3754–832.

75. Turnbull F. Blood Pressure Lowering Treatment Trialists C. Effects of different blood-pressure-lowering regimens on major cardiovascular events: results of prospectively-designed overviews of randomised trials. Lancet. 2003;362(9395):1527–35.

76. Verdecchia P, Reboldi G, Angeli F, et al. Angiotensin-converting enzyme inhibitors and calcium channel blockers for coronary heart disease and stroke prevention. Hypertension. 2005;46(2):386–92.

77. Lindholm LH, Carlberg B, Samuelsson O. Should beta blockers remain first choice in the treatment of primary hypertension? A meta-analysis. Lancet. 2005;366(9496):1545–53.

78. Dahlof B, Sever PS, Poulter NR, et al. Prevention of cardiovascular events with an antihypertensive regimen of amlodipine adding perindopril as required versus atenolol adding bendroflumethiazide as required, in the Anglo-Scandinavian Cardiac Outcomes Trial-Blood Pressure Lowering Arm (ASCOT-BPLA): a multicentre randomised controlled trial. Lancet. 2005;366(9489):895–906.

79. Poulter NR, Wedel H, Dahlof B, et al. Role of blood pressure and other variables in the differential cardiovascular event rates noted in the Anglo-Scandinavian Cardiac Outcomes Trial-Blood Pressure Lowering Arm (ASCOT-BPLA). Lancet. 2005;366(9489):907–13.

80. Medical Research Council trial of treatment of hypertension in older adults: principal results. MRC Working Party. BMJ. 1992;304(6824):405–12.

81. Webb AJ, Wilson M, Lovett N, Paul N, Fischer U, Rothwell PM. Response of day-to-day home blood pressure variability by antihypertensive drug class after transient ischemic attack or nondisabling stroke. Stroke. 2014;45(10):2967–73.

Chapter 14
A Review of Antihypertensive Drugs and Choosing the Right Antihypertensive for Recurrent Stroke Prevention

Domenic A. Sica

Considerable clinical trial evidence is available in support of antihypertensive therapy to lower blood pressure (BP) as relates to the primary reduction in stroke. More recently, findings have emerged to support an important role for antihypertensive therapy in recurrent stroke prevention [1]. To this end, guidelines now suggest the provision of BP-lowering medications to both normotensive and hypertensive patients with a prior stroke [2, 3].

Two large placebo-controlled trials have provided most of the supporting evidence for this recommendation [4, 5]. In the Poststroke Antihypertensive Study (PATS), indapamide decreased stroke rate by 29 % in a cohort of 5665 Chinese with a prior transient ischemic attack (TIA) or minor stroke [4]. Antihypertensive therapy also decreases the risk of a second stroke, a finding clearly shown by the Perindopril Protection Against Recurrent Stroke Study (PROGRESS), the second of these supporting studies [5]. Neither PATS nor PROGRESS specifies the level to which BP should be lowered in a poststroke/TIA population.

Core Principles of Antihypertensive Therapy

Pharmacodynamics Versus Pharmacokinetics

For most drugs and most patients, pharmacokinetic considerations are of marginal importance in that they are already reflected in the approved dose ranges and proposed dose intervals. Pharmacokinetic differences are most readily apparent in the use of certain drugs in subpopulations with reduced drug clearance. For example, a

D.A. Sica, M.D. (✉)
Division of Nephrology, Clinical Pharmacology and Hypertension, Virginia Commonwealth University Health System, MCV Station Box 980160, Richmond, VA 23298-0160, USA
e-mail: dsica@mcvh-vcu.edu

© Springer International Publishing Switzerland 2016
V. Aiyagari, P.B. Gorelick (eds.), *Hypertension and Stroke*, Clinical Hypertension and Vascular Diseases, DOI 10.1007/978-3-319-29152-9_14

water-soluble drug mainly eliminated by glomerular filtration/tubular secretion requires dosage reduction in patients with renal impairment as is the case for the β-blocker atenolol. Such drug accumulation with possible concentration-related side effects can be expected to occur in a relevant manner when the glomerular filtration rate (GFR) drops below the 30–40-mL/min range. Alternatively, it is the pharmacodynamic properties of an antihypertensive medication that are of the greatest importance in the efficiency of BP lowering.

Dose–response Counterregulatory Effects

Dose–response effects are present for all antihypertensive drug classes but incremental reductions in BP with dose titration are most evident with sympatholytics, peripheral α-blockers, and calcium channel blockers (CCBs). A major consideration in the pharmacodynamic dose–response relationship for an antihypertensive medication is the extent to which counterregulatory mechanisms activate with BP lowering. Acute and/or chronic BP reduction can be expected to set in motion a series of mechanisms that return BP towards starting values. Reflex increases in cardiac output, peripheral vasoconstriction, and salt/water retention can arise from baroreflex-mediated activation of the sympathetic and renin-angiotensin-aldosterone (RAA) systems. These counterregulatory responses are highly dose-dependent and most regularly seen with nonspecific vasodilating drugs (e.g., hydralazine or minoxidil), high-dose diuretics, or peripheral α-blockers.

It can prove difficult to approximate the extent to which counterregulatory systems are activated with antihypertensive medications and lead to "pseudotolerance." In that regard, a 10–20 % increase in heart rate should prompt either a lowering of the dose of the compound and/or addition of a pulse rate lowering compound — such as a β–blocker. Sodium (Na^+) retention, as a factor in loss of BP control, is most easily recognized if peripheral edema occurs/worsens, although a loss of BP control can still occur with volume expansion stopping short of peripheral edema. If volume expansion is suspected a diuretic can be given, or if one is in use the dose can be increased, to effect a weight loss of 1–2 % of body weight.

Blood Pressure Monitoring and Goals

Blood Pressure Goals

Treatment of hypertension is indicated for untreated patients with an ischemic stroke or a TIA, who after the first several days have an established BP >140 mmHg systolic and/or a diastolic value >90 mmHg. In addition, resumption of therapy is indicated for patients known to be hypertensive and who are beyond the first several days of an ischemic stroke or a TIA. Blood pressure goals and/or rate and extent of

BP reduction are yet to be clearly established. A systolic goal BP <140 mmHg and a diastolic BP goal of <90 mmHg would however be a sensible target and a systolic BP <130 mmHg for individuals having sustained a lacunar stroke would not be unreasonable as a target [2].

Blood Pressure Measurement

The accurate measurement of BP is a crucial issue in determining who should be viewed as being hypertensive and therein a candidate for treatment. In the patient having sustained a stroke or a TIA, there are several BP measurement considerations. First, atherosclerotic disease is not uncommon in the patient having sustained a stroke or a TIA. If one arm has sufficient plaque to lessen blood inflow more than in the other arm, then BP values will "lateralize" and the higher of the two measurements should be viewed as the value to "treat." Second, in patients having sustained a major stroke, muscle atrophy can develop on the affected side; thus, different side-to-side BP readings will occur as a measurement artifact if the cuff used on the non-atrophied arm is unwittingly used on the larger arm. Third, the scheduling of BP measurements, in the context of timing of medication administration, is of particular importance in that trough BP readings need to be shown to be near or at goal. Blood pressure measurements obtained at the time of peak antihypertensive medication effect can engender a false sense of security as to the overall adequacy of BP control.

Home Blood Pressure Monitoring

Conventional office BP measurement yields higher BP values than home-based readings, particularly for systolic BP [6, 7]. The level of home BP suggested to best correspond to a normal clinic BP of 140/90 mmHg is ≈ 135/85 mmHg. Home BP monitoring provides a large number of readings and thus adds to the precision of BP determination in any given patient over time [7, 8]. Home BP monitoring is useful for the long-term follow-up of patients with white coat hypertension and the evaluation of treatment efficacy in patients with sustained hypertension, which is of particular importance to the patient having experienced a stroke [9].

Technical, economic, and behavioral barriers have impeded the more widespread use of home monitoring in clinical practice. Low-cost monitors with memory and systems for telephonic transmission of readings, are of some utility in overcoming these barriers. The number of clinic visits may be reduced with home BP monitoring, making it a potentially cost-effective means for the management of hypertensive patient which is of particularly important in the patient having sustained a prior stroke and who is not particularly mobile. Studies have shown that adjustment of antihypertensive treatment based on home BP measurements instead of office BP readings can lead to less intensive drug treatment, which can then be expected to reduce side effect burden and minimize instances where there might be excessive reduction in BP and/or orthostatic hypotension. The latter is of some relevance to the poststroke patient whose postural BP changes can intensify based on their level of deconditioning.

Blood Pressure Goals and the J-curve

Progressive lowering of diastolic BP to values <60 mmHg can trigger ischemic events rather than provide incremental cardiovascular protection, particularly if critical arterial stenoses exist in the coronary circulation—the "J-curve" hypothesis [10]. Many examples of the J-curve relationship between BP and cardiovascular disease events reflect reverse causality, wherein underlying disease (e.g., reduced left ventricular function, poor general health, noncompliant arteries) is the basis for both the low BP and the increased risk of both CVD and non-CVD events [11].

In the presence of limited coronary flow reserve, as is seen in coronary artery disease (CAD), there is a J-curve relationship between treated diastolic BP and myocardial infarction, but not for stroke per se [12, 13]. Also, a wide pretreatment pulse pressure augurs an increased propensity for CVD sequelae of hypertension, which can be made more obvious by treatment [14]. Practically speaking, if systolic BP is controlled to <130 mmHg, there is marginal benefit, and even the potential for risk, in reducing diastolic BP to less than 80–85 mmHg.

There is some degree of variability in the specific target BP goal for recurrent stroke prevention, which to a certain degree reflects a variation on the J-curve theme. A meta-analysis that looked at impact of achieving tight versus usual systolic BP control on stroke prevention of randomized controlled trials found that achieving a systolic BP <130 mmHg compared with 130–139 mmHg seemed to provide additional stroke protection only among people with known vascular risk factors but not those with established or symptomatic vascular disease [15]. In point of fact, the J-curve hypothesis in the patient having sustained a stroke is untested in that most pertinent trials did not achieve recommended target systolic BP values <130 mmHg.

Need to Lower Blood Pressure Gradually

It is often recommended that BP be brought to goal gradually to avoid sudden and perhaps excessive reductions in cerebral or coronary blood flow. The rate of BP reduction is seldom a problem in the young hypertensive patient, but in the older patient with long-standing hypertension, rapid BP reduction may be poorly tolerated because of diminished cerebral or coronary artery autoregulatory ability [10, 13]. If BP drops below the autoregulatory range, symptoms of cerebral hypoperfusion such as dizziness, fatigue, and forgetfulness may arise. This is particularly the case in the elderly hypertensive patient, in whom the normal limits of cerebral autoregulation fall around a mean BP value of 100–110 mmHg. Concern about an "excessive" perceived BP drop in the elderly or the otherwise vulnerable patient should not, however, preclude attempting to reach recommended BP goals within a relatively short time (weeks rather than months) [16] since achieving rapid BP control offers significant benefits to the hypertensive patient who is at high CV risk [17]. Of note, certain antihypertensive compounds, such as ACE inhibitors, can effectively lower BP without adversely effecting regional cerebral blood flow [18].

Are the Preventive Effects of Antihypertensive Therapy Class-Specific Or Drug-Specific?

There are several drug classes used in the treatment of hypertension including diuretics, β-blockers, ACE inhibitors, ARBs, CCBs, peripheral α-adrenergic receptor antagonists, central α-agonists, aldosterone receptor antagonists amongst several other lesser used classes. There are several compounds within these drug classes and a modest degree of within class heterogeneity of a pharmacokinetic nature primarily relating to drug absorption and differing compound half-lives. Definitive evidence does not exist supporting a preferential positioning for a particular drug class in the primary or secondary prevention of stroke [19]. In that regard, the Blood Pressure Lowering Trialists' Collaboration has reported the effects of ACE inhibitors and CCBs on cardiovascular morbidity and mortality, including stroke [20–21]. As a matter of record, these overviews revealed a 30 % reduction in stroke risk with ACE inhibitors and a 39 % decrease with CCBs compared with placebo. Nonetheless, ACE inhibitors should be strongly considered as part of a treatment plan if even to gain benefit from their cardiovascular and cardiorenal protective effects.

Drug Classes

Diuretics: First Step Therapy

Thiazide-type diuretics are important primary and adjunctive therapies in the treatment of hypertension. They are of particular utility when administered, even in doses as low as 6.25 mg of hydrochlorothiazide (HCTZ) in the form of fixed-dose combination therapy [22]. In general, loop diuretics do not reduce BP as well as thiazide-type compounds when given as monotherapy. Loop diuretics find their greatest use as antihypertensive agents when they can correct clearly evident volume expanded states. The occurrence of metabolically negative side effects such as hypokalemia, hypomagnesemia, glucose intolerance, and hypercholesterolemia is much less common with low-dose diuretic therapy (e.g., 12.5–25 mg HCTZ once daily).

Diuretics are widely promoted for the control of hypertension because they have been shown in numerous controlled clinical trials to decrease hypertension-associated morbidity and mortality rates. The thiazide-type diuretic used in both the Systolic Hypertension in the Elderly Program (SHEP) and Antihypertensive and Lipid-Lowering Treatment to Prevent Heart Attack Trial (ALLHAT) was chlortha-lidone and the question arises as to how this compound might differ from HCTZ [23, 24]. In that regard, the extremely long half-life of 40–60 h for chlorthalidone clearly differentiates it from the relatively short-acting HCTZ, with a half-life rang-ing from 3.2–13.1 h. This half-life difference is marked by a significant difference in BP reduction when chlorthalidone is compared with HCTZ [25].

These BP and existing outcomes data with chlorthalidone suggest that this compound be used with more regularity in the patient with hypertension. Thiazide-type diuretic therapy has been suggested to offer additional benefits for stroke reduction above and beyond what might be expected from BP reduc-tion alone [26] with supporting data for this found in the PATS and PROGRESS trials [4, 5].

Angiotensin-Converting Enzyme Inhibitors: First Line Therapy

ACE inhibitors are considered a suitable first-step option in the treatment of hypertension in a wide range of patient types. Not all patients are *responders* to ACE inhibitor therapy but in those patients who are the dose–response curve for BP reduction is steep at low doses only to flatten thereafter at higher doses; thus, multiple dose titrations of an ACE inhibitor are seldom warranted to gain better BP control. Even modestly natriuretic doses (12.5-mg/day) of thiazide-type diuretics further reduce BP when combined with an ACE inhibitor [22]. Side effects associated with ACE inhibitors include cough, angioedema, and a distinc-tive form of functional renal insufficiency. · Cough and angioedema are *class effect* occurrences with ACE inhibitors; thus, the occurrence of either of these side effects prohibits the use of any ACE inhibitor. There is no specific level of renal function which precludes ACE inhibitor use unless significant hyperkale-mia (>5.5-mEq/L) arises with their use.

The enthusiasm for the use of ACE inhibitors goes beyond their effects on BP, since they are at best comparable with other drug classes, including diuretics, ARBs, and CCBs for BP control. These drugs reduce morbidity and mortality rates in patients with HF, post MI and proteinuric renal disease; however, it would now seem that BP reduction is of more importance in reducing end-organ event rates than might be the class of drugs [27]. The data/opinions supporting ACE inhibitors in specifically reducing stroke rate have been varied [28, 29]. The Heart Outcomes Prevention Evaluation (HOPE) trial results with the ACE inhibitor ramipril showed that the benefits of lowering BP on the risk of stroke are not confined to patients with hypertension, but they also extend to individuals with BP in the normotensive range. Compared with placebo, ramipril reduced the risk of any stroke by 32 % and that of fatal stroke by 61 %. Benefits were consistent across baseline BPs, drugs used, and subgroups defined by the presence or absence of previous stroke, peripheral arterial disease, diabetes or hypertension [30].

Additional data exists from the PROGRESS trial for the ACE inhibitor perindopril in the context of secondary stroke prevention [5]. These data are important since it has been a matter of some controversy as to whether the long-term lowering of BP, in patients who have sustained a prior cerebrovascular event, reduces recurrent stroke rate comparably to the benefit observed for primary stroke rate with BP reduction. In the PROGRESS trial, BP was reduced on average of 9/4 mmHg in the active treatment group, leading to a 28 % risk reduction of major stroke. This risk reduction extended to all forms of stroke (major disabling, hemorrhagic, ischemic, or unknown), was independent of BP and diabetes status. The most beneficial effect was seen in the group being given perindopril and indapamide in which BP decreased to 12/5 mmHg.

Angiotensin Receptor Blockers: First Line Therapy

For the most part the pharmacologic differences between the several compounds in this class are of little practical consequence including their ability to prevent new-onset diabetes in at risk patients. Angiotensin receptor blockers are pulse rate neutral and do not prompt salt and water retention or SNS activation. Increasing the dose of an ARB typically does not increase its peak effect; however, it can prolong the response. Response rates with ARBs range from 40 to 70 % in Stage 1 or 2 hypertension with Na^+ intake and ethnicity having some bearing on the overall effect. Although all ARBs are indicated for once-daily dosing, the effectiveness of an ARB may wane at the end of a dose interval, thereby necessitating a second dosing, which is often the case in poor to average responders. Even as there are no predictors of the magnitude of the BP reduction in response to an ARB, the coadministration of a diuretic oftentimes substantially further reduces BP [31]. Side effects are uncommon with ARBs with cough and angioedema being uncommon occurrences. ARBs can be safely used in patients with moderate to severely advanced stages of CKD with hyperkalemia being less likely than with ACE inhibitors [32].

It is this ease of use of these compounds that makes them particularly attractive candidates for the patient with hypertension. Unfortunately, there is a relative paucity of data with their use for primary or recurrent stroke prevention. In the Losartan Intervention for End-Points (LIFE) study, there were fewer strokes in the losartan-treated group than in the group treated with atenolol, which was an unexpected finding and one without an a priori specific reason for losartan to have decreased stroke rate [33]. In addition, in elderly hypertensive patients, a slightly more effective BP reduction with a candesartan-based regimen compared with control therapy, was followed by a greater reduction in the rate of nonfatal stroke [34].

Calcium Channel Blockers: First Line Therapy

Calcium channel blockers are a heterogeneous group of compounds, with distinctive structures and pharmacologic characteristics. There are two major classes of CCBs: dihydropyridines and nondihydropyridines, a subclass that includes verapamil and diltiazem. The latter two compounds reduce heart rate and cardiac contractility; whereas, the former can modestly increase heart rate in a dose-dependent manner and have little, if any, effect on contractility. The availability of CCBs in sustained-release delivery systems has improved tolerance and simplified the use of these drugs [35].

In considering CCB therapy, there are no significant differences in total major CV events between regimens based on ACE inhibitors, diuretics or β-blockers and these compounds other than for heart failure (HF), which occurs more commonly with a CCB-based regimen. Individual trials suggest a favorable effect of CCBs either given alone or together with other therapies on primary stroke prevention in diabetics [36]. A meta-regression analysis also suggests that CCBs provide more reduction in stroke rate than do diuretics or β-blockers. With this same meta-regression diltiazem compared with diuretics, β-blockers or both decreased the risk of stroke despite higher systolic pressure [19].

All patient subtypes are to some degree responsive to CCB monotherapy including elderly and low-renin, salt-sensitive, diabetic and black hypertensive patients. Calcium channel blockers have a steep dose–response curve for BP reduction, which simplifies their use since there are no reliable predictors of the magnitude of the BP reduction with a CCB. The degree to which BP drops with a CCB is a function of the pre-therapy BP; thus, the higher the BP when therapy begins the greater the fall in BP. Dihydropyridine CCBs can dose-dependently increase heart rate and in so doing diminish the accompanying BP lowering effect of these drugs. Calcium channel blockers have a mild natriuretic effect, which explains, in part, why their BP lowering effect is independent of Na$^+$ intake.

Most CCB-related side effects are class specific, with the exception of constipation and atrioventricular block, which occur most commonly with verapamil. Calcium channel blocker use, in general, can be associated with side effects, such as polyuria, gastroesophageal reflux, and/or gingival hyperplasia; however, peripheral edema is the side effect, which most commonly influences the use of these compounds. Calcium channel blocker-related edema is positional in nature and improves when a patient goes recumbent only to recur when a patient assumes an upright position; thus in the relatively bedbound stroke patient peripheral edema may only appear when a patient becomes more regularly upright.

Beta-Blockers: Second Line Therapy

The efficacy and side effect profile of β-blockers are both compound and delivery system dependent. β-blockers reduce BP without an accompanying decrease in peripheral vascular resistance and typically exhibit a relatively flat dose–response curve, a finding that should discourage their being "over-titrated." Beta-blockers had been first line therapy in the treatment of hypertension for a number of years. An early preferred status for these compounds was based on evidence suggesting a reduction in morbidity and mortality rates with their use in the patient with hypertension; however, more recent reviews of these data have found meager evidence to support the supposition that β-blocker based therapy, despite lowering BP, reduces the risk of heart attacks or strokes. Much of the debate on the proper place that β-blockers should have in hypertension management has focused on how effective the cardioselective β-blocker atenolol was in the treatment of hypertension and in providing specific outcomes benefits. The downfall of the β-blocker drug class (based on atenolol-related data) is premature and this drug class (and, in particular, the vasodilating β-blockers) still remains useful therapy choices.

Combined α-β-blockers are nonselective β-blockers without intrinsic sympathomimetic activity and their use has generally been reserved for the complicated hypertensive patient when an antihypertensive effect beyond that of β-blockade is desired. Labetalol, given either orally or intravenously, has been used to treat hypertensive urgencies and/or emergencies. In acutely hypertensive stroke patients, the CCB nicardipine has proven therapeutically superior to labetalol with each having been given intravenously [37]. Carvedilol has supplanted labetalol in the management of hypertension because of a cleaner side-effect profile and its being able to be given less frequently in a controlled-release delivery system. Carvedilol in its immediate release form does not adversely affect cerebral circulation parameters even as it reduces mean arterial pressure by $\approx 20\%$ [38]. Carvedilol has also proven more effective than metoprolol in a large heart failure study population as to reductions in stroke or fatal stroke — a finding attributed to the unique physicochemical features and not better β-blockade per se [39].

Two trials, totaling 2193 patients used the β-blocker atenolol, recording a small reduction in BP (5/3 mmHg) were neutral for secondary stroke protection [40, 41]. A recent Cochrane Database Review, relying mainly on these two trials, also concluded that there was no available evidence supporting the routine use of β-blockers for secondary protection after a stroke or a TIA [42]. In addition, a meta-analysis by Psaty et al. compared the relative benefits of high- and low-dose diuretics and β-blockers with respect to stroke and found the magnitude of effect was consistently greater with a diuretic, particularly with the low-dose regimen [43].

Aldosterone Receptor Antagonists: Second or Third Line Therapy

Although the most extensive antihypertensive treatment experience with aldosterone receptor antagonists (ARAs) exists with spironolactone, the ARA eplerenone is increasingly used because of a cleaner side-effect profile. The onset of action for spironolactone is characteristically slow, with a peak response at 48 h or more after the first dose. This may relate to a need for several days of spironolactone dosing for its active metabolites to reach steady-state plasma/tissue levels. Spironolactone and eplerenone have been used more recently as add-on therapy for resistant hypertension. The add-on effect of spironolactone occurs within days to weeks, persists for months, and is independent of ethnicity, plasma aldosterone values, and level of urinary aldosterone excretion. Hyperkalemia (>5.5 mEq/L) can also occur with ARAs and develops most typically in the setting of a reduced GFR and/or concomitant therapy with an ACE inhibitor or an ARB [44]. Aldosterone receptor antagonists are not indicated for stroke prevention; however, further studies seem warranted in stroke prevention based on emerging data with compounds in this drug class [45].

Peripheral Alpha-Adrenergic Blockers: Third Line Therapy

α_1-adrenergic-blocking drugs (α_1-blockers), such as doxazosin, terazosin, and prazosin, reduce BP comparable to other major drug classes. α_1 –blocker use has been simplified by the arrival of long-acting compounds in this class. These compounds are most effective in lowering both systolic and diastolic BPs in the upright position. α_1-blockers incrementally reduce BP when combined with most drug classes and are the only antihypertensive drug class to improve plasma lipid profiles and reduce insulin resistance [46]. In the difficult-to-treat hypertensive, these compounds reduce BP significantly when used as adjunctive therapy to ACE inhibitors or CCBs. Upward dose titration of an α_1-blocker can prompt renal Na^+ retention, and the ensuing volume expansion can lessen any BP lowering having occurred. Thus, α_1-blockers should be given with a diuretic unless doses are kept very low. In high-risk hypertensive patients, doxazosin has associated with a higher incidence of stroke and cardiovascular disease events, than was chlorthalidone [47].

First-dose hypotension or syncope although less common with doxazosin or terazosin than with shorter-acting α_1 -blockers nonetheless can still occur. Orthostatic hypotension can occur with these compounds, particularly in volume-contracted patients making this a drug class to be used thoughtfully in patients having had a prior stroke and who are deconditioned. Dizziness, headache, and drowsiness are other common side effects of α_1-blockers, symptoms that oftentimes can be misconstrued to represent sequelae to a cerebrovascular event.

Central Alpha-Agonists: Second or Third Line Therapy

Central α-agonists have a lengthy history in the treatment of hypertension; however, bothersome side effects have lessened the use of these compounds. Clonidine is the most commonly prescribed member of this drug class with other class members being guanfacine and alpha-methyldopa. A small dose of clonidine, in the order of 0.1–0.2 mg twice daily, adds to the BP lowering effect of most other agents and can be dependably used in this way. Dose titration of clonidine beyond 0.4 mg daily is commonly followed by compliance limiting side effects, including fatigue, sleepiness, and decreased salivary flow oftentimes described as "cotton mouth." Increasing the dose of clonidine frequently brings on salt and water retention; thus, diuretic add-on therapy is often viewed as being complementary therapy. Clonidine is available in a transdermal delivery system that has distinct therapeutic advantages but is limited in its use by issues of cost and local skin irritation. Transdermal clonidine is particularly useful in the management of the labile hypertensive patient, the hospitalized patient who cannot take medications by mouth, and the patient subject to early morning BP surges. At equivalent doses, transdermal clonidine is more apt to precipitate salt and water retention than does oral clonidine [48]. Clonidine is also useful second line therapy to aid in smoking cessation an important consideration in the patient with a prior stroke who remains a smoker.

Conclusions

Treatment of the patient with hypertension following a stroke begins at the time of a stroke. Typically, BP is allowed to permissively remain elevated in the immediate peri-stroke period. However, it is not uncommon for there to be a carryover effect such that the decision to either implement or proceed with aggressive chronic anti-hypertensive therapy is slow to occur. Blood pressure values in excess of national guidelines are common after stroke and/or TIAs. For this reason, long-term BP reduction in the poststroke patient should be in the hands of physicians comfortable with varying therapeutic goals and the numerous treatment options for BP control.

Lifestyle modifications should be considered in the treatment of hypertension including weight loss, limiting alcohol use, aerobic exercise, and consumption of a diet rich in fruit and vegetables. Clinicians should carry out an individualized selection of drug(s) process, based on demographic characteristics and comorbidities (cardiovascular disease, diabetes mellitus, and other chronic illnesses) among diuretics, ACE inhibitors, ARBs, or CCBs mindful of the frequent need for multi-drug combination therapy to effect hypertension control. An optimal drug regimen to achieve the recommended level of BP reduction is unclear in that head-to-head regimens have not occurred; available data would suggest that the combination of a diuretic and an ACE inhibitor or a CCB and an ACE inhibitor are useful.

References

1. Rashid P, Leonardi-Bee J, Bath P. Blood pressure reduction and secondary prevention of stroke and other vascular events. Stroke. 2003;34:2741–8.
2. Kernan WN, Ovbiagele B, Black HR, et al. Guidelines for the prevention of stroke in patients with stroke and ischemic attack. Stroke. 2014;45:2160–236.
3. Boan AD, Lackland DT, Ovbiagele B. Lowering of blood pressure for recurrent stroke prevention. Stroke. 2014;45:2506–13.

4. PATS Collaborating Group. Post-stroke antihypertensive treatment study. A Preliminary result. Chin Med J (Engl). 1995;108:710–7.
5. PROGRESS Collaborative Group. Randomized trial of a perindopril based blood pressure lowering regimen among 6,105 individuals with previous stroke or transient ischaemic attack. Lancet. 2001;358:1033–41.
6. Verberk WJ, Kroon AA, Kessels AG, de Leeuw PW. Home blood pressure measurement: a systematic review. J Am Coll Cardiol. 2005;46:743–51.
7. Pickering TG, Hall JE, Appel LJ, et al. Recommendations for blood pressure measurement in humans and experimental animals: part 1: blood pressure measurement in humans: a statement for professionals from the Subcommittee of Professional and Public Education of the American Heart Association Council on High Blood Pressure Research. Circulation. 2005;111:697–716.
8. O'Brien E, Asmar R, Beilin L, et al. European Society of Hypertension Working Group on Blood Pressure Monitoring. Practice guidelines of the European Society of Hypertension for clinic, ambulatory and self blood pressure measurement. J Hypertens. 2005;23:697–701.
9. Staessen JA, Den Hond E, Celis H, et al. Treatment of Hypertension Based on Home or Office Blood Pressure (THOP) Trial Investigators. Antihypertensive treatment based on blood pressure measurement at home or in the physician's office: a randomized controlled trial. JAMA. 2004;291:955–64.
10. Cruickshank JM. Coronary flow reserve and the J curve relation between diastolic blood pressure and myocardial infarction. BMJ. 1988;297:1227–30.
11. Cruickshank J. The J-curve in hypertension. Curr Cardiol Rep. 2003;5:441–52.
12. Farnett L, Mulrow CD, Linn WD, et al. The J-curve phenomenon and the treatment of hypertension: is there a point beyond which blood pressure reduction is dangerous? JAMA. 1991;265:489–95.
13. Jansen PA, Gribnau FW, Schulte BP, Pools EF. Contribution of inappropriate treatment for hypertension to pathogenesis of stroke in the elderly. Br Med J. 1986;293:914–7.
14. Kannel WB, Wilson PW, Nam BH, et al. A likely explanation for the J-curve of blood pressure cardiovascular risk. Am J Cardiol. 2004;94:380–4.
15. Lee M, Saver JL, Hong KS, et al. Does achieving an intensive versus usual blood pressure level prevent stroke. Ann Neurol. 2012;71:133–40.
16. Aries MJ, Elting JW, DeKeyser J, et al. Cerebral autoregulation in stroke. Stroke. 2010;41:2697–704.
17. Julius S, Kjeldsen SE, Weber M, et al. Outcomes in hypertensive patients at high cardiovascular risk treated with regimens based on valsartan or amlodipine: the VALUE randomised trial. Lancet. 2004;363:2022–31.
18. Waldemar G, Ibsen H, Strandgaard S, et al. The effect of fosinopril sodium on cerebral blood flow in moderate essential hypertension. Am J Hypertens. 1990;3:464–70.
19. Staessen JA, Wang JG, Thijs L. Cardiovascular protection and blood pressure reduction: a meta-analysis. Lancet. 2001;358:1303–15.
20. Blood Pressure Lowering Treatment Trialists Collaboration. Effects of different blood pressure lowering regimens on major cardiovascular events: results of prospectively-designed overviews of randomised trials. Lancet. 2003;362:1527–35.
21. Neal B, MacMahon S, Chapman N. Effect of ACE inhibitors, calcium antagonists, and other blood-pressure-lowering drugs: results of prospectively designed overviews of randomised trials: Blood Pressure Lowering Trialists' Collaboration. Lancet. 2000;356:1955–64.
22. Sica DA. Rationale for fixed-dose combinations in the treatment of hypertension: The Cycle Repeats. Drugs. 2002;62:243–62.
23. SHEP Cooperative Research Group. Prevention of stroke by antihypertensive drug treatment in older persons with isolated systolic hypertension: final results of the Systolic Hypertension in the Elderly Program (SHEP). JAMA. 1991;265:3255–64.
24. ALLHAT Officers and Coordinators for the ALLHAT Collaborative Research Group. The Antihypertensive and Lipid-Lowering Treatment to Prevent Heart Attack Trial. Major outcomes in high-risk hypertensive patients randomized to angiotensin-converting enzyme inhibitor or calcium channel blocker vs diuretic: The Antihypertensive and Lipid-Lowering Treatment to Prevent Heart Attack Trial (ALLHAT). JAMA. 2002;288:2981–97.

25. Ernst ME, Carter BL, Goerdt CJ, et al. Comparative antihypertensive effects of hydrochlorothiazide and chlorthalidone on ambulatory and office blood pressure. Hypertension. 2006;47:352–8.
26. Messerli FH, Grossman E, Lever AF. Do thiazide diuretics confer specific protection against strokes? Arch Intern Med. 2003;163:2557–660.
27. Sica DA. Do Pleiotropic effects of antihypertensive medications exist of is it all about the blood pressure. Curr Hypertens Rep. 2008;10:415–20.
28. Bath P. Blood-pressure lowering for the secondary prevention of stroke: ACE inhibition is not the key. Stroke. 2003;34:1334–5.
29. Davis SM, Donnan GA. Blood pressure reduction and ACE inhibition in secondary stroke prevention: mechanism uncertain. Stroke. 2003;34:1335–6.
30. Bosch J, Yusuf S, Pogue J, et al. Use of ramipril in preventing stroke: double blind randomised trial. BMJ. 2002;324:1–5.
31. Sica DA. Pharmacotherapy review: part 2. Angiotensin-receptor blockers. J Clin Hypertens (Greenwich). 2005;7:681–4.
32. Bakris GL, Siomos M, Richardson D, et al. ACE inhibition or angiotensin receptor blockade: impact on potassium in renal failure. Kidney Int. 2000;58:2084–92.
33. Dahlof B, Devereux RB, Kjeldsen SE, et al. Cardiovascular morbidity and mortality in the Losartan Intervention For Endpoint reduction in hypertension study (LIFE): a randomised trial against atenolol. Lancet. 2002;359:995–1003.
34. Lithell H, Hansson L, Skoog I, et al. The Study on Cognition and Prognosis in the Elderly (SCOPE): principal results of a randomized double-blind intervention trial. J Hypertens. 2003;21:875–86.
35. Sica DA. Calcium channel blocker class heterogeneity: select aspects of pharmacokinetics and pharmacodynamics. J Clin Hypertens (Greenwich). 2005;7 Suppl 1:21–6.
36. Tuomilehto J, Rastenyte D, Birkenhager WH, et al. Effects of calcium-channel blockade in older patients with diabetes and systolic hypertension. Systolic Hypertension in Europe Trial Investigators. N Engl J Med. 1999;340:677–84.
37. Liu-DeRyke X, Levy PD, Parker D, et al. A prospective evaluation of labetalol versus nicardipine for blood pressure management in patients with acute stroke. Neurocrit Care. 2013;19:41–7.
38. Kuriyama Y, Nakamura M, Kyougoku O, et al. European effects of carvedilol on cerebral blood flow and its autoregulation in previous stroke patients with hypertension. Eur J Clin Pharmacol. 1990;38:S120–1.
39. Remme WJ, Torp-Pedersen C, Cleland JGF, et al. Carvedilol protects better against vascular events than metoprolol in heart failure. Results from COMET. J Am Coll Cardiol. 2007;49:963–71.
40. The Dutch TIA Study Group. Trial of secondary prevention with atenolol after transient ischaemic attack or nondisabling ischaemic stroke. Stroke. 1993;24:543–8.
41. Eriksson S, Olofasson BP, Wester PO. Atenolol in secondary prevention after stroke. Cerebrovasc Dis. 1995;5:21–5.
42. De Lima LG, Saconato H, Atallah AN, et al. Beta-blockers for preventing stroke recurrence. Cochrane Database Syst Rev. 2014;10, CD007890.
43. Psaty BM, Smith NL, Siscovick DS, et al. Health outcomes associated with antihypertensive therapies used as first-line agent: a systematic review and meta-analysis. JAMA. 1997;277:739–45.
44. Sica DA. Pharmacokinetics and pharmacodynamics of mineralocorticoid blocking agents and their effects on potassium homeostasis. Heart Fail Rev. 2005;10:23–9.
45. Parviz Y, Iqbal J, Pitt B, et al. Emerging cardiovascular indications of mineralocorticoid receptor antagonists. Trends Endocrinol Metab. 2015;26:201–11.
46. Wykretowicz A, Guzik P, Wysocki H. Doxazosin in the current treatment of hypertension. Antihypertensive and Lipid-Lowering Treatment to Prevent Heart Attack Trial. Expert Opin Pharmacother. 2008;9:625–33.
47. Collaborative Research Group. Diuretic versus alpha-blocker as first-step antihypertensive therapy: final results from the Antihypertensive and Lipid-Lowering Treatment to Prevent Heart Attack Trial (ALLHAT). Hypertension. 2003;42:239–46.
48. Sica DA, Grubbs R. Transdermal clonidine: therapeutic considerations. J Clin Hypertens (Greenwich). 2005;7:558–62.

Part IV
Mechanisms and Sequelae of Elevated Blood Pressure on Brain Function and Cognition

Chapter 15
Vascular Cognitive Impairment and Alzheimer Disease: Are These Disorders Linked to Hypertension and Other Cardiovascular Risk Factors?

Fernando D. Testai and Philip B. Gorelick

Alzheimer disease (AD) and vascular forms of cognitive impairment (VCI) traditionally have been considered separate or divergent disorders [1]. AD, for example, has been defined as a "degenerative" disease characterized by neuritic plaque and neurofibrillary tangle pathology, neuronal loss, and deposition of amyloid in the brain parenchyma and brain blood vessels. On the other hand, VCI has been described as disorders caused by cerebrovascular brain injury which may vary from mild to severe cognitive dysfunction [2]. Practically, mixed neuropathology including both AD and VCI is common in the elderly, and vascular risk factors and atherosclerosis may be important in the genesis of both VCI and AD [3–6]. Furthermore, AD and stroke pathogenic mechanisms may be synergistic [7].

The pathophysiology and clinical manifestations of these disorders may be subtle as even the occurrence of stroke symptoms *without* a history of clinical stroke or TIA reported to a physician (referred to as "whispering strokes") may be associated with cognitive impairment, and the risk of this may increase with the presence of each additional cardiovascular factor [8, 9]. Overall, subclinical or "silent" strokes are the most common type of strokes with an estimated 9 million silent infarcts and 2 million silent hemorrhages compared to about 780,000 clinical strokes in the USA

F.D. Testai, M.D., Ph.D. (✉)
Department of Neurology and Rehabilitation, College of Medicine at Chicago, University of Illinois, 912 S Wood St, Chicago, IL 60612, USA
e-mail: Testai@uic.edu

P.B. Gorelick, M.D., M.P.H., F.A.C.P.
Professor, Department of Translational Science and Molecular Medicine,
College of Human Medicine, Michigan State University, 220 Cherry Street
SE Room H 3037, Grand Rapids, MI 49503, USA

Medical Director, Mercy Health Hauenstein Neurosciences, 220 Cherry Street SE Room H
3037, Grand Rapids, MI 49503, USA
e-mail: pgorelic@mercyhealth.com

© Springer International Publishing Switzerland 2016
V. Aiyagari, P.B. Gorelick (eds.), *Hypertension and Stroke*, Clinical
Hypertension and Vascular Diseases, DOI 10.1007/978-3-319-29152-9_15

[10]. "Silent" strokes are significant, therefore, as they may be associated with cognitive impairment and may be preventable.

The combination of AD neuropathology and hemispheric infarction may be sufficient to cause dementia [11]. This is important as the introduction of a vascular component to the process that causes cognitive impairment leads to the possibility of prevention. For example, the progression of cerebral white matter lesions and lacunar infarcts, the most common form of stroke lesions underlying VCI, may be associated with a variety of vascular risk factors such as cigarette smoking, elevated blood pressure, and baseline lesion load [12]. Lifestyle management and medical therapies have been shown to be effective ways to reduce or delay stroke and cardiovascular disease risk and possibly consequent cognitive complications [13].

In this chapter, we review pathophysiologic mechanisms and epidemiological evidence that link hypertension and other vascular risk factors to VCI and AD. We will show that these two disorders may have shared vascular risk factors and may be prevented by prevention or treatment of vascular factors.

Pathophysiologic Mechanisms and Epidemiological Evidence

Hypertension, VCI, and AD

Hypertension is a highly prevalent vascular risk factor, and the association of this condition with dementia or cognitive decline has been shown in many epidemiological studies. The Honolulu Asia Aging Study (HAAS), for example, clarified the association of midlife hypertension and risk of dementia in a cohort of 3703 Japanese-American men. Among individuals with untreated hypertension, the relative risk of dementia was about four times higher in subjects with SBP >160 mmHg compared with those with SBP 110–139 mmHg (OR 4.8; 95 % CI 2.0–11.0), and 3.8 times higher among individuals with DBP 90–94 mmHg compared with DBP of 80–89 mmHg (OR 3.8; 95 % CI 1.6–8.7). These results were consistent for patients with AD and VCI dementia subtypes [14]. Treated hypertension was not a risk factor for the occurrence of later-life dementia, however, suggesting a direct cause–effect phenomenon and highlighting the potential for early blood pressure management to delay or even prevent cognitive decline.

In the Atherosclerosis Risk in Communities (ARIC) study, cognitive assessments were administered to 10,963 subjects aged 45–64 years separated by 6 years. In this study, hypertension was defined by SBP ≥140 mmHg, DBP ≥90 mmHg, or use of antihypertensive medications. Hypertension or diabetes before the age of 60 years was independently associated with cognitive decline over 6 years as measured by the digit symbol subtest of the Wechsler Adult Intelligence Scale-Revised [15]. Other vascular risk factors at baseline such as smoking, carotid intima–media wall thickness, and hyperlipidemia, however, were not associated with cognitive changes. Epidemiological and population-based studies have consistently shown an association between cognitive decline and midlife hypertension. The data linking cognitive impairment to late-life hypertension, in comparison, is less robust. In the ARIC study, for example, 13,476 young adults aged 45–94 years were categorized based on blood pressure at entry as normal (SBP <120 mmHg and DBP <80 mmHg), prehypertension (SBP 120–139 mmHg or DBP 80–89 mmHg), and hypertension (SBP ≥140 mmHg or DBP ≥90 mmHg). Neurocognitive assessments exploring verbal learning and short-term memory (Delayed Word Recall Test), executive function and processing speed (Digit Symbol Substitution Test), and executive function and expressive language (Word Fluency Test) were performed at baseline and prespecified follow-up visits. Mean z scores for each test and global cognition were then calculated. In the median follow-up of 19.1 years, baseline hypertension was associated with a global z score decline of 0.056 (95 % CI −0.100 to −0.012). Among the group of patients with hypertension, change in global z score was less pronounced in individuals who received antihypertensives (−0.050 vs. 0.097). In this study, midlife but not late-life systolic BP was associated with a steeper cognitive decline over time [16].

These and other population-based studies, such as the Rotterdam, Göteborg, Uppsala, Finland, Canadian, and Framingham studies, provide additional evidence that supports hypertension as a vascular risk factor associated with late cognitive impairment or decline [17–21]. The interaction between both variables is complex and J- and U-shaped relationships have been described [22–24].

More recently, the Coronary Artery Risk Development in Young Adults (CARDIA) study provided additional information regarding the effect of blood pressure on cognition. In this study, 2,326 young adults aged 18–30 years underwent periodic blood pressure assessment. In the follow-up period of 25 years, blood pressure variability was associated with poor late cognitive performance independent of the cumulative exposure to blood pressure [25, 26]. In addition, cognitive function was further compromised in patients with nocturnal hypertension [27].

Different pathophysiological mechanisms have been proposed to explain the association of hypertension with cognitive impairment or decline. Hypertension may cause cerebrovascular damage in strategic areas of the brain involved in cognition. For example, the Rotterdam Scan Study has shown an association between the presence of silent brain infarcts and the risk of dementia and cognitive decline in individuals aged 60–90 years who were free of dementia and stroke at baseline. The presence of silent brain infarcts at baseline almost doubled the risk of dementia (HR 2.26; 95 % CI 1.09–4.70). Furthermore, the occurrence of subsequent infarcts was associated with a steeper decline in global cognitive function [28]. In a multivariate regression analysis, cerebrovascular risk factors such as older age, female sex, cigarette smoking, and elevated blood pressure, as well as baseline lesion load, predicted small vessel disease progression at 3 years which paralleled cognitive deterioration [12].

The location of the infarct may predict the cognitive domain affected and ultimately the type of dementia. In the Rotterdam Scan Study, thalamic infarcts were associated with decline in memory and non-thalamic infarcts with psychomotor slowing [28]. In another study done in African-Americans, the CT and MRI findings of patients with AD ($n=78$), vascular dementia ($n=66$), and stroke without dementia ($n=41$) were compared. On CT, white matter lesions, nonlacunar infarcts, and left subcortical infarcts were predictors of vascular dementia. Atrophy of the temporal sulci, dilated temporal horns and third ventricle, and right hemisphere infarcts on brain MRI distinguished AD from vascular dementia [29].

Pathological and biochemical studies have shown an association between hypertension and AD. In autopsy studies, the densities of neurofibrillary tangles and senile plaques, both hallmarks of AD, were elevated in hypertensive patients without dementia. In the Honolulu Heart Program/HAAS, SBP ≥160 mmHg in midlife was associated with brain atrophy and greater number of senile plaques in the neocortex and hippocampus [30, 31]. In addition, in the AD Neuroimaging Initiative, adults with elevated pulse pressure and no symptoms of cognitive impairment were more likely to have elevated levels of AD biomarkers in the cerebrospinal fluid, including amyloid-β and phosphorylated tau, and had a more rapid progression to dementia late in life [32, 33].

A similar association between hypertension and AD has been shown in neuroimaging studies. A study of 511 non-demented subjects aged 60–90 years showed that higher DBP 5 years before MRI predicted hippocampal atrophy, and that higher number of white matter lesions in MRI was associated with more severe atrophy of the hippocampus and amygdala as characteristically seen in individuals with AD [34]. Also, studies done using positron emission tomography (PET) have shown that hypertension and elevated pulse pressure are associated with increased cortical deposition of amyloid-β in cognitively normal adults. This association was more clearly demonstrated in individuals that carry at least one apolipoprotein E epsilon-4 (APOE ε4) allele suggesting a synergism between vascular and genetic factors [35]. Furthermore, Proton MR spectroscopy studies have shown a higher myoinositol/creatine ratio in cognitively intact hypertensive older patients compared to healthy age-matched controls. Interestingly, the myoinositol/creatine ratio in the hypertensive group was similar to that observed in early AD patients, providing further evidence of common pathophysiologic changes in both conditions [36].

Mechanistically, it has been suggested that chronic hypertension and other vascular risk factors lead to endothelial injury and blood–brain barrier dysfunction resulting in increased protein extravasation in the brain parenchyma. In return, this increased protein extravasation contributes to neuronal and synaptic dysfunction, impairs the clearance of cerebral amyloid-β, and facilitates the reentry of peripheral amyloid-β into the CNS [37, 38]. In addition, the chronic exposure to vascular risk factors induces hypoxia and oligemia which increase the amyloidogenic processing of the amyloid precursor protein and amyloid-β aggregation, enhance the phosphorylation of tau protein, and downregulate the amyloid-β degrading enzyme neprilysin [39–43] (Fig. 15.1).

Based on the epidemiological association between hypertension and cognitive decline, it has been proposed that blood pressure-lowering treatments could possibly prevent or ameliorate cognitive decline in patients with hypertension without a history of stroke. However, the results of several studies addressing this hypothesis have shown conflicting results. In a cross-sectional study of 2212 African-Americans aged over 65 years, antihypertensive treatment, excluding centrally acting sympatholytic drugs, was associated with a lower risk of diagnosis of cognitive impairment defined by the Community Screening Instrument for Dementia score (OR = 0.56; $p < 0.01$) [44].

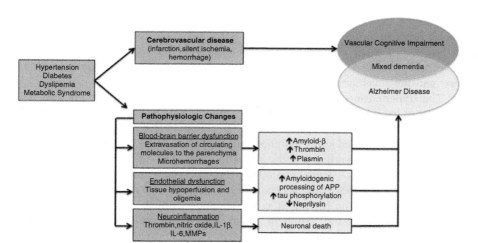

Fig. 15.1 Potential pathogenic processes linking vascular risk factors to vascular cognitive impairment and Alzheimer's disease. Vascular cognitive impairment is a disorder associated with both ischemic and hemorrhagic stroke. At the tissue level, the chronic exposure to vascular risk factors is associated with blood–brain barrier (BBB) dysregulation, endothelial dysfunction, and neuroinflammation. The BBB becomes increasingly permeable allowing the extravasation of blood cells and plasma macromolecules into the parenchyma. Some of these, such as thrombin and plasmin, have a direct effect on neuronal survival. In addition, there is an increased reentry of peripheral amyloid-β to the brain parenchyma. Endothelial dysfunction is associated with hypoperfusion and oligemia which facilitate the amyloidogenic processing of amyloid precursor protein (APP), downregulate the activity the enzymes that metabolize amyloid-β, such as neprilysin, and increase tau phosphorylation. In addition, vascular risk factors trigger an inflammatory response characterized by an increased production of multiple mediators including thrombin, nitric oxide, interleukins, and matrix metalloproteinases (MMPs), among others, which lead to neuronal cell death and further compromise BBB and endothelial function

Similar results were observed in the phase 2 of the Systolic Hypertension in Europe (Syst-Eur2) randomized trial. This study was a double-blind, placebo-controlled trial which included non-demented hypertensive patients aged above 60 years. Antihypertensive study intervention was started after randomization in the active treatment group and after termination in the control group. The median follow-up was 3.9 years, and the blood pressure in the placebo arm was 7.0/3.2 mmHg higher than in the active treatment arm. In this study, long-term antihypertensive therapy reduced the risk of dementia by 55 % ($p < 0.0001$) [45].

However, in the Systolic Hypertension in Elderly Prevention (SHEP) trial, antihypertensive treatment did not reduce the incidence of dementia in patients aged above 60 years with isolated systolic hypertension [46]. A subsequent analysis showed that cognitive and functional evaluations in this trial were biased toward the null effect due to differential dropout [47]. Similarly, the placebo-controlled Study on Cognition and Prognosis in the Elderly (SCOPE) failed to show a benefit in terms of cognitive decline associated with blood pressure lowering in elderly hypertensive patients [48]. The design of this trial allowed the use of open-label active antihypertensive therapy as needed. As a consequence, 84 % of the patients in the placebo group received antihypertensive treatment, significantly decreasing the blood pressure difference between the active treatment and the control groups. A recent systematic review comparing SHEP, Syst-Eur2, and SCOPE concluded that there is no convincing evidence from these trials that blood pressure lowering prevents the development of dementia [49].

The Hypertension in the Very Elderly (HYVET) trial investigated the risks and benefits of hypertension treatment among subjects aged 80 years or older with SBP 160–200 mmHg and DBP <110 mmHg. In this double-blind placebo-controlled trial, patients were randomly assigned to receive placebo or 1.5 mg of indapamide with the option of taking 2–4 mg of perindopril. The SBP treatment goal was 150 mmHg, and the DBP goal was 80 mmHg. Individuals enrolled in this study had no prior history of dementia, and cognitive function was assessed at baseline and annually with the Mini-Mental State Examination (MMSE). Patients with MMSE <24 points or a drop of 3 points in 1 year underwent expert evaluation and were classified as having cognitive decline or dementia. This study was stopped prematurely after an interim analysis showed a reduction in stroke and mortality in the active treatment group. A total of 3336 subjects had at least one annual follow-up examination. During the mean follow-up period of 2.2 years, the rates of dementia in the active treatment and placebo groups were not significantly different (HR 0.86; 95 % CI 0.67–1.09) [50]. Early termination, short follow-up, and inclusion of individuals with low MMSE at baseline have been suggested as confounders that might explain the lack of a beneficial effect of lowering blood pressure on the occurrence of dementia [51].

A meta-analysis including results obtained in HYVET and other placebo-controlled trials of blood pressure-lowering treatment showed decreased risk of dementia in the active treatment group (relative risk 0.87; $p=0.045$; 95 % CI 0.76–1.00) [50]. Overall, clinical equipoise exists in relation to the potential beneficial effects of blood pressure lowering on maintenance of cognitive vitality.

Different factors may account for the apparent discrepancy observed in the longitudinal and interventional studies, including short follow-up, differential dropout, and placebo patients receiving active treatment [49]. In addition, antihypertensive treatments may differ in their ability to prevent cognitive decline. In the HASS, for example, the use of β-blocker monotherapy but not other antihypertensive agents decreased the late development of cognitive impairment [52]. Interestingly, the protective effect of β-blocker was independent of hemodynamic variables such as SBP, pulse pressure, and heart rate suggesting that this drug class may influence amyloid-β deposition through pleiotropic mechanisms.

Other Cardiovascular Risk Factors, VCI, and AD

Diabetes Mellitus and Insulin

The possible influence of diabetes mellitus, glycemia, and insulin levels on demen-tia and cognitive decline has been a focus of interest [3]. In epidemiologic studies there has been controversy about the role of diabetes mellitus as a risk factor for AD, and clinically, there has been concern that tight control of glucose might lead to hypoglycemia and brain damage. Some of the latter concern has been allayed. In an average 18-year follow-up of 1144 patients with type 1 diabetes and mean age 27 years enrolled in the Diabetes Control and Complications Trial (DCCT) and its follow-up Epidemiology of Diabetes Interventions and Complications (EDIC) study, there were no substantial long-term declines in cognitive function despite relatively high rates of recurrent and severe hypoglycemia [53]. Forty percent of the subjects had at least one hypoglycemic coma or seizure event. Higher glycosylated hemoglobin levels, however, were associated with moderate and statistically signifi-cant declines in motor speed ($p=0.001$) and psychomotor efficiency ($p<0.001$). These DCCT/EDIC findings, however, cannot be generalized to older patients. In another study, exaggerated postprandial plasma glucose excursions in older type 2 diabetic persons were associated with impaired global, executive, and attention function, suggesting that tighter control of postprandial glucose might prevent cog-nitive decline in older diabetic patients [54].

A number of epidemiological studies have linked diabetes to dementia, impaired cognitive performance or risk of developing cognitive impairment, and vascular dementia, especially in the elderly and in subjects with severe systolic hypertension or heart disease [55–59]. In the Health Aging and Body Composition Study, patients with and without diabetes at entry completed modified MMSE and Digit Symbol Substitution at baseline and at prespecified intervals. In the 9-year follow-up period, patients with diabetes had an approximately 10 % decline in both measures compared to non-diabetic participants. Among diabetics, cognitive performance was particularly low in individuals with higher HbA1c levels, sug-gesting that optimal glucose control might be an effective strategy to preserve cognition [60]. In relation to AD, there has been controversy. The Framingham Study, for example, did not show that diabetes increased the risk of incident AD overall; however, it could be a risk factor for AD in those without other risk fac-tors such as elevated plasma homocysteine levels and the APOE ε4 genotype [61]. And in the Religious Orders Study, there was a relation between diabetes and cerebral infarction but not AD pathology [62].

Several pathogenic processes link diabetes to AD. First, both insulin and amyloid-β are metabolized by the insulin-degrading enzyme. Thus, from the mech-anistic standpoint, diabetic patients with hyperinsulinemia may have a decreased clearance of amyloid-β [63]. Second, diabetes and glucose intolerance are associ-ated with an increased production of advanced glycosylation end products (AGEs). These AGEs bind to AGE receptors (RAGEs) expressed in neuritic plaques, neurofibrillary tangles, neurons, and cerebral endothelium and modulate neuroinflammation, oxidative stress, and cellular damage. In addition, the binding of AGE to RAGE potentiates the toxicity of amyloid-β and facilitates its influx in the brain [64, 65]. Third, glycation of amyloid-β enhances its tendency to form aggregates [66]. Fourth, hyperinsulinemia is associated with increased production of adipokines (such as adiponectin and leptin) and cytokines which influence cognition. Studies done in animal models, for example, demonstrate that leptin has a beneficial effect on synaptic plasticity and memory [67, 68]. Also, in the Framingham study, elevated plasma levels of leptin were associated with improved cerebral volume and decreased risk of AD in non-demented adults [69]. Fifth, insulin receptors are located in the limbic system in high concentration and may affect cognitive performance [70]. In a small study, for example, insulin infusion was shown to improve cognitive function and mobilize amyloid-β from neurons or reduce its breakdown to an unfavorable form [71]. Furthermore, in the HAAS both low and high fasting insulin levels were associated with increased risk of developing dementia [72]; in the Columbia Aging Study hyperinsulinemia was associated with a higher risk of AD and memory decline [73]; and in the Uppsala Longitudinal Study of Adult Men, impaired acute insulin response in midlife was associated with increased risk of AD up to 35 years later [74]. Additionally, the Nurses' Health Study showed higher fasting insulin levels in subjects with cognitive decline, possibly independent of diabetes [75]. Finally, the insulin-degrading enzyme which has been implicated in the degradation of amyloid beta-protein and the intracellular amyloid precursor protein may act synergistically with APOE ε4 in increasing the risk of late-onset sporadic AD in Han Chinese [76].

In relation to brain structure and function, increased peripheral insulin has been associated with reduced AD-related brain atrophy, cognitive impairment, and dementia severity [77]. In addition, the combination of insulin and other diabetes medication has been associated with lower brain neuritic plaque density [78].

The effect of glycemic control on cognition has been controversial. In two small studies, the intranasal administration of insulin to patients with early AD or mild cognitive impairment improved attention, memory, and functional status supporting the trophic effect of insulin on cerebral function [79]. Peroxisome proliferator-activated receptor-gamma (PPAR-gamma) agonists have gained significant attention in the field as they have favorable pleiotropic functions, which include immunomodulation, neuroprotection, and enhanced processing of amyloid-β [80, 81]. In a small placebo-control study, the PPAR-gamma agonist rosiglitazone normalized plasma levels of amyloid-β and improved delayed recall and attention after 6 months of treatment [82]. These promising observations, however, were not reproduced in the Rosiglitazone in Alzheimer's Disease Study [83]. More recently, the Action to Control Cardiovascular Risk in Diabetes (ACCORD) study investigated the effect of two different glycemic control protocols on adult patients with type 2 diabetes and cardiovascular disease. Subjects were randomized to intense glycemic control (HbA1c goal <6.0 %) or standard therapy (HbA1c goal 7.0–7.9 %). The Memory in Diabetes (MIND) project was a sub-study embedded in ACCORD which investigated cognitive outcomes based on intensity of glycemic control. A total of 2977 individuals enrolled in ACCORD-MIND underwent neurocognitive assessment and brain imaging at baseline and 40 months. In this study, aggressive glycemic control reduced brain atrophy but did not sensibly affect cognitive outcomes [84, 85]. Intense glycemic control, in addition, reduced the 5-year rate of myocardial infarction but increased the 5-year mortality rate [86]. Furthermore, prolonged glycemic control has also yielded negative results. In the Finnish Diabetes Prevention Study, lifestyle intervention with the goal of preventing the occurrence of diabetes did not improve cognition in the 9-year follow-up period [87].

B Vitamins and Homocysteine

Homocysteine (Hcy) is a sulfur amino acid that may be elevated secondary to deficiencies of vitamin B_{12} and folate [88]. Hcy is associated with endothelial dysfunction, vascular disease, neuropsychiatric disorders, clinical stroke, silent stroke, and brain white matter disease. Homocysteine has also been linked to hippocampal neuronal loss, amyloid and glutamate neurotoxicity, and cognitive impairment and AD [88]. Administration of folic acid and vitamins B_6 and B_{12} can lower Hcy levels.

The literature is replete with epidemiological studies that link Hcy to cognitive decline or other important markers of cognition. We now explore a few examples. In the Framingham Study, increased plasma Hcy was an independent risk factor for developing dementia and AD [89]. In the Hordaland Homocysteine Study, increased plasma Hcy was an independent risk factor for memory dysfunction, and a "favorable" change in folate or Hcy concentrations over time led to better memory performance [90]. In the Northern Manhattan Study, cross-sectional data provided evidence that Hcy was a risk for white matter disease [91]. In the Baltimore Memory Study, higher Hcy levels were associated with worse cognitive function across a broad range of domains [92]. In the Northern Manhattan Study, in persons older than 65 years, elevated Hcy was independently associated with decreased cognition [93]. Other studies such as the Columbia Aging Project and one early report from the Rotterdam Study showed no link between high Hcy and AD or total Hcy and cognitive impairment, respectively [94, 95].

Several more recently published epidemiological studies have suggested the following relationships between Hcy and cognition. In the population-based prospective Three-City Study, the association of high Hcy and low cognition in elderly persons was observed only in those with low folate levels [96]. In the Framingham Offspring Study, higher Hcy levels were associated with smaller brain volumes and silent brain infarcts on magnetic resonance imaging (MRI), even in healthy, middle-aged adults [97]. In the Oxford Project to Investigate Memory and Aging, decrease in brain volume was greater among those with lower vitamin B_{12} and holotranscobalamin levels and higher plasma Hcy and methylmalonic acid levels at baseline [98].

Clinical trials of vitamin supplementation to lower Hcy and improve cognition, thus far, have been disappointing. In one such study, supplementation with daily folate (1000 μg) and vitamins B_{12} (500 μg) and B_6 (10 mg) failed to improve cogni-

Table 15.1 Key relationships of select cardiovascular risk factors and cognition

Metabolic syndrome (MetS), Body mass index (BMI), and related factors
1. MetS is associated with every grade of leukoaraiosis, AD, and may not be associated with cognitive decline in the oldest old [100–103]
2. BMI is associated with AD pathology in persons with and without dementia and word-list learning and Digit symbol Substitution Test and word-list learning in healthy, non-demented, middle-aged men and women, and declining BMI is associated with increased risk of AD [104–106]
3. Central obesity and older age are negatively associated with hippocampal volumes and positively associated with white matter hyperintensities and vascular risk factors including obesity cluster and increase the risk of AD or dementia [107–109]
4. Diabetes type 2 duration and hyperglycemia may contribute to brain atrophy [110]
Dietary factors: risks and benefits on cognition and cognitive decline
1. *Dietary factors which may increase risk of cognitive impairment*: high intake of calories and fats may be associated with a higher risk of AD in persons carrying the APOE ε4 allele; saturated fats may increase risk of cognitive impairment; and saturated or *trans*-unsaturated fats may increase risk of AD [127–129]
2. *Dietary factors which may decrease risk of cognitive impairment*: fatty fish and marine omega-3 polyunsaturated fatty acids (PUFAs) reduce risk of cognitive impairment [128]; high intake of unsaturated, unhydrogenated fats may protect from AD [129]; n-3 fatty acids and weekly consumption of fish may reduce risk of AD [130]; fatty fish may reduce risk of AD and dementia for those without APOE ε4 allele [131]; DASH (Dietary Approach to Stop Hypertension) and Mediterranean diets slow down the progression of cognitive decline and AD-associated mortality [147–149]; MIND diet, a hybrid of the Mediterranean and DASH diets, decreases the risk of AD [191]; plasma phosphatidylcholine reduces risk of all-cause dementia; and higher folate intake may decrease the risk of AD [132–134]
3. *Dietary factors which may influence cognitive decline*: a diet high in saturated or *trans*-saturated fat or low in nonhydrogenated unsaturated fats may be associated with cognitive decline; vitamin E from foods or supplements may be associated with less cognitive decline as may fish consumption, vegetables, and high intake of folate; and high dietary intake of copper in conjunction with a diet high in saturated and *trans*-fats may be associated with accelerated cognitive decline [135–141]
4. *Dietary factors which may not be associated with increased or decreased risk on cognition or decline*: high intake of total, saturated, and *trans*-fat and cholesterol and low intake of monounsaturated fatty acids (MUFAs), PUFAs, n-6 PUFA, and n-3 PUFA on risk of dementia or its subtypes; dietary, supplemental, or total intake of carotenes and vitamins C and E on risk of AD, antioxidants vitamins C, E and beta carotene and zinc or copper on cognition; vitamin E had a weak or no protective effect on cognitive impairment; and omega-3 fatty acids in patients with mild to moderate AD did not delay the rate of cognitive decline [142–146]

tion in healthy persons 65 years of age or older with plasma Hcy concentrations of at least 13 μmol/L [99]. Similarly, a high-dose regimen of B vitamin supplements did not slow cognitive decline in persons with mild to moderate AD [88].

Metabolic Syndrome, Body Mass Index, and Related Factors

A number of epidemiologic studies provide a link between metabolic syndrome, BMI or related factors, and cognitive impairment. Key findings from these studies are summarized in Table 15.1 [100–110]. In addition, more recently published studies have provided further verification of some of the findings in Table 15.1. Specifically, midlife central obesity was shown to independently increase the risk of dementia in later life [111], and increased BMI in midlife was associated with MR spectroscopic findings consistent with neuronal or myelin abnormalities primarily in the frontal lobes [112]. Finally, impaired insulin secretion as early as midlife was shown to increase the risk of AD up to 35 years later [74]. Metabolic syndrome, obesity, BMI, and related factors serve as targets for intervention to reduce the risk of cognitive impairment and decline.

Cholesterol

Cholesterol and other lipid substances play an important role in normal brain function [113]. Abnormal central nervous system cholesterol homeostasis likely plays a role in the pathogenesis of AD via complex interactions of membrane cholesterol, ox sterols, APOE, amyloid precursor protein (APP) processing, and amyloid-β peptide aggregation and toxicity [113]. Membrane cholesterol, for example, may be an important regulator of APP processing and may promote amyloidogenic processing through beta- and gamma-secretase instead of nonamyloidogenic processing via alpha-secretase.

Despite all of the interest in cholesterol as a risk for cognitive impairment and decline and the possible role of statin agents to reduce these risks [114], epidemiological studies have provided mixed results about cholesterol as a risk factor for dementia or cognitive decline and the role of statin agents [115–120]. These studies also highlight the possible importance of APOE when dealing with cholesterol relationships and cognition and emphasize that elevated cholesterol in midlife may be a risk for later cognitive impairment, but this relationship may not hold in late life as cholesterol may decrease due to aging or as a result of cognitive decline [121–123]. Finally, clinical trials of statin agents have not conclusively shown a benefit in prevention of cognitive impairment or decline [124, 125].

Diet and Related Factors

Diet may be a factor which increases or decreases risk of cognitive impairment and decline. Oxidative stress is one of the mechanisms whereby this may happen [126]. There are many publications which address this topic. In Table 15.1, we highlight the results of select studies which show risks or benefits of diet on cognition and cognitive decline [127–149]. In addition, a recently published clinical trial of cognitively healthy persons 65 years of age and older showed no overall effect of 26 weeks of eicosapentaenoic and docosahexaenoic acid supplementation (fish oil) on cognitive performance [150].

Hormonal Factors

Estrogens may exert beneficial effects on the aging brain by inhibiting beta-amyloid formation, stimulating cholinergic activity, reducing oxidative stress, and protecting against vascular risks [151]. Although some observational epidemiological studies have suggested a benefit of hormonal replacement therapy on a number of important outcomes such as cognition and cardiovascular disease [151, 152], an important clinical trial, the Women's Health Initiative Memory Study, has shown that estrogen therapy did *not* reduce the incidence of dementia or mild cognitive impairment, and when pooling the results of estrogen alone and estrogen plus progestin, there were increased risks of both endpoints [153]. These results were consistent for middle age (50–55 years) or older (65–79 years) women [153–155]. In addition, there was an adverse effect on global cognition in those treated with estrogen [154]. In another randomized controlled clinical trial, estrogen therapy administered for 1 year to women with mild to moderate AD did not slow disease progression nor improve global cognition or functional outcomes [156].

The North American Menopause Society issued a position statement in 2012 recommending that health-care professionals weigh the risks and benefits of estrogen and progestogen administration for use around the time of menopause for certain disorders (e.g., osteoporosis or fractures). This statement highlights the paucity of data supporting the use of hormonal treatment at any age for prevention or treatment of cognitive decline or dementia [157]. It is believed that timing and duration of use of postmenopausal hormone replacement may hold the key to effective and safe administration of these medications.

Compared to hormone replacement therapy for women, there is a paucity of information about the efficacy and safety of testosterone and androgens to improve cognition or prevent cognitive impairment in men [158, 159].

Exercise and Other Lifestyle Factors

A healthy lifestyle is believed to prevent cognitive impairment [2–5, 13, 160]. One of the components of healthy lifestyle is exercise. Exercise may have beneficial effects which could prevent cognitive decline such as lowering of blood pressure, improving the lipid profile, cerebral blood flow, glucose utilization, and oxygen extraction, protective effects on the vascular endothelium, and other benefits. Overall, physical activity may oppose functional and structural changes of the brain that occur with aging [161], and epidemiologic observational studies suggest a benefit of exercise for prevention of cognitive impairment and decline [162–166]. For example, increased cardiorespiratory fitness might reduce brain atrophy in AD and reduce the formation of senile plaques [161, 167].

A clinical trial including subjects with a mean age of 68.6 years with subjective memory impairment showed that a 6-month program of exercise provided a modest improvement in cognitive function over an 18-month follow-up period [166]. For those who can partake in exercise and other healthy lifestyle choices, provision of habitual exercise, social interaction, adequate nutrition, and educational activities are reasonable prescriptions to improve well-being in later life, for stroke and cardiovascular disease prevention, and possibly for prevention of cognitive impairment or decline [3, 13, 168]. A meta-analysis including 11 randomized studies with healthy subjects older than 55 years showed that aerobic exercise is associated with an improvement in cognition [169]. Similarly, a modest alcohol consumption might prevent cognitive impairment or at least do no harm [3], whereas heavier alcohol consumption may be associated with smaller brain volume [170].

Whereas case–control trials have been inconsistent in relation to smoking, pooled analysis from cohort studies shows a substantial association with dementia (RR of 1.99; 95 % CI 1.33–2.98) [171, 172]. The effect of smoking on the risk of dementia may be age-dependent and more deleterious at younger ages [172]. This observation may be explained, at least in part, by selection bias due to censoring by death in the elderly [172].

In a meta-analysis of 19 prospective studies and 17,023 participants, current smokers had a greater yearly decline in MMSE than those who never smoked, and current smokers had increased cognitive decline compared to former smokers [173]. In another epidemiological study of 10,211 men aged 40–59 years at baseline and followed by 40 years, the hazard ratio (HR) of death from dementia among heavy smokers was 1.58 (95 % CI 1.03–2.43) compared to nonsmokers [174].

Inflammation and Nonsteroidal Anti-inflammatory Drugs

Cytokine-mediated mechanisms may be involved in the pathogenesis of AD and other forms of cognitive impairment in the elderly [175]. Observational epidemiological studies have suggested a possible protective relationship of NSAIDs on cognition [176, 177]. Despite the encouraging but not confirmatory observational study evidence pointing to the possible benefits of NSAIDs on cognitive function, clinical trials have not verified the observational study findings. In a study of mild to moderate AD patients who were about 74 years of age, neither rofecoxib (25 mg/day) nor low-dose naproxen (220 mg twice daily), compared to placebo, slowed cognitive decline [178]. In another clinical trial study, men and women aged 70 years and older with a family history of AD received either celecoxib (200 mg twice a day), naproxen (220 mg twice a day), or placebo [175]. Neither celecoxib nor naproxen improved cognitive function, and there was some evidence to suggest a detrimental effect of naproxen. More recently, a meta-analysis including 14 randomized controlled trials concluded that neither aspirin, steroids, traditional NSAIDs, nor cyclooxygenase-2 inhibitors sensibly modify the natural history of AD [179].

Possible Novel or Emerging Factors

Several possible novel or emerging cardiovascular risk factors for cognitive function include cystatin C, serum uric acid (UA), and cerebral microbleeds. Cystatin C, a measure of kidney function, co-localizes with brain beta-amyloid, and high levels of cystatin C may be associated with cognitive impairment [180]. Serum UA may be associated with cognitive impairment; however, this relationship may be mediated by severity of cerebral ischemia such as brain white matter hyperintensities [181]. Cerebral microbleeds have been associated with white matter disease, particularly in APOE ε4 carriers, and may portend an increased risk of cognitive impairment [182, 183]. In Rotterdam Scan Study and in the Singapore Study, for example, microbleeds were associated with poor neurocognitive performance independently of vascular risk factors [184, 185].

Finally, it has been suggested that the presence of atherosclerosis or atrial fibrillation may be linked to AD [186, 187]. Linkage of these factors to AD could provide new avenues for prevention.

Conclusion

Our approach to dementia and cognitive impairment has shifted. Now, cognitive impairment is conceptualized along a continuum of milder to more severe forms whereby we have moved our focus from effects to causes of cognitive impairment. The latter approach is well suited for prevention of dementia and cognitive impairment and for the maintenance of cognitive vitality as a mechanistic-based approach to the prevention of these disorders when they manifest at early stages is likely to be prudent. Whereas observational epidemiological studies provide evidence of benefit for control of traditional cardiovascular disease risk factors for the maintenance of cognitive vitality, such hypotheses need to be tested in large-scale clinical trials to provide more definitive proof of efficacy and safety. We anticipate that the lifecycle stage of intervention will be an important factor to consider. The American Heart Association and the American Stroke Association issued a position statement in 2011 related to the contribution of vascular diseases and risk factors to cognitive impairment and dementia. This document emphasizes that early modification of vascular risk factors may be required to prevent or postpone the onset of VCI or AD [188]. However, once cognitive impairment is present, cerebrovascular brain injury may either be too extensive or may require a different strategy for successful remediation.

The pathophysiologic distinction between AD and VCI has been challenged and has become somewhat blurred given the possible shared risks and mechanisms for these disorders [189, 190] (Fig. 15.1). By better understanding underlying mechanisms we may be able to better prevent and treat these important disorders of later life.

References

1. Gorelick PB, Mangone CA. Vascular dementias in the elderly. Clin Geriatr Med. 1991;7(3):599–615.
2. Gorelick PB. Risk factors for vascular dementia and Alzheimer disease. Stroke. 2004;35(11 Suppl 1):2620–2.
3. Gorelick PB, William M. Feinberg Lecture: cognitive vitality and the role of stroke and cardiovascular disease risk factors. Stroke. 2005;36(4):875–9.
4. Gorelick PB. Can we save the brain from the ravages of midlife cardiovascular risk factors? Neurology. 1999;52(6):1114–5.
5. Gorelick PB, Erkinjuntti T, Hofman A, Rocca WA, Skoog I, Winblad B. Prevention of vascular dementia. Alzheimer Dis Assoc Disord. 1999;13 Suppl 3:S131–9.
6. Gorelick PB, Freels S, Harris Y, Dollear T, Billingsley M, Brown N. Epidemiology of vascular and Alzheimer's dementia among African Americans in Chicago, IL: baseline frequency and comparison of risk factors. Neurology. 1994;44(8):1391–6.
7. Iadecola C, Gorelick PB. Converging pathogenic mechanisms in vascular and neurodegenerative dementia. Stroke. 2003;34(2):335–7.
8. Wadley VG, McClure LA, Howard VJ, Unverzagt FW, Go RC, Moy CS, et al. Cognitive status, stroke symptom reports, and modifiable risk factors among individuals with no diagnosis of stroke or transient ischemic attack in the REasons for Geographic and Racial Differences in Stroke (REGARDS) Study. Stroke. 2007;38(4):1143–7.
9. Gorelick PB, Bowler JV. Advances in vascular cognitive impairment 2007. Stroke. 2008;39(2):279–82.
10. Hachinski V. World Stroke Day 2008: "little strokes, big trouble". Stroke. 2008;39(9):2407–20.
11. Troncoso JC, Zonderman AB, Resnick SM, Crain B, Pletnikova O, O'Brien RJ. Effect of infarcts on dementia in the Baltimore longitudinal study of aging. Ann Neurol. 2008;64(2):168–76.
12. van Dijk EJ, Prins ND, Vrooman HA, Hofman A, Koudstaal PJ, Breteler MM. Progression of cerebral small vessel disease in relation to risk factors and cognitive consequences: Rotterdam Scan study. Stroke. 2008;39(10):2712–9.
13. Gorelick PB. Primary prevention of stroke: impact of healthy lifestyle. Circulation. 2008;118(9):904–6.
14. Launer LJ, Ross GW, Petrovitch H, Masaki K, Foley D, White LR, et al. Midlife blood pressure and dementia: the Honolulu-Asia aging study. Neurobiol Aging. 2000;21(1):49–55.
15. Knopman D, Boland LL, Mosley T, Howard G, Liao D, Szklo M, et al. Cardiovascular risk factors and cognitive decline in middle-aged adults. Neurology. 2001;56(1):42–8.
16. Gottesman RF, Schneider AL, Albert M, Alonso A, Bandeen-Roche K, Coker L, et al. Midlife hypertension and 20-year cognitive change: the atherosclerosis risk in communities neurocognitive study. JAMA Neurol. 2014;71(10):1218–27.

17. Breteler MM, van Swieten JC, Bots ML, Grobbee DE, Claus JJ, van den Hout JH, et al. Cerebral white matter lesions, vascular risk factors, and cognitive function in a population-based study: the Rotterdam Study. Neurology. 1994;44(7):1246–52.
18. Skoog I, Lernfelt B, Landahl S, Palmertz B, Andreasson LA, Nilsson L, et al. 15-year longitudinal study of blood pressure and dementia. Lancet. 1996;347(9009):1141–5.
19. Kilander L, Nyman H, Boberg M, Hansson L, Lithell H. Hypertension is related to cognitive impairment: a 20-year follow-up of 999 men. Hypertension. 1998;31(3):780–6.
20. Elias MF, Elias PK, Sullivan LM, Wolf PA, D'Agostino RB. Lower cognitive function in the presence of obesity and hypertension: the Framingham heart study. Int J Obes Relat Metab Disord. 2003;27(2):260–8.
21. Kivipelto M, Helkala EL, Hanninen T, Laakso MP, Hallikainen M, Alhainen K, et al. Midlife vascular risk factors and late-life mild cognitive impairment: a population-based study. Neurology. 2001;56(12):1683–9.
22. Waldstein SR, Giggey PP, Thayer JF, Zonderman AB. Nonlinear relations of blood pressure to cognitive function: the Baltimore Longitudinal Study of Aging. Hypertension. 2005; 45(3):374–9.
23. Glynn RJ, Beckett LA, Hebert LE, Morris MC, Scherr PA, Evans DA. Current and remote blood pressure and cognitive decline. JAMA. 1999;281(5):438–45.
24. Okumiya K, Matsubayashi K, Wada T, Osaki Y, Doi Y, Ozawa T. J-curve relation between blood pressure and decline in cognitive function in older people living in community. Japan J Am Geriatr Soc. 1997;45(8):1032–3.
25. Yano Y, Bakris GL, Inokuchi T, Ohba Y, Tamaki N, Nagata M, et al. Association of cognitive dysfunction with cardiovascular disease events in elderly hypertensive patients. J Hypertens. 2014;32(2):423–31.
26. Yano Y, Ning H, Allen N, Reis JP, Launer LJ, Liu K, et al. Long-term blood pressure variability throughout young adulthood and cognitive function in midlife: the Coronary Artery Risk Development in Young Adults (CARDIA) study. Hypertension. 2014;64(5):983–8.
27. Yano Y, Ning H, Muntner P, Reis JP, Calhoun DA, Viera AJ, et al. Nocturnal blood pressure in young adults and cognitive function in midlife: The Coronary Artery Risk Development in Young Adults (CARDIA) Study. Am J Hypertens. 2015;28(10):1240–7.
28. Vermeer SE, Prins ND, den Heijer T, Hofman A, Koudstaal PJ, Breteler MM. Silent brain infarcts and the risk of dementia and cognitive decline. N Engl J Med. 2003;348(13): 1215–22.
29. Charletta D, Gorelick PB, Dollear TJ, Freels S, Harris Y. CT and MRI findings among African-Americans with Alzheimer's disease, vascular dementia, and stroke without dementia. Neurology. 1995;45(8):1456–61.
30. Sparks DL, Scheff SW, Liu H, Landers TM, Coyne CM. Hunsaker JC,3rd. Increased incidence of neurofibrillary tangles (NFT) in non-demented individuals with hypertension. J Neurol Sci. 1995;131(2):162–9.
31. Petrovitch H, White LR, Izmirilian G, Ross GW, Havlik RJ, Markesbery W, et al. Midlife blood pressure and neuritic plaques, neurofibrillary tangles, and brain weight at death: the HAAS. Honolulu-Asia aging Study. Neurobiol Aging. 2000;21(1):57–62.
32. Nation DA, Edland SD, Bondi MW, Salmon DP, Delano-Wood L, Peskind ER, et al. Pulse pressure is associated with Alzheimer biomarkers in cognitively normal older adults. Neurology. 2013;81(23):2024–7.
33. Nation DA, Edmonds EC, Bangen KJ, Delano-Wood L, Scanlon BK, Han SD, et al. Pulse pressure in relation to Tau-mediated neurodegeneration, cerebral amyloidosis, and progression to dementia in very old adults. JAMA Neurol. 2015;72(5):546–53.
34. den Heijer T, Launer LJ, Prins ND, van Dijk EJ, Vermeer SE, Hofman A, et al. Association between blood pressure, white matter lesions, and atrophy of the medial temporal lobe. Neurology. 2005;64(2):263–7.
35. Rodrigue KM, Rieck JR, Kennedy KM, Devous MDS, Diaz-Arrastia R, Park DC. Risk factors for beta-amyloid deposition in healthy aging: vascular and genetic effects. JAMA Neurol. 2013;70(5):600–6.

36. Catani M, Mecocci P, Tarducci R, Howard R, Pelliccioli GP, Mariani E, et al. Proton magnetic resonance spectroscopy reveals similar white matter biochemical changes in patients with chronic hypertension and early Alzheimer's disease. J Am Geriatr Soc. 2002; 50(10):1707–10.
37. Akinyemi RO, Mukaetova-Ladinska EB, Attems J, Ihara M, Kalaria RN. Vascular risk factors and neurodegeneration in ageing related dementias: Alzheimer's disease and vascular dementia. Curr Alzheimer Res. 2013;10(6):642–53.
38. Sengillo JD, Winkler EA, Walker CT, Sullivan JS, Johnson M, Zlokovic BV. Deficiency in mural vascular cells coincides with blood-brain barrier disruption in Alzheimer's disease. Brain Pathol. 2013;23(3):303–10.
39. Wang X, Xing A, Xu C, Cai Q, Liu H, Li L. Cerebrovascular hypoperfusion induces spatial memory impairment, synaptic changes, and amyloid-beta oligomerization in rats. J Alzheimers Dis. 2010;21(3):813–22.
40. Koike MA, Green KN, Blurton-Jones M, Laferla FM. Oligemic hypoperfusion differentially affects tau and amyloid-{beta}. Am J Pathol. 2010;177(1):300–10.
41. Hiltunen M, Makinen P, Peraniemi S, Sivenius J, van Groen T, Soininen H, et al. Focal cerebral ischemia in rats alters APP processing and expression of Abeta peptide degrading enzymes in the thalamus. Neurobiol Dis. 2009;35(1):103–13.
42. Fisk L, Nalivaeva NN, Boyle JP, Peers CS, Turner AJ. Effects of hypoxia and oxidative stress on expression of neprilysin in human neuroblastoma cells and rat cortical neurones and astrocytes. Neurochem Res. 2007;32(10):1741–8.
43. Li L, Zhang X, Yang D, Luo G, Chen S, Le W. Hypoxia increases Abeta generation by altering beta- and gamma-cleavage of APP. Neurobiol Aging. 2009;30(7):1091–8.
44. Richards SS, Emsley CL, Roberts J, Murray MD, Hall K, Gao S, et al. The association between vascular risk factor-mediating medications and cognition and dementia diagnosis in a community-based sample of African-Americans. J Am Geriatr Soc. 2000;48(9):1035–41.
45. Forette F, Seux ML, Staessen JA, Thijs L, Babarskiene MR, Babeanu S, et al. The prevention of dementia with antihypertensive treatment: new evidence from the Systolic Hypertension in Europe (Syst-Eur) study. Arch Intern Med. 2002;162(18):2046–52.
46. SHEP Cooperative Research Group. Prevention of stroke by antihypertensive drug treatment in older persons with isolated systolic hypertension. Final results of the Systolic Hypertension in the Elderly Program (SHEP). JAMA. 1991;265(24):3255–64.
47. Di Bari M, Pahor M, Franse LV, Shorr RI, Wan JY, Ferrucci L, et al. Dementia and disability outcomes in large hypertension trials: lessons learned from the systolic hypertension in the elderly program (SHEP) trial. Am J Epidemiol. 2001;153(1):72–8.
48. Lithell H, Hansson L, Skoog I, Elmfeldt D, Hofman A, Olofsson B, et al. The Study on Cognition and Prognosis in the Elderly (SCOPE): principal results of a randomized double-blind intervention trial. J Hypertens. 2003;21(5):875–86.
49. McGuinness B, Todd S, Passmore P, Bullock R. Blood pressure lowering in patients without prior cerebrovascular disease for prevention of cognitive impairment and dementia. Cochrane Database Syst Rev. 2009;4, CD004034.
50. Peters R, Beckett N, Forette F, Tuomilehto J, Clarke R, Ritchie C, et al. Incident dementia and blood pressure lowering in the Hypertension in the Very Elderly Trial cognitive function assessment (HYVET-COG): a double-blind, placebo controlled trial. Lancet Neurol. 2008;7(8):683–9.
51. Skoog I. Antihypertensive treatment and dementia prevention. Lancet Neurol. 2008;7(8): 664–5.
52. Gelber RP, Ross GW, Petrovitch H, Masaki KH, Launer LJ, White LR. Antihypertensive medication use and risk of cognitive impairment: the Honolulu-Asia Aging Study. Neurology. 2013;81(10):888–95.
53. Diabetes Control and Complications Trial/Epidemiology of Diabetes Interventions and Complications Study Research Group, Jacobson AM, Musen G, Ryan CM, Silvers N, Cleary P, et al. Long-term effect of diabetes and its treatment on cognitive function. N Engl J Med. 2007;356(18):1842–52.

54. Abbatecola AM, Rizzo MR, Barbieri M, Grella R, Arciello A, Laieta MT, et al. Postprandial plasma glucose excursions and cognitive functioning in aged type 2 diabetics. Neurology. 2006;67(2):235–40.
55. Beeri MS, Schmeidler J, Silverman JM, Gandy S, Wysocki M, Hannigan CM, et al. Insulin in combination with other diabetes medication is associated with less Alzheimer neuropathology. Neurology. 2008;71(10):750–7.
56. Yaffe K, Blackwell T, Kanaya AM, Davidowitz N, Barrett-Connor E, Krueger K. Diabetes, impaired fasting glucose, and development of cognitive impairment in older women. Neurology. 2004;63(4):658–63.
57. Xu WL, Qiu CX, Wahlin A, Winblad B, Fratiglioni L. Diabetes mellitus and risk of dementia in the Kungsholmen project: a 6-year follow-up study. Neurology. 2004;63(7):1181–6.
58. Kumari M, Marmot M. Diabetes and cognitive function in a middle-aged cohort: findings from the Whitehall II study. Neurology. 2005;65(10):1597–603.
59. Xiong GL, Plassman BL, Helms MJ, Steffens DC. Vascular risk factors and cognitive decline among elderly male twins. Neurology. 2006;67(9):1586–91.
60. Yaffe K, Falvey C, Hamilton N, Schwartz AV, Simonsick EM, Satterfield S, et al. Diabetes, glucose control, and 9-year cognitive decline among older adults without dementia. Arch Neurol. 2012;69(9):1170–5.
61. Akomolafe A, Beiser A, Meigs JB, Au R, Green RC, Farrer LA, et al. Diabetes mellitus and risk of developing Alzheimer disease: results from the Framingham Study. Arch Neurol. 2006;63(11):1551–5.
62. Arvanitakis Z, Schneider JA, Wilson RS, Li Y, Arnold SE, Wang Z, et al. Diabetes is related to cerebral infarction but not to AD pathology in older persons. Neurology. 2006;67(11):1960–5.
63. Willette AA, Johnson SC, Birdsill AC, Sager MA, Christian B, Baker LD, et al. Insulin resistance predicts brain amyloid deposition in late middle-aged adults. Alzheimers Dement. 2015;11(5):504–10.
64. Chen C, Li XH, Tu Y, Sun HT, Liang HQ, Cheng SX, et al. Abeta-AGE aggravates cognitive deficit in rats via RAGE pathway. Neuroscience. 2014;257:1–10.
65. Deane R, Du Yan S, Submamaryan RK, LaRue B, Jovanovic S, Hogg E, et al. RAGE mediates amyloid-beta peptide transport across the blood-brain barrier and accumulation in brain. Nat Med. 2003;9(7):907–13.
66. Yamagishi S, Nakamura K, Inoue H, Kikuchi S, Takeuchi M. Serum or cerebrospinal fluid levels of glyceraldehyde-derived advanced glycation end products (AGEs) may be a promising biomarker for early detection of Alzheimer's disease. Med Hypotheses. 2005;64(6):1205–7.
67. Li XL, Aou S, Oomura Y, Hori N, Fukunaga K, Hori T. Impairment of long-term potentiation and spatial memory in leptin receptor-deficient rodents. Neuroscience. 2002;113(3):607–15.
68. Perez-Gonzalez R, Alvira-Botero MX, Robayo O, Antequera D, Garzon M, Martin-Moreno AM, et al. Leptin gene therapy attenuates neuronal damages evoked by amyloid-beta and rescues memory deficits in APP/PS1 mice. Gene Ther. 2014;21(3):298–308.
69. Lieb W, Beiser AS, Vasan RS, Tan ZS, Au R, Harris TB, et al. Association of plasma leptin levels with incident Alzheimer disease and MRI measures of brain aging. JAMA. 2009;302(23):2565–72.
70. Strachan MW. Insulin and cognitive function. Lancet. 2003;362(9392):1253.
71. Watson GS, Peskind ER, Asthana S, Purganan K, Wait C, Chapman D, et al. Insulin increases CSF Abeta42 levels in normal older adults. Neurology. 2003;60(12):1899–903.
72. Peila R, Rodriguez BL, White LR, Launer LJ. Fasting insulin and incident dementia in an elderly population of Japanese-American men. Neurology. 2004;63(2):228–33.
73. Luchsinger JA, Tang MX, Shea S, Mayeux R. Hyperinsulinemia and risk of Alzheimer disease. Neurology. 2004;63(7):1187–92.
74. Ronnemaa E, Zethelius B, Sundelof J, Sundstrom J, Degerman-Gunnarsson M, Berne C, et al. Impaired insulin secretion increases the risk of Alzheimer disease. Neurology. 2008;71(14):1065–71.

75. van Oijen M, Okereke OI, Kang JH, Pollak MN, Hu FB, Hankinson SE, et al. Fasting insulin levels and cognitive decline in older women without diabetes. Neuroepidemiology. 2008; 30(3):174–9.
76. Bian L, Yang JD, Guo TW, Sun Y, Duan SW, Chen WY, et al. Insulin-degrading enzyme and Alzheimer disease: a genetic association study in the Han Chinese. Neurology. 2004;63(2): 241–5.
77. Burns JM, Donnelly JE, Anderson HS, Mayo MS, Spencer-Gardner L, Thomas G, et al. Peripheral insulin and brain structure in early Alzheimer disease. Neurology. 2007; 69(11):1094–104.
78. Schnaider Beeri M, Goldbourt U, Silverman JM, Noy S, Schmeidler J, Ravona-Springer R, et al. Diabetes mellitus in midlife and the risk of dementia three decades later. Neurology. 2004;63(10):1902–7.
79. Claxton A, Baker LD, Hanson A, Trittschuh EH, Cholerton B, Morgan A, et al. Long-acting intranasal insulin detemir improves cognition for adults with mild cognitive impairment or early-stage Alzheimer's disease dementia. J Alzheimers Dis. 2015;44(3):897–906.
80. d'Abramo C, Massone S, Zingg JM, Pizzuti A, Marambaud P, Dalla Piccola B, et al. Role of peroxisome proliferator-activated receptor gamma in amyloid precursor protein processing and amyloid beta-mediated cell death. Biochem J. 2005;391(Pt 3):693–8.
81. Jiang Q, Heneka M, Landreth GE. The role of peroxisome proliferator-activated receptor-gamma (PPARgamma) in Alzheimer's disease: therapeutic implications. CNS Drugs. 2008;22(1):1–14.
82. Watson GS, Cholerton BA, Reger MA, Baker LD, Plymate SR, Asthana S, et al. Preserved cognition in patients with early Alzheimer disease and amnestic mild cognitive impairment during treatment with rosiglitazone: a preliminary study. Am J Geriatr Psychiatry. 2005; 13(11):950–8.
83. Risner ME, Saunders AM, Altman JF, Ormandy GC, Craft S, Foley IM, et al. Efficacy of rosiglitazone in a genetically defined population with mild-to-moderate Alzheimer's disease. Pharmacogenomics J. 2006;6(4):246–54.
84. Launer LJ, Miller ME, Williamson JD, Lazar RM, Gerstein HC, Murray AM, et al. Effects of intensive glucose lowering on brain structure and function in people with type 2 diabetes (ACCORD MIND): a randomised open-label substudy. Lancet Neurol. 2011;10(11):969–77.
85. Williamson JD, Launer LJ, Bryan RN, Coker LH, Lazar RM, Gerstein HC, et al. Cognitive function and brain structure in persons with type 2 diabetes mellitus after intensive lowering of blood pressure and lipid levels: a randomized clinical trial. JAMA Intern Med. 2014;174(3):324–33.
86. ACCORD Study Group, Gerstein HC, Miller ME, Genuth S, Ismail-Beigi F, Buse JB, et al. Long-term effects of intensive glucose lowering on cardiovascular outcomes. N Engl J Med. 2011;364(9):818–28.
87. Luchsinger JA, Lehtisalo J, Lindstrom J, Ngandu T, Kivipelto M, Ahtiluoto S, et al. Cognition in the Finnish diabetes prevention study. Diabetes Res Clin Pract. 2015;108(3):63–6.
88. Aisen PS, Schneider LS, Sano M, Diaz-Arrastia R, van Dyck CH, Weiner MF, et al. High-dose B vitamin supplementation and cognitive decline in Alzheimer disease: a randomized controlled trial. JAMA. 2008;300(15):1774–83.
89. Seshadri S, Beiser A, Selhub J, Jacques PF, Rosenberg IH, D'Agostino RB, et al. Plasma homocysteine as a risk factor for dementia and Alzheimer's disease. N Engl J Med. 2002;346(7):476–83.
90. Nurk E, Refsum H, Tell GS, Engedal K, Vollset SE, Ueland PM, et al. Plasma total homocysteine and memory in the elderly: the Hordaland Homocysteine Study. Ann Neurol. 2005;58(6):847–57.
91. Wright CB, Paik MC, Brown TR, Stabler SP, Allen RH, Sacco RL, et al. Total homocysteine is associated with white matter hyperintensity volume: the Northern Manhattan Study. Stroke. 2005;36(6):1207–11.

92. Schafer JH, Glass TA, Bolla KI, Mintz M, Jedlicka AE, Schwartz BS. Homocysteine and cognitive function in a population-based study of older adults. J Am Geriatr Soc. 2005;53(3):381–8.
93. Wright CB, Lee HS, Paik MC, Stabler SP, Allen RH, Sacco RL. Total homocysteine and cognition in a tri-ethnic cohort: the Northern Manhattan Study. Neurology. 2004;63(2):254–60.
94. Luchsinger JA, Tang MX, Shea S, Miller J, Green R, Mayeux R. Plasma homocysteine levels and risk of Alzheimer disease. Neurology. 2004;62(11):1972–6.
95. Kalmijn S, Launer LJ, Lindemans J, Bots ML, Hofman A, Breteler MM. Total homocysteine and cognitive decline in a community-based sample of elderly subjects: the Rotterdam Study. Am J Epidemiol. 1999;150(3):283–9.
96. Vidal JS, Dufouil C, Ducros V, Tzourio C. Homocysteine, folate and cognition in a large community-based sample of elderly people--the 3C Dijon Study. Neuroepidemiology. 2008;30(4):207–14.
97. Seshadri S, Wolf PA, Beiser AS, Selhub J, Au R, Jacques PF, et al. Association of plasma total homocysteine levels with subclinical brain injury: cerebral volumes, white matter hyperintensity, and silent brain infarcts at volumetric magnetic resonance imaging in the Framingham Offspring Study. Arch Neurol. 2008;65(5):642–9.
98. Vogiatzoglou A, Refsum H, Johnston C, Smith SM, Bradley KM, de Jager C, et al. Vitamin B12 status and rate of brain volume loss in community-dwelling elderly. Neurology. 2008;71(11):826–32.
99. McMahon JA, Green TJ, Skeaff CM, Knight RG, Mann JI, Williams SM. A controlled trial of homocysteine lowering and cognitive performance. N Engl J Med. 2006;354(26):2764–72.
100. Park K, Yasuda N, Toyonaga S, Yamada SM, Nakabayashi H, Nakasato M, et al. Significant association between leukoaraiosis and metabolic syndrome in healthy subjects. Neurology. 2007;69(10):974–8.
101. Razay G, Vreugdenhil A, Wilcock G. The metabolic syndrome and Alzheimer disease. Arch Neurol. 2007;64(1):93–6.
102. Vanhanen M, Koivisto K, Moilanen L, Helkala EL, Hanninen T, Soininen H, et al. Association of metabolic syndrome with Alzheimer disease: a population-based study. Neurology. 2006;67(5):843–7.
103. van den Berg E, Biessels GJ, de Craen AJ, Gussekloo J, Westendorp RG. The metabolic syndrome is associated with decelerated cognitive decline in the oldest old. Neurology. 2007;69(10):979–85.
104. Buchman AS, Schneider JA, Wilson RS, Bienias JL, Bennett DA. Body mass index in older persons is associated with Alzheimer disease pathology. Neurology. 2006;67(11):1949–54.
105. Cournot M, Marquie JC, Ansiau D, Martinaud C, Fonds H, Ferrieres J, et al. Relation between body mass index and cognitive function in healthy middle-aged men and women. Neurology. 2006;67(7):1208–14.
106. Buchman AS, Wilson RS, Bienias JL, Shah RC, Evans DA, Bennett DA. Change in body mass index and risk of incident Alzheimer disease. Neurology. 2005;65(6):892–7.
107. Jagust W, Harvey D, Mungas D, Haan M. Central obesity and the aging brain. Arch Neurol. 2005;62(10):1545–8.
108. Luchsinger JA, Reitz C, Honig LS, Tang MX, Shea S, Mayeux R. Aggregation of vascular risk factors and risk of incident Alzheimer disease. Neurology. 2005;65(4):545–51.
109. Kivipelto M, Ngandu T, Fratiglioni L, Viitanen M, Kareholt I, Winblad B, et al. Obesity and vascular risk factors at midlife and the risk of dementia and Alzheimer disease. Arch Neurol. 2005;62(10):1556–60.
110. Tiehuis AM, van der Graaf Y, Visseren FL, Vincken KL, Biessels GJ, Appelman AP, et al. Diabetes increases atrophy and vascular lesions on brain MRI in patients with symptomatic arterial disease. Stroke. 2008;39(5):1600–3.
111. Whitmer RA, Gustafson DR, Barrett-Connor E, Haan MN, Gunderson EP, Yaffe K. Central obesity and increased risk of dementia more than three decades later. Neurology. 2008;71(14):1057–64.

112. Gazdzinski S, Kornak J, Weiner MW, Meyerhoff DJ. Body mass index and magnetic reso-nance markers of brain integrity in adults. Ann Neurol. 2008;63(5):652–7.
113. Benarroch EE. Brain cholesterol metabolism and neurologic disease. Neurology. 2008;71(17):1368–73.
114. Wolozin B, Kellman W, Ruosseau P, Celesia GG, Siegel G. Decreased prevalence of Alzheimer disease associated with 3-hydroxy-3-methyglutaryl coenzyme A reductase inhibi-tors. Arch Neurol. 2000;57(10):1439–43.
115. Li G, Shofer JB, Kukull WA, Peskind ER, Tsuang DW, Breitner JC, et al. Serum cholesterol and risk of Alzheimer disease: a community-based cohort study. Neurology. 2005;65(7):1045–50.
116. Dufouil C, Richard F, Fievet N, Dartigues JF, Ritchie K, Tzourio C, et al. APOE genotype, cholesterol level, lipid-lowering treatment, and dementia: the Three-City Study. Neurology. 2005;64(9):1531–8.
117. Reitz C, Luchsinger J, Tang MX, Manly J, Mayeux R. Impact of plasma lipids and time on memory performance in healthy elderly without dementia. Neurology. 2005;64(8):1378–83.
118. Evans RM, Hui S, Perkins A, Lahiri DK, Poirier J, Farlow MR. Cholesterol and APOE geno-type interact to influence Alzheimer disease progression. Neurology. 2004;62(10):1869–71.
119. Rea TD, Breitner JC, Psaty BM, Fitzpatrick AL, Lopez OL, Newman AB, et al. Statin use and the risk of incident dementia: the Cardiovascular Health Study. Arch Neurol. 2005;62(7):1047–51.
120. Bernick C, Katz R, Smith NL, Rapp S, Bhadelia R, Carlson M, et al. Statins and cognitive function in the elderly: the Cardiovascular Health Study. Neurology. 2005;65(9):1388–94.
121. Hall K, Murrell J, Ogunniyi A, Deeg M, Baiyewu O, Gao S, et al. Cholesterol, APOE geno-type, and Alzheimer disease: an epidemiologic study of Nigerian Yoruba. Neurology. 2006;66(2):223–7.
122. Stewart R, White LR, Xue QL, Launer LJ. Twenty-six-year change in total cholesterol levels and incident dementia: the Honolulu-Asia Aging Study. Arch Neurol. 2007;64(1):103–7.
123. Solomon A, Kareholt I, Ngandu T, Winblad B, Nissinen A, Tuomilehto J, et al. Serum cho-lesterol changes after midlife and late-life cognition: twenty-one-year follow-up study. Neurology. 2007;68(10):751–6.
124. Sparks DL, Sabbagh MN, Connor DJ, Lopez J, Launer LJ, Browne P, et al. Atorvastatin for the treatment of mild to moderate Alzheimer disease: preliminary results. Arch Neurol. 2005;62(5):753–7.
125. Jones RW, Kivipelto M, Feldman H, Sparks L, Doody R, Waters DD, et al. The Atorvastatin/Donepezil in Alzheimer's Disease Study (LEADe): design and baseline characteristics. Alzheimers Dement. 2008;4(2):145–53.
126. Markesbery WR. The role of oxidative stress in Alzheimer disease. Arch Neurol. 1999;56(12):1449–52.
127. Luchsinger JA, Tang MX, Shea S, Mayeux R. Caloric intake and the risk of Alzheimer dis-ease. Arch Neurol. 2002;59(8):1258–63.
128. Kalmijn S, van Boxtel MP, Ocke M, Verschuren WM, Kromhout D, Launer LJ. Dietary intake of fatty acids and fish in relation to cognitive performance at middle age. Neurology. 2004;62(2):275–80.
129. Morris MC, Evans DA, Bienias JL, Tangney CC, Bennett DA, Aggarwal N, et al. Dietary fats and the risk of incident Alzheimer disease. Arch Neurol. 2003;60(2):194–200.
130. Morris MC, Evans DA, Bienias JL, Tangney CC, Bennett DA, Wilson RS, et al. Consumption of fish and n-3 fatty acids and risk of incident Alzheimer disease. Arch Neurol. 2003;60(7):940–6.
131. Huang TL, Zandi PP, Tucker KL, Fitzpatrick AL, Kuller LH, Fried LP, et al. Benefits of fatty fish on dementia risk are stronger for those without APOE epsilon4. Neurology. 2005;65(9):1409–14.
132. Scarmeas N, Luchsinger JA, Mayeux R, Stern Y. Mediterranean diet and Alzheimer disease mortality. Neurology. 2007;69(11):1084–93.

133. Schaefer EJ, Bongard V, Beiser AS, Lamon-Fava S, Robins SJ, Au R, et al. Plasma phosphatidylcholine docosahexaenoic acid content and risk of dementia and Alzheimer disease: the Framingham Heart Study. Arch Neurol. 2006;63(11):1545–50.
134. Luchsinger JA, Tang MX, Miller J, Green R, Mayeux R. Relation of higher folate intake to lower risk of Alzheimer disease in the elderly. Arch Neurol. 2007;64(1):86–92.
135. Morris MC, Evans DA, Bienias JL, Tangney CC, Wilson RS. Dietary fat intake and 6-year cognitive change in an older biracial community population. Neurology. 2004;62(9):1573–9.
136. Morris MC, Evans DA, Bienias JL, Tangney CC, Wilson RS. Vitamin E and cognitive decline in older persons. Arch Neurol. 2002;59(7):1125–32.
137. Morris MC, Evans DA, Tangney CC, Bienias JL, Wilson RS. Fish consumption and cognitive decline with age in a large community study. Arch Neurol. 2005;62(12):1849–53.
138. Kang JH, Ascherio A, Grodstein F. Fruit and vegetable consumption and cognitive decline in aging women. Ann Neurol. 2005;57(5):713–20.
139. Morris MC, Evans DA, Tangney CC, Bienias JL, Wilson RS. Associations of vegetable and fruit consumption with age-related cognitive change. Neurology. 2006;67(8):1370–6.
140. Morris MC, Evans DA, Bienias JL, Tangney CC, Hebert LE, Scherr PA, et al. Dietary folate and vitamin B12 intake and cognitive decline among community-dwelling older persons. Arch Neurol. 2005;62(4):641–5.
141. Morris MC, Evans DA, Tangney CC, Bienias JL, Schneider JA, Wilson RS, et al. Dietary copper and high saturated and trans fat intakes associated with cognitive decline. Arch Neurol. 2006;63(8):1085–8.
142. Engelhart MJ, Geerlings MI, Ruitenberg A, Van Swieten JC, Hofman A, Witteman JC, et al. Diet and risk of dementia: Does fat matter?: The Rotterdam Study. Neurology. 2002;59(12):1915–21.
143. Luchsinger JA, Tang MX, Shea S, Mayeux R. Antioxidant vitamin intake and risk of Alzheimer disease. Arch Neurol. 2003;60(2):203–8.
144. Yaffe K, Clemons TE, McBee WL, Lindblad AS. Age-Related Eye Disease Study Research Group. Impact of antioxidants, zinc, and copper on cognition in the elderly: a randomized, controlled trial. Neurology. 2004;63(9):1705–7.
145. Dunn JE, Weintraub S, Stoddard AM, Banks S. Serum alpha-tocopherol, concurrent and past vitamin E intake, and mild cognitive impairment. Neurology. 2007;68(9):670–6.
146. Freund-Levi Y, Eriksdotter-Jonhagen M, Cederholm T, Basun H, Faxen-Irving G, Garlind A, et al. Omega-3 fatty acid treatment in 174 patients with mild to moderate Alzheimer disease: OmegAD study: a randomized double-blind trial. Arch Neurol. 2006;63(10):1402–8.
147. Tangney CC, Li H, Wang Y, Barnes L, Schneider JA, Bennett DA, et al. Relation of DASH- and Mediterranean-like dietary patterns to cognitive decline in older persons. Neurology. 2014;83(16):1410–6.
148. Feart C, Samieri C, Rondeau V, Amieva H, Portet F, Dartigues JF, et al. Adherence to a Mediterranean diet, cognitive decline, and risk of dementia. JAMA. 2009;302(6):638–48.
149. Scarmeas N, Luchsinger JA, Schupf N, Brickman AM, Cosentino S, Tang MX, et al. Physical activity, diet, and risk of Alzheimer disease. JAMA. 2009;302(6):627–37.
150. van de Rest O, Geleijnse JM, Kok FJ, van Staveren WA, Dullemeijer C, Olderikkert MG, et al. Effect of fish oil on cognitive performance in older subjects: a randomized, controlled trial. Neurology. 2008;71(6):430–8.
151. Zandi PP, Carlson MC, Plassman BL, Welsh-Bohmer KA, Mayer LS, Steffens DC, et al. Hormone replacement therapy and incidence of Alzheimer disease in older women: the Cache County Study. JAMA. 2002;288(17):2123–9.
152. Col NF, Pauker SG. The discrepancy between observational studies and randomized trials of menopausal hormone therapy: did expectations shape experience? Ann Intern Med. 2003;139(11):923–9.
153. Shumaker SA, Legault C, Kuller L, Rapp SR, Thal L, Lane DS, et al. Conjugated equine estrogens and incidence of probable dementia and mild cognitive impairment in postmenopausal women: Women's Health Initiative Memory Study. JAMA. 2004;291(24):2947–58.

154. Espeland MA, Rapp SR, Shumaker SA, Brunner R, Manson JE, Sherwin BB, et al. Conjugated equine estrogens and global cognitive function in postmenopausal women: Women's Health Initiative Memory Study. JAMA. 2004;291(24):2959–68.
155. Espeland MA, Shumaker SA, Leng I, Manson JE, Brown CM, LeBlanc ES, et al. Long-term effects on cognitive function of postmenopausal hormone therapy prescribed to women aged 50 to 55 years. JAMA Intern Med. 2013;173(15):1429–36.
156. Mulnard RA, Cotman CW, Kawas C, van Dyck CH, Sano M, Doody R, et al. Estrogen replacement therapy for treatment of mild to moderate Alzheimer disease: a randomized controlled trial. Alzheimer's Disease Cooperative Study. JAMA. 2000;283(8):1007–15.
157. North American Menopause Society. The 2012 hormone therapy position statement of: The North American Menopause Society. Menopause. 2012;19(3):257–71.
158. Cherrier MM, Matsumoto AM, Amory JK, Asthana S, Bremner W, Peskind ER, et al. Testosterone improves spatial memory in men with Alzheimer disease and mild cognitive impairment. Neurology. 2005;64(12):2063–8.
159. Emmelot-Vonk MH, Verhaar HJ, Nakhai Pour HR, Aleman A, Lock TM, Bosch JL, et al. Effect of testosterone supplementation on functional mobility, cognition, and other parameters in older men: a randomized controlled trial. JAMA. 2008;299(1):39–52.
160. Floel A, Witte AV, Lohmann H, Wersching H, Ringelstein EB, Berger K, et al. Lifestyle and memory in the elderly. Neuroepidemiology. 2008;31(1):39–47.
161. Burns JM, Cronk BB, Anderson HS, Donnelly JE, Thomas GP, Harsha A, et al. Cardiorespiratory fitness and brain atrophy in early Alzheimer disease. Neurology. 2008;71(3):210–6.
162. Heyn P, Abreu BC, Ottenbacher KJ. The effects of exercise training on elderly persons with cognitive impairment and dementia: a meta-analysis. Arch Phys Med Rehabil. 2004;85(10): 1694–704.
163. Weuve J, Kang JH, Manson JE, Breteler MM, Ware JH, Grodstein F. Physical activity, including walking, and cognitive function in older women. JAMA. 2004;292(12):1454–61.
164. Abbott RD, White LR, Ross GW, Masaki KH, Curb JD, Petrovitch H. Walking and dementia in physically capable elderly men. JAMA. 2004;292(12):1447–53.
165. Larson EB, Wang L, Bowen JD, McCormick WC, Teri L, Crane P, et al. Exercise is associated with reduced risk for incident dementia among persons 65 years of age and older. Ann Intern Med. 2006;144(2):73–81.
166. Lautenschlager NT, Cox KL, Flicker L, Foster JK, van Bockxmeer FM, Xiao J, et al. Effect of physical activity on cognitive function in older adults at risk for Alzheimer disease: a randomized trial. JAMA. 2008;300(9):1027–37.
167. Liang KY, Mintun MA, Fagan AM, Goate AM, Bugg JM, Holtzman DM, et al. Exercise and Alzheimer's disease biomarkers in cognitively normal older adults. Ann Neurol. 2010; 68(3):311–8.
168. Larson EB. Physical activity for older adults at risk for Alzheimer disease. JAMA. 2008;300(9):1077–9.
169. Angevaren M, Aufdemkampe G, Verhaar HJ, Aleman A, Vanhees L. Physical activity and enhanced fitness to improve cognitive function in older people without known cognitive impairment. Cochrane Database Syst Rev. 2008; 3:CD005381.
170. Paul CA, Au R, Fredman L, Massaro JM, Seshadri S, Decarli C, et al. Association of alcohol consumption with brain volume in the Framingham study. Arch Neurol. 2008;65(10): 1363–7.
171. Almeida OP, Hulse GK, Lawrence D, Flicker L. Smoking as a risk factor for Alzheimer's disease: contrasting evidence from a systematic review of case-control and cohort studies. Addiction. 2002;97(1):15–28.
172. Hernan MA, Alonso A, Logroscino G. Cigarette smoking and dementia: potential selection bias in the elderly. Epidemiology. 2008;19(3):448–50.

173. Anstey KJ, von Sanden C, Salim A, O'Kearney R. Smoking as a risk factor for dementia and cognitive decline: a meta-analysis of prospective studies. Am J Epidemiol. 2007;166(4): 367–78.
174. Alonso A, Jacobs Jr DR, Menotti A, Nissinen A, Dontas A, Kafatos A, et al. Cardiovascular risk factors and dementia mortality: 40 years of follow-up in the Seven Countries Study. J Neurol Sci. 2009;280(1-2):79–83.
175. ADAPT Research Group, Martin BK, Szekely C, Brandt J, Piantadosi S, Breitner JC, et al. Cognitive function over time in the Alzheimer's Disease Anti-inflammatory Prevention Trial (ADAPT): results of a randomized, controlled trial of naproxen and celecoxib. Arch Neurol. 2008;65(7):896–905.
176. Etminan M, Gill S, Samii A. Effect of non-steroidal anti-inflammatory drugs on risk of Alzheimer's disease: systematic review and meta-analysis of observational studies. BMJ. 2003;327(7407):128.
177. Szekely CA, Thorne JE, Zandi PP, Ek M, Messias E, Breitner JC, et al. Nonsteroidal anti-inflammatory drugs for the prevention of Alzheimer's disease: a systematic review. Neuroepidemiology. 2004;23(4):159–69.
178. Aisen PS, Schafer KA, Grundman M, Pfeiffer E, Sano M, Davis KL, et al. Effects of rofecoxib or naproxen vs placebo on Alzheimer disease progression: a randomized controlled trial. JAMA. 2003;289(21):2819–26.
179. Jaturapatporn D, Isaac MG, McCleery J, Tabet N. Aspirin, steroidal and non-steroidal anti-inflammatory drugs for the treatment of Alzheimer's disease. Cochrane Database Syst Rev. 2012;2, CD006378.
180. Yaffe K, Lindquist K, Shlipak MG, Simonsick E, Fried L, Rosano C, et al. Cystatin C as a marker of cognitive function in elders: findings from the health ABC study. Ann Neurol. 2008;63(6):798–802.
181. Vannorsdall TD, Jinnah HA, Gordon B, Kraut M, Schretlen DJ. Cerebral ischemia mediates the effect of serum uric acid on cognitive function. Stroke. 2008;39(12):3418–20.
182. Gorelick PB. Cerebral microbleeds: evidence of heightened risk associated with aspirin use. Arch Neurol. 2009;66(6):691–3.
183. Kester MI, Goos JD, Teunissen CE, Benedictus MR, Bouwman FH, Wattjes MP, et al. Associations between cerebral small-vessel disease and Alzheimer disease pathology as measured by cerebrospinal fluid biomarkers. JAMA Neurol. 2014;71(7):855–62.
184. Poels MM, Ikram MA, van der Lugt A, Hofman A, Niessen WJ, Krestin GP, et al. Cerebral microbleeds are associated with worse cognitive function: the Rotterdam Scan Study. Neurology. 2012;78(5):326–33.
185. Hilal S, Saini M, Tan CS, Catindig JA, Koay WI, Niessen WJ, et al. Cerebral microbleeds and cognition: the epidemiology of dementia in Singapore study. Alzheimer Dis Assoc Disord. 2014;28(2):106–12.
186. Muqtadar H, Testai FD, Gorelick PB. The dementia of cardiac disease. Curr Cardiol Rep. 2012;14(6):732–40.
187. Casserly IP, Topol EJ. Convergence of atherosclerosis and Alzheimer's disease: Cholesterol, inflammation, and misfolded proteins. Discov Med. 2004;4(22):149–56.
188. Gorelick PB, Scuteri A, Black SE, Decarli C, Greenberg SM, Iadecola C, et al. Vascular contributions to cognitive impairment and dementia: a statement for healthcare professionals from the American Heart Association/American Stroke Association. Stroke. 2011;42(9):2672–713.
189. Vagnucci Jr AH, Li WW. Alzheimer's disease and angiogenesis. Lancet. 2003; 361(9357):605–8.
190. Birns J, Kalra L. Cognitive function and hypertension. J Hum Hypertens. 2009;23(2): 86–96.
191. Morris MC, Tangney CC, Wang Y, Sacks FM, Bennett DA, Aggarwal NT. MIND diet associated with reduced incidence of Alzheimer's disease. Alzheimers Dement. 2015;11(9): 1007–14.

Chapter 16
Hypertension, Cerebral Small Vessel Disease, and Cognitive Function

David L. Nyenhuis

Vascular Cognitive Impairment (VCI) is caused by a heterogeneous group of neurovascular pathologies, including large vessel ischemic infarction, hemorrhage, and the combination of cerebrovascular and Alzheimer's pathology [1]. However, VCI is primarily associated with subcortical gray and white matter pathology arising from small vessel disease. Hypertension is a major factor in the development of small vessel disease. This chapter will focus on linkages between hypertension, small vessel disease, cognitive decline, and dementia.

Pathophysiology of Small Vessel Disease

Small vessel disease is not a unitary entity. It is associated with both focal lacunar infarction in subcortical regions of gray and white matter and more diffuse, less well-defined white matter pathology. The "small vessels" consist of intracerebral end-arteries and arterioles, most often located in border zone areas that are vulnerable to ischemic changes associated with aging [2, 3] and exacerbated by chronic hypertension [4]. These changes include microvascular fibrosis and basement membrane thickening, which in turn lead to a narrowing of the arteriole lumen [5].

Lacunar infarctions are most often found in basal ganglia structures, in periventricular white matter, and in other subcortical gray matter structures, such as the thalamus [6]. The advent of modern neuroimaging techniques such as MRI has resulted in a proliferation of studies examining the presence, severity, and effects of white matter hyperintensities (WMH) and its underlying pathologic substrate.

D.L. Nyenhuis, Ph.D. (✉)
Hauenstein Neuroscience Center, Mercy Health Saint Mary's Health Care,
245 Cherry St. SE, Suite 104, Grand Rapids, MI 49503, USA
e-mail: nyenhuda@mercyhealth.com

© Springer International Publishing Switzerland 2016
V. Aiyagari, P.B. Gorelick (eds.), *Hypertension and Stroke*, Clinical
Hypertension and Vascular Diseases, DOI 10.1007/978-3-319-29152-9_16

The underlying white matter lesions (WML) that show as WMH on MRI are thought to consist of the combination of demyelination, lacunar infarction, and axonal loss [7]. The histopathology of WML includes diffuse pallor of the white matter and rarefaction of the myelin sheaths. This demyelination tends to spare subcortical U-fibers [8]. Reactive gliosis consistent with ischemic injury and cell death is also seen [9]. The total volume of WMH is inversely related to brain volume, as measured by brain parenchymal fraction (BPF). This supports the hypothesis that axonal loss and cell death are associated with WMH. Vascular abnormalities such as microangiopathy of penetrating vessels, tortuosity of hyalinized vessels, and more focal fibrinous necrosis accompany white matter lesions [8].

Hypertension and Small Vessel Disease

The relationship between hypertension and small vessel disease is complex, involving an interaction between extensive cardiovascular/cerebrovascular autonomic systems. While this relationship is covered more extensively in other chapters in this text, in the simplest forms, hypertension induces vascular hypertrophy, which in turn leads to increased vascular resistance [4]. After an acute rise in pressure, stretch receptors in arterial walls feed back to "reset" the system, thereby attempting to lower blood pressure. Small vessel disease is thought to occur because of cerebral arteriosclerosis of the penetrating vessels or episodic hypoperfusion secondary to hypertension [6]. Some have suggested that venular-based ischemia also has a role in small vessel disease [5]. Similar to a fluid-filled balloon which is squeezed on one end causing a displacement of fluid toward the distal zone, when pressure is released, that same distal area of previously high volume experiences a dramatic drop in volume. In older adults whose arteries may be less elastic and "brittle," such dramatic shifts require more time for recovery, leaving areas transiently under-perfused. Likewise, in the cerebrovascular system, given their size and location, smaller diameter vascular distributions or border zone areas appear most vulnerable to ischemic changes associated with hypertension. Periventricular white matter regions are also particularly vulnerable to hypoxic injury following sudden changes in blood pressure as these areas are perfused by long and small diameter medullary arteries.

White Matter Hyperintensities and Cognition

WMH are commonly viewed in T2-weighted MRI images of the elderly; 92 % of the community sample enrolled in the Rotterdam Scan Study [10] and 95 % of the Cardiovascular Health Study sample [11] showed at least a mild degree of WMH. However, WMH may not be associated with cognitive decline in everyone, and many consider these changes to be relatively benign. Questions arise to how or to what degree white matter pathology affects cognition. The presence of WMH has been associated with cognitive impairment and dementia [12, 13]. While severity of the disease burden inversely relates to cognitive performance, the relationship of reduced cognitive performance can be observed even when burden is relatively small [14]. The Cardiovascular Health Study reported on 3301 community elderly with no history of stroke or transient ischemic attack who underwent MRI and two measures of cognitive function. Using templates, radiologists graded WMH on a scale from 0 (none) to 9. Higher grades were associated with older age, silent stroke on MRI, and higher systolic blood pressure (SBP). The grade of WMH was also found to correlate with cognitive impairment; the higher the grade, the greater the likelihood of cognitive dysfunction [11]. The investigators concluded that asymptomatic white matter findings might not be clinically insignificant or benign. In a separate study, Gouw et al. [15] examined the relationship between cognition and WMH in 639 non-demented elderly subjects 65–84 years of age. The volume of WMH correlated with decreased performance on the Mini-mental State Examination (MMSE), a widely used cognitive screening test that has been criticized for its failure to assess executive functioning (i.e., initiation, planning, higher-order problem-solving behaviors) or processing speed domains. That the correlation was found despite the relative insensitivity of the outcome measure supports a robust relationship between volume of WMH and cognition.

Pattern of Cognitive Dysfunction in Patients with White Matter Hyperintensities

Compared to Alzheimer's disease, which presents with prominent impairments in episodic memory, the heterogeneous nature of VCI makes it more difficult to characterize a prototypic cognitive presentation. Often, executive function is labeled as a core VCI deficit. Executive function is the term used to describe an array of cognitive functions believed dependent on frontal lobe and related subcortical function. Behaviors such as nonverbal reasoning, planning, initiation, problem-solving, working memory, and higher-order aspects of attention fall under the "executive" rubric. These behaviors are assumed to be supported by many distributed and parallel neural networks and various "executive functions" can be disrupted, dependent on the extent and nature of the network disruption. Several studies have suggested a pattern of deficits in VCI marked by executive dysfunction, slowed information processing, inconsistent new learning and memory, bradykinesia, and disturbances in affect or emotional regulation [16, 17]. This pattern is linked with the presence and severity of WMH in patients with and without other subtypes of VCI-related pathology, such as large artery infarction [16]. However, the presence of executive dysfunction *in vivo* may not be strongly predictive of the presence of underlying cerebrovascular pathology assessed at autopsy [18], and persons with cerebrovascular disease show a more diverse set of cognitive deficits than persons with probable Alzheimer's disease [17]. This raises questions of the specificity of executive dysfunction to VCI, especially in patients with mixed cerebrovascular and Alzheimer's pathology.

Location of White Matter Hyperintensities and Cognition

The location of white matter changes appears to have a differential effect on cognitive functioning. WML in periventricular regions may disrupt bundles of cholinergic fibers resulting in cholinergic denervation [19], which could contribute to the development of cognitive decline and executive dysfunction. In a study examining the role of WMH and executive function, Oosterman et al. [20] examined the performance of 151 subjects with WMH on several tasks of executive functioning. The authors found significant correlations with WMH and performance on tasks of inhibition, planning, and working memory. Of interest, periventricular WMH correlated with inhibition and working memory, while diffuse WMH correlated with planning ability.

The Rotterdam Scan Study was a prospective population-based cohort study examining age-related changes to the brains of cognitively intact elderly people across seven years. Using 1077 participants from this study cohort, Prins et al. [21] determined that over the course of the study, more severe periventricular WML, but not subcortical WML, increased the risk of dementia. The association between periventricular WML and dementia was independent of the presence of cerebral infarcts, incident stroke, or generalized brain atrophy. De Groot et al. [13] reported similar findings.

Debette et al. [22] examined the relationship between subcortical and periventricular WMH on MMSE and Dementia Rating Scale performance over two assessments (mean duration three years) in 170 patients with mild cognitive impairment (MCI). Relative to patients whose cognitive scores did not change or improved over the assessments, individuals who demonstrated cognitive decline had a higher number of periventricular and subcortical white matter hyperintensities at baseline. The rate of global cognitive decline was also associated with a higher number and an increase in the amount of white matter abnormalities. This was especially apparent when comparing periventricular hyperintensities and decline in the executive function domain. Another study by Bombois et al. [23] reported that presence of subcortical hyperintensities was also associated with executive dysfunction, regardless of MCI subtype.

Prins et al. [24] examined 1440 non-demented subjects from the original Rotterdam Scan Study on imaging and neuropsychological variables at three time intervals. The authors evaluated the relationship between cerebral small vessel disease and rate of decline in select domains of cognitive function. They found that periventricular lesions, infarcts, and generalized atrophy correlated with the rate of decline in global cognitive function. Increasing severity of periventricular and subcortical white matter lesions was associated with steeper declines on tasks of information processing speed while subcortical lesions alone were significantly associated with declines on a task of executive function (i.e., verbal fluency). It could be that damage to the long association efferent fibers in the periventricular regions has relative importance in impacting connectivity and thus cognitive function. The presence of periventricular lesions may signal the loss of functional integrity in frontal-subcortical systems. Indeed, the periventricular region has a high number of long association fibers which connect subcortical to cortical regions. While some have questioned whether the periventricular and deep subcortical WMH arise from similar processes [25], others have noted more severe and varied cognitive deficits associated with deep versus periventricular WMH [26]. It is therefore not yet clear whether cognitive differences are due to location or the severity of white matter pathology.

Volume of White Matter Hyperintensities and Cognition

Questions remain whether a critical volume of WMH must be reached before there is a disruption in cognitive function. Visual rating scales have historically been employed to estimate the amount of WMH volume [11]. Using these methods, higher graded WMH severity has negatively correlated with cognitive performance. Studies which have utilized computerized quantification show similar inverse relationships between WMH volume and cognitive performance, particularly in the domains of visual scanning and motor speed [27], visuospatial memory [27], verbal recognition memory [28], working memory [28], and new learning [27]. Wright et al [29] examined 656 subjects from the Northern Manhattan Study (NOMAS); they calculated WMH volume using semi-automated MRI methods. Examining WMH volume both as a continuous variable and by quartiles, the authors found that WMH volume was inversely related to cognitive performance on tasks of sensorimotor ability, cognitive flexibility, and mental sequencing. Further, they determined that having WMH volume of 0.75 % of cranial volume or greater was associated with poorer cognitive performance, which the authors concluded provides evidence of a threshold effect.

Lacunar Infarction and Cognition

Based on extensive functional neuroanatomic connectivity, subcortical structures interact with frontal regions in a distributed neural network. The smaller penetrating arteries such as the anterior and posterior choroidal, lenticulostriate, Heubner's, and tuberothalamic arteries that perfuse subcortical gray matter and white matter are especially vulnerable to occlusive change and subsequent brain ischemia following increases in blood pressure. Given that these structures receive their blood supply through deep penetrating arteries, subcortical structures such as the thalamus and basal ganglia are vulnerable to vascular injury secondary to hypertension. Indeed, studies have shown abnormal blood flow in basal ganglia and related frontal regions (e.g., anterior cingulate) in patients with high blood pressure who did not otherwise demonstrate cognitive impairment or other signs of cerebrovascular disease [30].

Five frontal-subcortical loops have been identified [31], three of which have direct relevance to cognitive function. A disconnection hypothesis offers that lesions at various points within these parallel networks can result in three somewhat distinct neurobehavioral syndromes. Damage to the dorsolateral prefrontal circuit results in a dysexecutive syndrome. A compromised orbitofrontal circuit results in social disinhibition. Disruption in the anterior cingulate medial frontal circuit manifests in marked apathy. Given the role of subcortical nuclei in integrating information and modulating output, a strategic lacunar infarct may result in a more pronounced frontal-subcortical behavioral syndrome, but general compromise of white matter pathways could also serve to disrupt the functioning of one or all three of these pathways.

Basal Ganglia, Thalamus, and Cognition

Stroke confined to the basal ganglia impacts cognitive function in almost all domains assessed [32]. Basal ganglia nuclei have been extensively studied in their role in movement. Lesions of basal ganglia nuclei result in alterations in muscle tone, abnormal movements, ideomotor apraxia, reduced spontaneous movement, and slowing of movements. A line of research has focused on the role of the basal ganglia in larger neural networks including those involving cognition, emotion, and behavior. These studies have implicated the basal ganglia in mood regulation, goal-directed behavior, and higher-order cognitive function [33–35]. The basal ganglia also have a relationship with core limbic structures including the hippocampus and amygdala that are critical to drive-related behaviors associated with reward and reinforcement. The extent of direct and reciprocal connections suggests that the basal ganglia facilitate the integration of complex affective, social, and cognitive processes, and thereby influence the affective or motivational salience of the input reaching the prefrontal systems [31, 36–38]. The basal ganglia appear key to many cognitive functions including implicit or procedural memory, motor learning, sequencing, stimulus-response based learning, and attention [35, 39], and contribute to higher-order cognitive function, including working memory [40–42], response inhibition, response generation, and cognitive flexibility [39, 43].

The thalamus comprises many functionally distinct nuclei involved in parallel and reciprocal cortical-subcortical neural loops. The thalamus exists as an important relay station with rich connections to the basal ganglia and frontal lobes. Individual thalamic nuclei are involved in many cognitive functions including language, memory, response inhibition, working memory, and attention [44–46].

The thalamus receives its blood supply from several vessels. Specific nuclei and various neurobehavioral syndromes are observed following strategic infarcts confined to these vessels. The paramedian thalamic artery arises from the basilar artery and supplies bilateral anteromedial regions involved in memory systems, specifically the mediodorsal nucleus of the thalamus. Bilateral infarction of the distribution of the paramedian thalamic artery not surprisingly is associated with a dementia syndrome [47] and may also present with personality changes including apathy, disinhibition, and psychosis [48]. As the principle target of output for basal ganglia and thalamus is the frontal lobes, localized lesions in these regions result in widespread disruption of frontal-striatal circuits. Carrera et al. [49] examined 71 patients with MRI and document stroke confined to four "classic" thalamic territories. They compared each on tests of cognition, and found that patients with strokes confined to three of the territories (the anterior, paramedian, and inferolateral thalamus) all demonstrated some degree of cognitive impairment, most consistently in areas related to executive functions. Deficits in verbal fluency, initiation, and anterograde memory with better recognition performance were observed in patients with anteromedian territory involvement. As such, the cognitive changes usually observed in patients with subcortical white matter hyperintensities and/or lacunar infarctions resemble a frontal-subcortical disconnection syndrome.

Small Vessel Disease and Mood

While poststroke depression is found after either large vessel stroke or subcortical lacunes [50, 51], the data on the relationship between small vessel disease (SVD) and depression is mixed [52, 53]. There is support for a very modest relationship between SVD and depression. For example, in a group of nondisabled elderly, O'Brien et al. [54] found a weak correlation between the presence of lacunar infarctions and depression symptoms. In this same study, WMH showed a more robust relationship to depressive symptoms than lacunar infarction. It is critical to note that symptoms associated with depression may actually be indicative of other neurobehavioral syndromes, rather than a primary mood disturbance. Turning again to the basal ganglia lesion literature, in individuals with basal ganglia dysfunction, one often observes apathy, loss of motivation and diminished spontaneity, reduced verbal output, paucity of facial expression, diminished motor behavior, and increased response latency [36, 37]. These symptoms are observed in depression, but are not always indicative of a primary depressive episode [55]. Given the psychiatric changes associated with frontal-subcortical disruption, especially the medial frontal system, it may be that individuals who present as depressed actually demonstrate abulia, anhedonia, or other forms of mood dysregulation instead of low mood.

Hypertension and Cognitive Dysfunction

NHANES (2011–2012) [56] reports that hypertension prevalence is 65 % in individuals aged 60 and older. Hypertension and small vessel disease are long established risk factors for stroke and vascular dementia (VaD) [57]. It is also well documented that lowering blood pressure in hypertensive patients decreases the risk of stroke and cerebral white matter disease [6]. It is less clear if lowering blood pressure will have similar protective effects on cognition and the prevention of dementia. The relationship between hypertension and cognition is not likely to be linear. Beyond hypertension-specific variables (i.e., how well hypertension is controlled, duration, systolic blood pressure [SBP]/diastolic blood pressure [DBP] level), other determinants such as age and ApoE4 allele status play a role in the development and extent of subcortical white matter lesions [6] and possibly cognitive decline.

Cross-sectional Studies

Significant research has been dedicated to exploring the relationship between hypertension and cognitive change. The findings are often mixed. The interpretation of study results is complicated by differences across investigations in methodology such as the definition of hypertension, marker of hypertension (e.g., SBP versus DBP), cognitive domains assessed, sample variables (i.e., age, gender, race), treatment with antihypertensives (e.g., yes or no, specific type of medication), and presence of comorbid conditions or other risk factors for cognitive decline. Cross-sectional studies using outcome measures more sensitive to white matter changes (and presumably changes associated with elevated blood pressure) have inconsistently demonstrated a relationship between elevated blood pressure and cognitive decline and dementia [58–63].

Cross-sectional studies have extensively examined the effects of hypertension on domain-specific cognitive measures. Hypertension at an earlier age, of more chronic duration, and more poorly controlled tends to adopt a linear, inverted "U"-shaped [64, 65] or "J"-shaped [66] relationship with cognition. Hypertension has been demonstrated to adversely impact simple attention [67, 68], executive function [66, 68], and psychomotor speed [66, 68–71]. Thus, the cognitive domains impacted (i.e., executive functions, processing speed) are similar to those affected in patients with cerebral white matter disease and VCI. However, other cross-sectional studies with detailed neuropsychological batteries find no relationship between hypertension and cognition [72–74]. Some argue that age-effects contribute to these conflicting findings. Qiu et al. [59], in their review of this literature, hypothesize that a minimum level of blood pressure is necessary to support cognitive functions. Additionally, low blood pressure in the elderly could in itself serve as a marker for cognitive impairment.

Longitudinal Observational Studies

Despite methodological differences, longitudinal studies with detailed neuropsychological protocols consistently demonstrate that midlife hypertension increases the risk for cognitive dysfunction later in life. Birns and Kalra [16] review

22 longitudinal studies, 15 of which include domain-specific cognitive measures. All 22 studies report a relationship with cognitive dysfunction and chronic hypertension (i.e., inverse relationship, J- and U-shaped, quadratic). One study found that individuals who demonstrated a reduction of blood pressure over the course of the study evidenced decreased performance on speeded tasks, but individuals within this blood pressure subgroup tended to be taking medication with possible sedating effects [75]. The specific cognitive domains vulnerable to the effects of chronic hypertension are executive functions [68, 75], attention [76], psychomotor speed [77], and verbal memory [75]. The interpretation of many longitudinal studies is complicated by differing antihypertensive treatments, with potentially differential impact on remediating or preventing cognitive decline.

Using data from the Honolulu Asia Aging Study, Peila et al. [78] examined the cognitive performance of hypertensive middle-aged cognitively intact men at three time periods over a total of 12 years. The authors found that normotensive adults and persons being treated with antihypertensives showed less cognitive decline compared to persons who were never treated for hypertension. Moreover, for each year of treatment with antihypertensives, there was a reduction in the risk of incident dementia. Murray et al. [79] conducted a longitudinal analysis of the effects of antihypertensive medications on cognition in 1617 cognitively intact African-American participants over three time periods: baseline, 2 years, and 5 years. They found that antihypertensive medication reduced the odds of demonstrating cognitive impairment by 38 % compared to individuals who did not use medication. In participants with uncontrolled hypertension who did not use medication, incident cognitive impairment was 6 % higher compared to participants with controlled blood pressure who were continuously taking medication.

Randomized Placebo-Controlled Clinical Trials

Lowering blood pressure has been demonstrated to reduce stroke risk. It is less clear if lowering blood pressure can reduce white matter disease burden or alter the trajectory of cognition over time. Birns and Kalra [16] detail eight clinical trials that focus on the effects of antihypertensives on cognition. The findings across trials are mixed. It would appear that lowering blood pressure with various therapeutic agents does not impair cognition, but there is only inconsistent evidence that reducing blood pressure improves cognition or prevents dementia [80, 81]. Table 16.1 summarizes these findings. Studies which do support a positive association with antihypertensive treatment and cognition suggest that the effect may depend on the type of antihypertensive drug used (e.g., calcium channel blocker, diuretic, angiotensin receptor antagonist) and the benefits appear to affect global functioning as measured by the MMSE versus individual cognitive domains [82–84]. In studies with more rigorous cognitive outcome measures, it appears that ACE inhibitors and calcium channel blockers may be associated with fewer deleterious effects on cognitive function [85] than other medications such as thiazide, which may have sedating effects [86, 87].

Table 16.1 Studies examining effects of antihypertensives on cognitive outcome

Type of agent	Impact on cognitive outcome variable			Domain specific
	Positive impact	Negative impact	No significant impact on cognitive function	
ACE inhibitor	82		86	
Alpha agonist hypotensive		85		Increased processing speed/ reaction time on vigilance task (i.e., sedating)
Alpha blocker			87	
Angiotensin receptor blocker			83	
Beta blocker			80, 81, 86, 87	
Calcium channel blocker	84, 85			Increased vigilance/attention (i.e., alerting), 85
Thiazide diuretic	84	86, 87	80, 81	

In a study of 2902 non-demented patients randomized to antihypertensive treatment with nitrendipine with possible additional enalapril maltese and hydrochlorothiazide versus no medication, Forette et al. [88] in the extended follow-up of the Systolic Hypertension in Europe (Syst-Eur) trial found that the incidence of dementia was reduced by 55 % in the treatment group. While the authors originally hypothesized that antihypertensives would reduce the risk of VaD, the follow-up study found that the incidence of dementia was reduced for all dementia subtypes, predominantly Alzheimer's disease (AD). The authors speculate that the protective benefits of calcium channel blockers may be in areas of shared pathology in AD, VaD, and mixed AD + cerebrovascular disease presentations.

A secondary analysis of the Perindopril Protection Against Recurrent Stroke Study (PROGRESS) study examined if lowering blood pressure would reduce the risk of dementia and cognitive decline among individuals with cerebrovascular disease [82]. The study included 6105 participants with a history of TIA or ischemic stroke in a randomized double-blind, placebo-controlled study. Cognitive decline was assessed at baseline, 6 months, 12 months, and annually using the MMSE, with decline being a reduction of three or more points between two visits. Active treatment reduced the risk of "cognitive decline with recurrent stroke" by 19 % and a risk reduction of 31 % for developing dementia in participants with no cognitive impairment at the baseline assessment. However, active treatment did not appear to impact participants classified as cognitively impaired at the outset of the study. The authors concluded that the benefits of treatment are primarily the consequence of stroke prevention rather than a direct effect on dementia or cognitive decline. A follow-up substudy comprising 192 individuals who had a baseline and follow-up (mean duration 36 months) MRI, supported this conclusion as the risk of developing new WMH was reduced by 43 % in the active treatment group [89].

Skoog et al. [12] in the Study on Cognition and Prognosis in the Elderly (SCOPE) examined the effects of antihypertensives on cognition as measured by MMSE in a randomized placebo-controlled study of 4937 patients aged 70–89 years with mild to moderate hypertension followed over the course of three to five years. This study compared subjects with slightly lower baseline MMSE scores to those with higher scores. Despite a reduction in blood pressure, individuals with lower cognitive functioning scores at baseline were at a higher risk of significant cognitive decline and dementia.

In the Systolic Hypertension in the Elderly Program (SHEP) trial (1985–1990), the original findings did not show any antihypertensive benefit on cognitive function. The original study compared the incidence of cognitive decline between participants receiving low-dose diuretic and/or β (beta) blocker and those who received a placebo. Di Bari et al. [90] reexamined the findings after considering the rates of differential dropout in the groups. In the original SHEP trial, 4736 participants with isolated systolic hypertension were randomized to active treatment or placebo and followed over 5 years. All participants were administered the short-Comprehensive Assessment and Referral Evaluation and a dementia score was determined based on performance on the cognitive component score and on subjects' reported basic activities of daily living. When the authors examined the dropout rates, they determined that individuals with a high number of nonfatal cardiovascular events were more likely to dropout. The authors concluded that only the healthiest subjects in both groups returned for follow-up cognitive assessment, which may have attenuated the recognition of a benefit of antihypertensives on cognition.

Meta-Analytic Studies

In recent years, a number of investigators have explored relationships between hypertension and cognition using meta-analytic techniques. Birns and colleagues [91] pooled clinical trial data to form a sample of 19,501 subjects. They found that modest reductions in blood pressure were associated with improved MMSE scores, as well as improvements on some measures of memory. However, McGuinness et al [92], in a Cochran review using a similar but not identical data set, found no relationship between lowered blood pressure and either dementia incidence or cognitive decline. Together, these studies highlight both the tenuous relationship between lowered blood pressure and cognitive function within the confines of clinical trials (e.g., relatively brief study period), and the impact of study selection criteria on meta-analytic outcomes.

Two other recent meta-analyses examined relationships between antihypertensive medication use, cognitive decline, and dementia. Chang-Quan et al. [93] calculated pooled relative risk using fixed- and random-effects models with data from 14 longitudinal studies. Pooled study subjects totaled 32,528 who used antihypertensive medication and 36,905 who did not use antihypertensive medication. They found a lower incidence of vascular dementia and all-cause dementia in patients who used antihypertensive medication, but no differences between the two groups in the incidence of Alzheimer's disease or in cognitive decline. Marpillat et al [94] examined the effect of antihypertensive classes on cognitive decline and dementia incidence. They found that antihypertensive use, regardless of class, showed benefit in overall cognitive function, as well as in the specific cognitive areas of attention, memory, visuospatial skills, and executive functions. Moreover, using network meta-analytic techniques, they showed that angiotensin II receptor blockers (ARBs) showed larger overall cognitive effects than β-blockers, diuretics, and angiotensin-converting enzyme inhibitors.

Summary

The relationships between cerebral small vessel disease, hypertension, and cognitive functioning is complex. Evidence to date suggests that WMH on MRI are not "benign" insignificant incidental findings. Just as they serve as markers for cerebrovascular disease and increased risk for stroke, the cumulative impact of WMH and poorly controlled hypertension raise the risk for cognitive deterioration, dementia, and mood and behavior disturbance due to frontal-subcortical disconnection. It is less clear, however, what later-life treatment can be used to preserve cognitive functioning or to prevent cognitive decline or behavioral change. Additional well-designed clinical trials of blood pressure lowering in those at risk of cognitive decline or dementia are needed to guide clinicians in the treatment of these patients.

References

1. Gorelick PB, Scuteri A, Black SE, et al. Vascular contributions to cognitive impairment and dementia: a statement for healthcare professionals from the American Heart Association/American Stroke Association. Stroke. 2011;42:2672–713.
2. Bouras C, Kövari E, Herrmann F, et al. Stereologic analysis of microvascular morphology in the elderly: Alzheimer disease pathology and cognitive status. J Neuropathol Exp Neurol. 2006;65:235–44.
3. Wardlaw J. What causes lacunar stroke? J Neurol Neurosurg Psychiatry. 2005;76:617–9.
4. Palatini P, Julius S. The role of cardiac autonomic function in hypertension and cardiovascular disease. Curr Hypertens Rep. 2009;11:199–205.
5. Black S, Gao F, Bilbao J. Understanding white matter disease: imaging-pathological correlations in vascular cognitive impairment. Stroke. 2009;40(Suppl):S48–52.
6. Pantoni L. Cerebral small vessel disease: from pathogenesis and clinical characteristics to therapeutic challenges. Lancet Neurol. 2010;9:689–70.
7. Englund E. Neuropathology of white matter lesions in vascular cognitive impairment. Cerebrovasc Dis. 2002;2:11–5.
8. Jellinger K. The enigma of vascular cognitive disorder and vascular dementia. Acta Neuropathol. 2007;446:348–88.
9. Chui H. Subcortical ischemic vascular dementia. Neurol Clin. 2007;25:717–40.
10. de Leeuw F, de Groot J, Oudkerk M, et al. Hypertension and cerebral white matter lesions in a prospective cohort study. Brain. 2002;125:765–72.

11. Longstreth W, Manolio T, Arnold A, et al. Clinical correlates of white matter findings on cranial magnetic resonance imaging of 3301 elderly people: the Cardiovascular Health Study. Stroke. 1996;27:1274–82.
12. Skoog I, Lithell H, Hansson L, et al. Effect of baseline cognitive function and antihypertensive treatment on cognitive and cardiovascular outcomes: study on cognition and prognosis in the elderly (SCOPE). Am J Hypertens. 2005;18:1052–9.
13. DeGroot J, de Leeuw F, Oudkerk M, et al. Periventricular cerebral white matter lesions predict rate of cognitive decline. Ann Neurol. 2002;52:335–41.
14. Birns J, Kalra L. Cognitive function and hypertension. J Hum Hypertens. 2009;23:86–96.
15. Gouw A, Van der Flier W, van Straaten E, et al. Simple versus complex assessment of white matter hyperintensities in relation to physical performance and cognition: the LADIS study. J Neurol. 2006;253:1189–96.
16. Nyenhuis D, Gorelick PB, Geenen EJ, et al. The pattern of neuropsychological deficits in Vascular Cognitive Impairment-No Dementia (Vascular CIND). Clin Neuropsychol. 2004;18:41–9.
17. Zhou A, Jia J. Different cognitive profiles between mild cognitive impairment due to cerebral small vessel disease and mild cognitive impairment of Alzheimer's disease origin. J Int Neuropsychol Soc. 2009;15:898–905.
18. Reed B, Mungas DM, Kramer JH, et al. Profiles of neuropsychological impairment in autopsy-defined Alzheimer's disease and cerebrovascular disease. Brain. 2007;130:731–9.
19. Selden N, Gitelman DR, Salamon-Murayama N, et al. Trajectories of cholinergic pathways within the cerebral hemispheres of the human brain. Brain. 1998;121:2249–57.
20. Oosterman J, Vogels R, van Harten B, et al. The role of white matter hyperintensities and medial temporal lobe atrophy in age-related executive dysfunctioning. Brain Cogn. 2008;68:128–33.
21. Prins N, van Dijk EJ, den Heijer T, et al. Cerebral white matter lesions and the risk of dementia. Arch Neurol. 2004;61:1531–4.
22. Debette S, Bombois E, Bruandet A, et al. Subcortical hyperintensities are associated with cognitive decline in patients with mild cognitive impairment. Stroke. 2007;38:2924–30.
23. Bombois S, Debette S, Delbeuck X, et al. Prevalence of subcortical vascular lesions and association with executive function in mild cognitive impairment subtypes. Stroke. 2007;38:2595–7.
24. Prins N, van Dijk EJ, de Heijer T, et al. Cerebral small-vessel disease and decline in information processing speed, executive function and memory. Brain. 2005;128:2034–41.
25. DeCarli C, Fletcher E, Ramey V, et al. Anatomical mapping of white matter hyperintensities (WMH): exploring the relationships between periventricular WMH, deep WMH, and total WMH burden. Stroke. 2005;36:50–5.
26. Soriano-Raya JJ, Miralbell J, López-Cancio E, et al. Deep versus periventricular white matter lesions and cognitive function in a community sample of middle-aged participants. J Int Neuropsychol Soc. 2012;18:874–85.
27. Au R, Massaro J, Wolf P, et al. Association of white matter hyperintensity volume with decreased cognitive functioning. The Framingham Heart Study. Arch Neurol. 2006;63:246–50.
28. Libon D, Price C, Giovannetti T, et al. Linking MRI hyperintensities with patterns of neuropsychological impairment. Evidence of a threshold effect. Stroke. 2008;39:806–13.
29. Wright C, Festa J, Paik M, et al. White matter hyperintensities and subclinical infarction. Associations with psychomotor speed and cognitive flexibility. Stroke. 2008;39:800–5.
30. Dai W, Lopez O, Carmichael O, et al. Abnormal regional blood flow in cognitively normal elderly subjects with hypertension. Stroke. 2008;39:349–54.
31. Cummings J. Frontal subcortical circuits and human behavior. Arch Neurol. 1993;50:873–80.
32. Su C, Chen HM, Kwan AL, et al. Neuropsychological impairment after hemorrhagic stroke in basal ganglia. Arch Clin Neuropsychol. 2007;22:465–74.

33. Ring H, Serra-Mestres J. Neuropsychiatry of the basal ganglia. J Neurol Neurosurg Psychiatry. 2001;72:12–21.
34. Ho B, Andreasen N, Nopoulos P, et al. Progressive structural brains abnormalities and their relationship to clinical outcome. A longitudinal magnetic resonance imaging study in early schizophrenia. Arch Gen Psychiatry. 2003;60:585–94.
35. Bodkin J, Cohen B, Salomon M, et al. Treatment of negative symptoms in schizophrenia and schizoaffective disorders by selegiline augmentation of antipsychotic medication: a pilot study examining the role of dopamine. J Nerv Ment Dis. 1996;184:295–301.
36. Ongur D, Price J. The organization of networks within the orbital frontal and medial prefrontal cortex in rats, monkeys and humans. Cereb Cortex. 2000;10:206–19.
37. Carmichael S, Price J. Limbic connections of the orbital and medial prefrontal cortex in macaque monkeys. J Comp Neurol. 1995;363:615–41.
38. Burruss J, Hurley R, Taber K, et al. Functional neuroanatomy of the frontal lobe circuits. Radiology. 2000;214:227–30.
39. Graybiel A. The basal ganglia and cognitive pattern generators. Schizophr Bull. 1997;23:459–69.
40. Postle B, D'Esposito M. Dissociation of human caudate nucleus activity in spatial and nonspatial working memory: an event-related fMRI study. Cogn Brain Res. 1999;8:107–15.
41. Lewis S, Cools R, Robbins T, et al. Using executive heterogeneity to explore the nature of working memory deficits in Parkinson's disease. Neuropsychologia. 2003;41:645–54.
42. Cohen J, Forman S, Braver T, et al. Activation of the prefrontal cortex in a nonspatial working memory task with functional MRI. Hum Brain Mapp. 1994;1:293–304.
43. Schroeder U, Kuehler A, Haslinger B, et al. Subthalamic nucleus stimulation affects striato-anterior cingulate cortex in a response conflict task: a PET study. Brain. 2002;125:1995–2004.
44. Seidenberg M, Hermann B, Pulsipher D, et al. Thalamic atrophy and cognition in unilateral temporal lobe epilepsy. J Int Neuropsychol Soc. 2008;14:384–93.
45. Rees G. Visual attention: the thalamus at the centre? Curr Biol. 2009;19:213–4.
46. De Witte L, Verhoeven J, Engelborghs S, et al. Crossed aphasia and visuo-spatial neglect following a right thalamic stroke: a case study and review of the literature. Behav Neurol. 2008;19:177–94.
47. Stuss D, Gubermann A, Nelson R, et al. The neuropsychology of paramedian thalamic infarction. Brain Cogni. 1988;8:348–78.
48. Carrera E, Bogousslavsky J. The thalamus and behavior: effects of anatomically distinct strokes. Neurology. 2006;66:1817–23.
49. Carrera E, Michel P, Bogousslavsky J. Anteromedian, central, and posterolateral infarcts of the thalamus: three variant types. Stroke. 2004;35:2826–31.
50. Chen Y, Chen X, Mok V, et al. Poststroke depression in patients with small subcortical infarcts. Clin Neurol Neurosurg. 2009;111:256–60.
51. Hackett ML, Yapa C, Parag V, Anderson CS. Frequency of depression after stroke: a systematic review of observational studies. Stroke. 2005;36:1330–40.
52. Lyness J, Caine E, Cox C, et al. Cerebrovascular risk factors and later-life major depression. Testing a small-vessel brain disease model. Am J Geriatr Psychiatry. 1998;6:5–13.
53. Luijendijk H, Stricker B, Hofman A, et al. Cerebrovascular risk factors and incident depression in community-dwelling elderly. Acta Psychiatr Scand. 2008;118:139–48.
54. O'Brien J, Firbank M, Krishnan M, et al. LADIS Group. White matter hyperintensities rather than lacunar infarcts are associated with depressive symptoms in older people: the LADIS study. Am J Geriatr Psych. 2006;14:834–41.
55. Levy M, Cummings J, Fairbanks L, et al. Apathy is not depression. J Neuropsychiatry Clin Neurosci. 1998;10:314–9.
56. NHANES. http://www.cdc.gov/nchs/data/databriefs/db133.htm#x2013;2012. Accessed 26 July 2015.
57. Gottesman RF, Schneider AL, Albert M, et al. Midlife hypertension and 20-year cognitive change: the atherosclerosis risk in communities neurocognitive study. JAMA Neurol. 2014;71:1218–27.

58. Shah K, Qureshi SU, Johnson M, et al. Does use of antihypertensive drugs affect the incidence or progression of dementia? A systematic review. Am J Geriatr Pharmacother. 2009;7:250–61.
59. Qiu C, Winblad B, Fratiglioni L. The age-dependent relation of blood pressure to cognitive function and dementia. Lancet Neurol. 2005;4:487–99.
60. Stewart R, Richards M, Brayne C, et al. Vascular risk and cognitive impairment in an older, British, African-Caribbean population. J Am Geriatr Soc. 2001;48:263–9.
61. Harrington F, Saxby B, McKeith I, et al. Cognitive performance in hypertensive and normotensive older subjects. Hypertension. 2000;36:1079–82.
62. Budge M, de Jager C, Hogervorst E, et al. Oxford Project To Investigate Memory and Ageing (OPTIMA). Total plasma homocysteine, age, systolic blood pressure, and cognitive performance in older people. J Am Geriatr Soc. 2002;50:2014–8.
63. Andre-Petersson L, Hagberg B, Janzon L, et al. A comparison of cognitive ability in normotensive and hypertensive 68-year-old mean; results from population study 'men born in 1914', in Malmo, Sweden. Exp Ageing Res. 2001;27:319–40.
64. Paran E, Anson O, Reuveni H. Blood pressure and cognitive functioning among independent elderly. Am J Hypertens. 2003;16:818–26.
65. Morris M, Scherr P, Hebert L, et al. Association between blood pressure and cognitive function in a biracial community population of older persons. Neuroepidemiology. 2002;21:123–30.
66. Waldstein S, Giggey PP, Thayer JF, et al. Nonlinear relations of blood pressure to cognitive function. The Baltimore longitudinal aging study. Hypertension. 2005;45:374–9.
67. Scherr P, Hebert LE, Smith LA, et al. Relation of blood pressure to cognitive function in the elderly. Am J Epidemiol. 1991;134:1303–15.
68. Elias M, Robbins M, Schultz Jr N, et al. Is blood pressure an important variable in research on aging and neuropsychological test performance? J Gerontol. 1990;45:P128–35.
69. Van Boxtel M, Gaillard C, Houx PJ, et al. Can the blood pressure predict task performance in a healthy population sample? J Hypertens. 1997;15:1069–76.
70. Kuo H, Sorond F, Iloputaife I, et al. Effect of blood pressure on cognitive functions in elderly persons. J Gerontol A Biol Sci Med Sci. 2004;59:1191–4.
71. Cerhan J, Folsom A, Mortimer J, et al. Correlates of cognitive function in middle-aged adults. Atherosclerosis Risk in Communities (ARIC) Study Investigators. Gerontology. 1998;44:94–105.
72. Izquierdo-Porrera A, Waldstein S. Cardiovascular risk factors and cognitive function in African Americans. J Gerontol B Psychol Sci Soc Sci. 2002;57:P377–80.
73. Farmer M, White L, Abbott R, et al. Blood pressure and cognitive performance. The Framingham Study. Am J Epidemiol. 1987;126:1103–14.
74. Desmond D, Tatemichi T, Paik M, et al. Risk factors for cerebrovascular disease as correlates of cognitive function in a stroke-free cohort. Arch Neurol. 1993;50:162–6.
75. Swan G, Carmelli D, Larue A. Systolic blood pressure tracking over 25 to 30 years and cognitive performance in older adults. Stroke. 1998;29:2334–40.
76. Kilander L, Nyman H, Boberg M, et al. Hypertension is related to cognitive impairment: a 20-year follow-up of 999 men. Hypertension. 1998;31:780–6.
77. Knopman D, Boland L, Mosley T, et al. Cardiovascular risk factors and cognitive decline in middle-aged adults. Neurology. 2001;56:42–8.
78. Peila R, White LR, Masaki K, et al. Reducing the risk of dementia: Efficacy of long-term treatment of hypertension. Stroke. 2006;37:1165–71.
79. Murray M, Lane KA, Gao S, et al. Preservation of cognitive function with antihypertensive medications: a longitudinal analysis of a community-based sample of African-Americans. Arch Intern Med. 2002;162:2090–6.
80. Prince M, Bird A, Blizard R, et al. Is the cognitive function of older patients affected by antihypertensive treatment? Results from 54 months of the Medical Research Council's trial of hypertension in older adults. Br Med J. 1996;312:801–5.

81. Applegate W, Pressels S, Wittes J, et al. Impact of the treatment of isolated systolic hypertension on behavioral variables: results from the Systolic Hypertension in the Elderly Program. Arch Intern Med. 1994;154:2154–60.
82. Tzourio C, Anderson C, Chapman N, et al. Effects of blood pressure lowering with perindopril and indapamide therapy on dementia and cognitive decline in patients with cerebrovascular disease. Arch Intern Med. 2003;163:1069–75.
83. Lithell H, Hansson L, Skoog I, et al. The Study on Cognition and Prognosis in the Elderly (SCOPE): principal results of a randomized double-blind intervention trial. J Hypertens. 2003;21:875–86.
84. Forette F, Seux M, Staessen J, et al. Prevention of dementia in randomised double-blind placebo-controlled Systolic Hypertension in Europe (Syst-Eur) trial. Lancet. 1996;352:2046–52.
85. Denolle T, Sassano P, Allain H, et al. Effects of nicardipine and clonidine on cognitive functions and electroencephalography in hypertensive patients. Fundam Clin Pharmacol. 2002;16:527–35.
86. McCovery Jr E, Wright Jr J, Culbert J, et al. Effect of hydrochlorothiazide, enalapril, and propranolol on quality of life and cognitive and motor function in hypertensive patients. Clin Pharm. 1993;12:300–5.
87. Lasser N, Nash J, Lasser V, et al. Effects of antihypertensive therapy on blood pressure control, cognition, and reactivity. A placebo-controlled comparison of prazosin, propranolol, and hydrochlorothiazide. Am J Med. 1989;86:98–103.
88. Forette F, Seux M, Staessen J, et al. The prevention of dementia with antihypertensive treatment: new evidence from the Systolic Hypertension in Europe (Syst-Eur) study. Arch Intern Med. 2002;162:2046–52.
89. Dufouil C, Chalmers J, Coskun O, et al. Effects of blood pressure lowering on cerebral white matter hyperintensities in patients with stroke. The PROGRESS (Perindopril Protection Against Recurrent Stroke Study) Magnetic Resonance Imaging Substudy. Circulation. 2005;112:1644–50.
90. Di Bari M, Pahor M, Franse L, et al. Dementia and disability outcomes in large hypertension trials: lessons learned from the Systolic Hypertension in the Elderly Program (SHEP) trial. Am J Epidemiol. 2001;153:72–8.
91. Birns J, Morris R, Donaldson N, Kalra L. The effects of blood pressure reduction on cognitive function: a review of effects based on pooled data from clinical trials. J Hypertens. 2006;24:1907–14.
92. McGuinness B, Todd S, Passmore P, Bullock R. Blood pressure lowering in patients without prior cerebrovascular disease for prevention of cognitive impairment and dementia. Cochrane Database Syst Rev. 2009;4, CD004034.
93. Chang-Quan H, Hui W, Chao-Min W, et al. The association of antihypertensive medication use with risk of cognitive decline and dementia: a meta-analysis of longitudinal studies. Int J Clin Pract. 2011;65:1295–305.
94. Marpillat N, Macquin-Mavier I, Tropeano AI, et al. Antihypertensive classes, cognitive decline and incidence of dementia: a network meta-analysis. J Hypertens. 2013;31:1073–82.

Chapter 17
Cerebral Microbleeds, Small-Vessel Disease of the Brain, Hypertension, and Cognition

Anand Viswanathan, Hugues Chabriat, and Steven M. Greenberg

Cerebral microbleeds (CMB) have been increasingly recognized on neuroimaging since the widespread application of magnetic resonance imaging (MRI) techniques tailored to detect foci of magnetic susceptibility. CMB are most often clinically asymptomatic and are a result of rupture of small blood vessels in basal ganglia or subcortical white matter [1–4].

CMB were first described after the clinical use of gradient-echo (GRE) or T2*-weighted MRI [1, 5, 6]. GRE MRI is a technique highly sensitive in the detection of old and recent cerebral hemorrhage [1, 6]. The reduction of the signal on GRE sequences is caused by hemosiderin, a blood breakdown product which causes magnetic susceptibility-induced dephasing leading to T2* signal loss. CMB appear larger on GRE sequences as compared to the actual tissue lesions because of the so-called *blooming effect* of the MR signal at the border of these lesions [7, 8]. GRE MRI can detect millimeter-sized paramagnetic blood products (including hemosiderin) in brain parenchyma [9]. As hemosiderin remains in macrophages for many years after hemorrhage [10, 11], GRE sequences allow for reliable assessment of an individual's hemorrhagic burden over time. Furthermore, more recent technical

A. Viswanathan, M.D., Ph.D. (✉)
Stroke Service and Memory Disorders Unit, Department of Neurology,
Massachusetts General Hospital Stroke Research Center, Harvard Medical School,
175 Cambridge Street, Suite 300, Boston, MA 02114, USA
e-mail: aviswanathan1@partners.org

H. Chabriat, M.D., Ph.D.
Department of Neurology, CHU Lariboisière, Assistance Publique des Hôpitaux de Paris,
14 Rue Vesale, Paris 75005, France

S.M. Greenberg, M.D., Ph.D.
Stroke Service, Department of Neurology, Massachusetts General Hospital Stroke Research
Center, Harvard Medical School, 175 Cambridge Street, Suite 300, Boston, MA 02114, USA

© Springer International Publishing Switzerland 2016
V. Aiyagari, P.B. Gorelick (eds.), *Hypertension and Stroke*, Clinical
Hypertension and Vascular Diseases, DOI 10.1007/978-3-319-29152-9_17

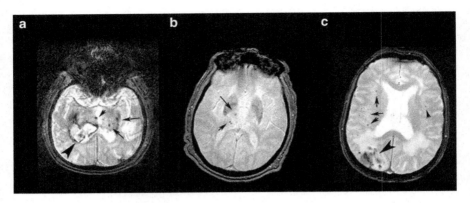

Fig. 17.1 Examples of CMB in different populations. Gradient-echo MRI sequences (**a**) in a patient with long-standing history of hypertension with deep intracerebral hemorrhage (*large arrowhead*). This patient also has CMB in contralateral deep structures including the thalamus (*arrows*). (**b**) In a patient with CADASIL. Multiple CMB are seen in the thalamus, a common location for CMB in CADASIL (**c**) In a patient with probable CAA demonstrating a parietal lobar intracerebral hemorrhage (*large arrowhead*) and numerous CMB in the frontal lobe (*arrows*)

advances in MRI software and hardware have yielded significant improvements in sensitivity, which has led to increased detection of CMB in different populations [12–15]. Novel techniques such as susceptibility-weighted imaging (SWI) have considerably increased CMB detection rates [13].

CMB are defined as small rounded foci which appear hypointense and distinct from vascular flow voids, leptomeningeal hemosiderosis, or nonhemorrhagic subcortical mineralization [1, 16] (Fig. 17.1). Choice of precise size parameters does not appear to have a major effect on CMB detection [2].

Radiopathologic studies have demonstrated that these areas of GRE hypointensity correlate well with brain parenchymal areas of hemosiderin-laden macrophages [1, 8, 17]. These pathologic data suggests that CMB result from specific underlying small-vessel pathologies such as hypertensive vasculopathy [18], cerebral amyloid angiopathy (CAA) [19–21], or cerebral autosomal dominant arteriopathy with subcortical infarcts and leukoencephalopathy (CADASIL) [22–25]. Their presence and number may also reflect the severity of these small-vessel pathologies and thus predict clinical outcome (including risk of dementia and cognitive decline) in these diseases.

In this chapter, we discuss the pathophysiology, prevalence, and risk factors for CMB in different populations. We also discuss the potential clinical implications of CMB in relation to cognition and disability in individuals harboring these lesions.

Cerebral Microbleeds in Specific Cerebral Small-Vessel Diseases

Cerebral Microbleeds in Hypertension-Related Vasculopathy and Cerebrovascular Disease

Evidence suggests that cerebral microbleeds are common in patients with hypertension-related cerebral vasculopathy, although few studies have restricted analyses exclusively to this group [26, 27]. Copenhaver et al. evaluated microbleeds in black patients with ICH (a high proportion having hypertension). Compared to white subjects, black subjects had greater number of microbleeds in multiple territories and 93 % had hypertension compared to 62 % of white subjects [26]. More recently, Zhang et al., examined the association between kidney function biomarkers and CMB in patients with hypertension. They found that several biomarkers of kidney function including serum cystatin C were associated with the presence of CMB in hypertensive patients.

Elevated blood pressure is common in patients with cerebrovascular disease and incidence of stroke rises with increasing blood pressure levels [28, 29]. The reported prevalence of CMB in these stroke populations or patients undergoing MRI is highly variable (range 18–68 %) [30–36]. This is likely due to limitations surrounding many of these studies, including nonselective clinical criteria, inclusion of multiple stroke subtypes, and variable size-based definition of microbleeds.

Chronic blood pressure elevation may increase an individual's risk for CMB. In order to investigate this, Lee et al. evaluated the relationship between CMB and cardiac damage induced by chronic hypertension. Left ventricular hypertrophy was evaluated in 102 consecutive survivors of acute stroke (72 with ischemic stroke, 30 with ICH) [36]. Left ventricular mass index was measured by transthoracic echocardiography. CMB were detected in 64 % of patients. In multivariable analysis, history of previous stroke and the number of CMB were associated with left ventricular hypertrophy, suggesting that poorly controlled blood pressure may increase the number of CMB.

CMB have been well described in patients with ICH [6, 10, 16, 17, 37, 38]. The presence of CMB has been shown to be nearly tenfold more common in this population than in healthy elderly [37]. Several studies examining patients presenting with primary ICH (deep and lobar) have reported prevalence of CMB to range between 54 and 70 % with the majority of subjects having multiple CMB [37, 39]. Individuals with CMB were more likely to be hypertensive, have a previous history of stroke, have more lacunar infarcts and more extensive white matter lesions. Roob et al. found there to be a correlation between cerebral microbleed distribution and the location of primary ICH. Individuals with deep ICH tended to have CMB in the basal ganglia and thalamus as compared to individuals with lobar ICH.

Cerebral Microbleeds in CAA

CMB have been extensively studied in CAA [2, 10, 14, 16, 40], the disease which accounts for the majority of primary lobar ICH in the elderly [41]. The Boston criteria are a set of validated criteria and have been established to identify those lobar ICHs caused by CAA [41]. The presence of multiple, strictly lobar hemorrhages (including microbleeds) detected by gradient-echo MRI sequences has been shown to be highly specific for severe CAA in elderly patients with no other definite cause of ICH (termed *probable* CAA-related ICH) [41]. These criteria have been compared against the established gold-standard of CAA, examination of histologic specimens from autopsy, hematoma evacuation, or cortical biopsy [41]. Thirty-nine primary lobar ICH patients aged ≥55 years with available pathologic tissue were diagnosed on clinical and radiologic grounds with possible or probable CAA. Thirteen patients were diagnosed with probable CAA, and all demonstrated pathological evidence of CAA in cerebral blood vessels. Eleven of these patients underwent GRE imaging, and 73 % showed evidence of multiple hemorrhagic lesions, including microbleeds. Sixteen of 26 patients (63 %) with the diagnosis of possible CAA (single lobar macro- or microhemorrhage) demonstrated pathologic evidence of CAA. These criteria have been recently shown to have high specificity and high positive predictive value for CAA even for patients harboring multiple lobar microbleeds without ICH [42]. Interestingly, in patients with probable or possible CAA there was no association between number of microbleeds and age, sex, APOE genotype or other vascular risk factors including hypertension, coronary artery disease, diabetes, or previous stroke [16].

The distribution of microbleeds in CAA shows a posterior cortical predominance [43] as has been reported previously in lobar macrohemorrhages [44, 45]. In 59 patients with probable CAA, microbleeds occurred more frequently in the temporal and occipital lobes when taking into account the relative size of each lobe [43]. The lesions also tended to cluster in the same lobe in subjects with multiple lesions. The distribution of new microhemorrhages at follow-up correlated with the distribution of baseline microbleeds [43]. Finally, in those patients who experience recurrent lobar ICH, the location of the hematoma is positively associated with the distribution of baseline microbleeds [16]. This is supported by pathologic data which show that CAA pathology favors the posterior cortical regions, particularly the occipital lobe [46, 47].

Cerebral Microbleeds in CADASIL

In patients with CADASIL, the reported frequency of microbleeds has ranged from 25 to 69 % with one large prospective cohort study finding that CMB occur in approximately 35 % of patients with the disease [22–25]. The main clinical manifestations of CADASIL include attacks of migraine with aura, mood disturbances, recurrent ischemic strokes, and progressive cognitive decline [48]. In various studies, CMB were most commonly found in the thalamus, subcortical white matter, basal ganglia, and brain stem [22–24]. There is minimal overlap between regions of CMB and regions of lacunar infarction or prominent WMH in CADASIL [22, 23].

Dichgans et al. performed a pathological examination of CMB in CADASIL. The investigators examined seven autopsy cases of CADASIL and found evidence of hemosiderin-laden macrophages in six out of seven cases [23]. In all cases, macrophages were found in the vicinity of 100–300 μ diameter blood vessels with characteristic degenerative changes of CADASIL. There was no evidence of amyloid deposition or vascular malformations, supporting the involvement of CADASIL-related ultrastructural modifications of the vessel walls in these lesions.

An ongoing two-center prospective cohort study has investigated risk factors for CMB, and the impact of CMB on clinical outcome in CADASIL [22]. The study showed that CMB are independently associated with blood pressure levels and HbA1c. The number of CMB was also associated with lacunar infarct volume, and extent of WMH. CMB were found to be an independent predictor of neurologic disability.

Until recently, blood pressure had not been thought to play a significant role in the pathophysiology of genetic small-vessel diseases [23, 24, 49]. In the above-described CADASIL study, CMB were independently associated with blood pressure levels. However, the average blood pressure values in subjects with CMB and in those without were found to be in the normal range (<140/90). When hypertensive patients (those individuals with blood pressure >140/90) were removed from the analysis, the association between CMB and blood pressure remained highly significant [22]. This suggests that small increases in blood pressure may contribute to CMB in CADASIL through an additive effect on the ultrastructural vessel wall modifications caused by Notch3 mutations [23, 50]. In support of this possibility, a recent small study in patients with the NOTCH3 R544C mutation showed that CMB occurred more frequently in deep brain regions (e.g., basal ganglia, thalamus, brain stem) in presence of hypertension. Furthermore in this study, CADASIL patients with CMB were more likely to have symptomatic stroke [51]. Further studies are needed to determine which factors (pulsatility, cerebrovascular resistance, or vessel wall stiffness) most strongly influence the rupture of the cerebral microvessel wall in the setting of CADASIL and moderate elevations of blood pressure. Acceptable blood pressure values in the setting of an existent cerebral microangiopathy may well differ from established normal ranges recommended for the general population.

Specialized Methods for Improved Detection of Cerebral Microbleeds

A variety of MRI factors (including sequence parameters, spatial resolution, magnetic field strength, and post-processing techniques) can lead to improved CMB detection [2]. For example, application of 3D T2*-weighted MRI at submillimeter spatial resolution has recently been shown to detect more CMB when compared to conventional 2D GRE at lower resolution [52]. Another study found that individual CMB identified in CAA subjects had approximately double the contrast index (a measure of conspicuity) when imaged with 1.5 mm slices compared to 5 mm slices [14]. Susceptibility-weighted imaging (SWI), which is becoming more widespread in clinical practice and research, has been shown to have greater sensitivity and increased reliability for CMB compared to conventional GRE imaging [53, 54].

Microbleeds in Population-Based Studies: The Role of Location

CMB have been noted in numerous healthy populations [15, 55–60]. Most [15, 55–58, 60], but not all [59, 61], of these studies showed hypertension to be a risk factor for CMB. Results from a pooled analysis of many of these studies demonstrated an increased risk of CMB in subjects with hypertension (OR 3.9 95 % CI 2.4–6.4) [4]. Overall, these investigators also found an increased risk of CMB with diabetes in these populations (OR 2.2, 95 % CI 1.2–4.2) [4]. The earlier studies were not able to distinguish the risk associated with specific location of CMB (lobar versus deep CMB).

However, more recent population-based data from the Rotterdam Scan study [15], the AGES-Reykjavik study [61], and the Framingham study [60] provide further evidence to support a potential etiologic distinction between lobar and deep CMB. In the Rotterdam study, Vernooij et al. demonstrated that APOE ε4 carriers more often had strictly lobar CMB than noncarriers. In contrast, cardiovascular risk factors (including elevated systolic blood pressure) and presence of lacunes and white matter lesions were associated with CMB in deep, but not lobar, locations The study included 1062 subjects with a mean age of 69.6 years. In this study, rates of CMB were increased compared to prior studies (ranging from 17.8 to 38.3 %). The higher prevalence of CMB compared to previous studies is likely due to both the higher mean age of the cohort (69.6 years) and the study's use of specialized high-resolution GRE sequences. In the AGES-Reykjavik study (1962 subjects with a mean age of 76 years), 61 % had CMB located in the cerebral lobes and greater than a third were located in posterior regions (parietal or occipital lobes), a pattern suggestive of CAA [43]. Furthermore, APOE ε4ε4 genotype was associated with increased likelihood of having a cerebral microbleed. These findings are supported by more recent work from the Framingham study (1965 subjects with a mean age of 67 years). CMB occurred in 8.8 % of subjects and were located in lobar regions in 63 % [60]. The investigators found that hypertension increased the risk of CMB in any location while low total cholesterol and *APOE* ε4 increased the risk of lobar CMB. Interestingly, after adjusting for cholesterol levels or concomitant medication use, statin use increased the risk of CMB in lobar and mixed locations (CMB in lobar plus deep areas), but not in exclusively deep locations. While these data are provocative, further studies are needed to more definitively address whether statins should be avoided in patients with lobar CMB.

Recent work from the Rotterdam study suggests that the incidence of new CMB in the general population is considerable (10.2 %). In this study, microbleeds at baseline predicted development of new microbleeds (OR, 5.38; 95 % CI, 3.34–8.67). Incident deep microbleeds were associated with cardiovascular risk factors, lacunar infarcts, and larger white matter lesion load at baseline, and incident microbleeds in strictly lobar areas were associated with the apolipoprotein E ε4/ε4 genotype or larger white matter lesion volume [62].

To summarize, there are several lines of evidence supporting the hypothesis that CMB in strictly lobar locations are due primarily to CAA and those involving deep hemispheric or brain stem structures are due primarily to hypertension-related vasculopathy. Therefore, CMB in strictly lobar locations may be a result of underlying subclinical CAA pathology and not related to traditional cardiovascular risk factors such as hypertension. These findings are consistent with previous studies in CAA which demonstrate that hypertension and other vascular risk factors are not associated with the number of CMB. In addition, vascular risk factors do not seem to independently influence outcome [16]. Finally, the association between strictly lobar CMB and the APOE ε4 allele in the above population-based studies is consistent with previous studies which demonstrate this association in subjects with probable or possible CAA [63]. By contrast, CMB located in deep regions (such as the basal ganglia or thalamus) are associated with high systolic blood pressure and wider pulse pressures. CMB in deep locations were not associated with APOE genotype [15, 60].

This hypothesis is further supported by histopathologic studies which examine CMB and associated vascular pathologies [1, 17, 41]. In these studies, CMB associated with hypertensive vasculopathy more commonly occurred in basal ganglia, thalamus, brain stem, and cerebellum [1], whereas CAA-associated CMB had a lobar (or less commonly, cerebellar) distribution [41].

Cerebral Microbleeds and Clinical Impairment

In addition to the potential role of CMB as markers of specific small-vessel disease, they also may have direct effects on cognition and disability. Neuropathological studies demonstrate tissue damage associated with CMB [17, 41, 64], thus providing a potential mechanism for clinical impairment.

Microbleeds in CAA have been shown to be related to disease progression, recurrent ICH, and CAA-related clinical impairment [16, 65]. Microbleeds are more common than macrohemorrhages and tend to accumulate over time. Greenberg and colleagues evaluated 94 elderly patients (≥55 years) presenting with lobar ICH for number of baseline hemorrhages [16]. Among those patients who underwent MRI 16-months later, 50 % experienced new, frequently multiple microbleeds. Predictors of new microbleeds included larger number of hemorrhages at baseline and the presence of the APOE ε2 or ε4 allele. Both the number of hemorrhages at baseline and the number of new microbleeds at follow-up were associated with increased risk of recurrent hemorrhage (3-year cumulative risk 14%, 17%, 38%, and 51% in subjects with 1, 2, 3–5, or ≥6 baseline hemorrhages, respectively). In individuals with cognitive impairment, there was a trend toward increased number of baseline hemorrhages. Finally, the incidence of cognitive impairment, functional dependence, or death at follow-up was increased by the number of hemorrhages at baseline (mean 27.9 months, HR 1.9 95% CI 1.2–2.8 for each increase in category of baseline hemorrhages).

CMB have also been associated with clinical disability in CADASIL [22, 66]. In a two-center cohort study of 147 patients with CADASIL, the number of CMB was independently associated with functional dependence (defined as modified Rankin score ≥3) with an odds ratio per additional microbleed of 1.16 (95% confidence interval 1.01–1.34, p, $p=0.034$) after adjustment for other confounding variables [22]. However, multivariable analysis did not demonstrate that the overall burden of CMB was associated with cognitive function.

For patients with cerebrovascular disease, a small case–control study of patients with ischemic stroke or TIA found that individuals with CMB performed significantly worse than those without them on standard tests of executive function [67].

Finally, CMB may have an impact on mortality in patients with cognitive impairment or dementia. A large longitudinal study has recently demonstrated that CMB were the strongest predictor of mortality in a memory clinic population (HR = 1.5; 95% CI, 1.1–2.0) [68]. This may suggest that CMB vascular pathology acts in synergy with neurodegenerative mechanisms associated with Alzheimer's disease to increase mortality in these patients.

If CMB have direct effects on brain function rather than simply marking the presence of other cerebrovascular pathologies, one would expect the specific location of CMB to play a role. In analyses of the two-center CADASIL cohort, CMB in the caudate were independently associated with lower global cognitive scores (based on the Mattis dementia rating scale; $p=0.027$), and CMB in the frontal lobes showed a trend toward lower global cognitive scores ($p=0.056$) [66]. Similarly, a small study of stroke or TIA patients suggested CMB in the frontal lobes and basal ganglia were associated with executive dysfunction [67]. Finally, a recent population-based study has suggested that CMB in deep regions (basal ganglia, thalamus, and infratentorial areas) were associated with impaired cognitive function as measured by mini-mental status examination (MMSE). The investigators found that individuals with deep CMB were more likely to have an MMSE score more than 1.5 standard deviations below the age and education-related mean (OR, 3.34; 95% CI, 1.24–8.99) [69]. These findings need further confirmation in large well-controlled studies of different populations including in individuals without prior stroke.

Microbleeds, Hypertension, and Cognition

Hypertension has been established as a risk factor for cognitive impairment and dementia in numerous studies. An association between high blood pressure and the risk of Alzheimer's disease was also reported in cohort studies with a 15- to 21-year

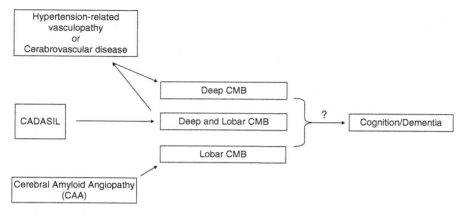

Fig. 17.2 The influence of cerebrovascular pathology on CMB location and its relationship to cognition. As depicted in the diagram, small-vessel diseases such as hypertension-related vasculopathy, cerebral amyloid angiopathy, and CADASIL can predispose an individual to developing CMB. Hypertension-related vasculopathy most commonly leads to development of CMB in deep areas, while cerebral amyloid angiopathy predisposes individuals to lobar CMB. In CADASIL, CMB develop in both deep and lobar locations (see text for details). *CMB* cerebral microbleeds

long follow-up [70, 71]. Furthermore, the presence of hypertension has been shown to be associated with a greater rate of cognitive decline in patients with Alzheimer's disease [72]. Finally, higher blood pressures have been associated with greater cognitive decline in patients after stroke in the PROGRESS trial [73]. There is some suggestion that the blood pressure effect may be related to attenuation of progression of white matter hyperintensities or brain atrophy [74–76]. Recent evidence suggests that CMB may be associated with subjective cognitive complaints in patients with hypertension [77] or in patients with cerebral small-vessel disease [78]. Whether the influence of hypertension on cognition is mediated, at least in part, through CMB requires further study (Fig. 17.2).

Future therapeutic trials should examine the specific effects of blood pressure reduction on cerebral microbleed burden to more precisely define the relationship between hypertension, CMB, and cognition. Studies such as these should help define the clinical impact of CMB and consequently influence future treatment decisions in individuals harboring these lesions.

Acknowledgment The authors have no financial disclosures to report.

References

1. Fazekas F, Kleinert R, Roob G, et al. Histopathologic analysis of foci of signal loss on gradient-echo T2*-weighted MR images in patients with spontaneous intracerebral hemorrhage: evidence of microangiopathy-related microbleeds. AJNR Am J Neuroradiol. 1999;20:637–42.

2. Greenberg SM, Vernooij MW, Cordonnier C, et al. Cerebral microbleeds: a guide to detection and interpretation. Lancet Neurol. 2009;8:165–74.
3. Viswanathan A, Chabriat H. Cerebral microhemorrhage. Stroke. 2006;37:550–5.
4. Cordonnier C, Al-Shahi Salman R, Wardlaw J. Spontaneous brain microbleeds: systematic review, subgroup analyses and standards for study design and reporting. Brain. 2007;130:1988–2003.
5. Scharf J, Brauherr E, Forsting M, Sartor K. Significance of haemorrhagic lacunes on MRI in patients with hypertensive cerebrovascular disease and intracerebral haemorrhage. Neuroradiology. 1994;36:504–8.
6. Offenbacher H, Fazekas F, Schmidt R, Koch M, Fazekas G, Kapeller P. MR of cerebral abnormalities concomitant with primary intracerebral hematomas. AJNR Am J Neuroradiol. 1996;17:573–8.
7. Alemany Ripoll M, Stenborg A, Sonninen P, Terent A, Raininko R. Detection and appearance of intraparenchymal haematomas of the brain at 1.5 T with spin-echo, FLAIR and GE sequences: poor relationship to the age of the haematoma. Neuroradiology. 2004;46:435–43.
8. Ripoll MA, Siosteen B, Hartman M, Raininko R. MR detectability and appearance of small experimental intracranial hematomas at 1.5 T and 0.5 T. A 6-7-month follow-up study. Acta Radiol. 2003;44:199–205.
9. Atlas SW, Mark AS, Grossman RI, Gomori JM. Intracranial hemorrhage: gradient-echo MR imaging at 1.5 T. Comparison with spin-echo imaging and clinical applications. Radiology. 1988;168:803–7.
10. Greenberg SM, Finklestein SP, Schaefer PW. Petechial hemorrhages accompanying lobar hemorrhage: detection by gradient-echo MRI. Neurology. 1996;46:1751–4.
11. Roob G, Fazekas F. Magnetic resonance imaging of cerebral microbleeds. Curr Opin Neurol. 2000;13:69–73.
12. Haacke EM, DelProposto ZS, Chaturvedi S, et al. Imaging cerebral amyloid angiopathy with susceptibility-weighted imaging. AJNR Am J Neuroradiol. 2007;28:316–7.
13. Haacke EM, Mittal S, Wu Z, Neelavalli J, Cheng YC. Susceptibility-weighted imaging: technical aspects and clinical applications, part 1. AJNR Am J Neuroradiol. 2009;30:19–30.
14. Nandigam RN, Viswanathan A, Delgado P, et al. MR imaging detection of cerebral microbleeds: effect of susceptibility-weighted imaging, section thickness, and field strength. AJNR Am J Neuroradiol. 2009;30(2):338–43.
15. Vernooij MW, van der Lugt A, Ikram MA, et al. Prevalence and risk factors of cerebral microbleeds: the Rotterdam Scan Study. Neurology. 2008;70:1208–14.
16. Greenberg SM, Eng JA, Ning M, Smith EE, Rosand J. Hemorrhage burden predicts recurrent intracerebral hemorrhage after lobar hemorrhage. Stroke. 2004;35:1415–20.
17. Tanaka A, Ueno Y, Nakayama Y, Takano K, Takebayashi S. Small chronic hemorrhages and ischemic lesions in association with spontaneous intracerebral hematomas. Stroke. 1999;30:1637–42.
18. Fisher CM. Pathological observations in hypertensive cerebral hemorrhage. J Neuropathol Exp Neurol. 1971;30:536–50.
19. Vinters HV, Natte R, Maat-Schieman ML, et al. Secondary microvascular degeneration in amyloid angiopathy of patients with hereditary cerebral hemorrhage with amyloidosis, Dutch type (HCHWA-D). Acta Neuropathol. 1998;95:235–44.
20. Vonsattel JP, Myers RH, Hedley-Whyte ET, Ropper AH, Bird ED, Richardson Jr EP. Cerebral amyloid angiopathy without and with cerebral hemorrhages: a comparative histological study. Ann Neurol. 1991;30:637–49.
21. Vinters HV. Cerebral amyloid angiopathy. A critical review. Stroke. 1987;18:311–24.
22. Viswanathan A, Guichard JP, Gschwendtner A, et al. Blood pressure and haemoglobin A1c are associated with microhaemorrhage in CADASIL: a two-centre cohort study. Brain. 2006;129:2375–83.

23. Dichgans M, Holtmannspotter M, Herzog J, Peters N, Bergmann M, Yousry TA. Cerebral microbleeds in CADASIL: a gradient-echo magnetic resonance imaging and autopsy study. Stroke. 2002;33:67–71.
24. Lesnik Oberstein SA, van den Boom R, van Buchem MA, et al. Cerebral microbleeds in CADASIL. Neurology. 2001;57:1066–70.
25. van den Boom R, Lesnik Oberstein SA, Ferrari MD, Haan J, van Buchem MA. Cerebral autosomal dominant arteriopathy with subcortical infarcts and leukoencephalopathy: MR imaging findings at different ages--3rd-6th decades. Radiology. 2003;229:683–90.
26. Copenhaver BR, Hsia AW, Merino JG, et al. Racial differences in microbleed prevalence in primary intracerebral hemorrhage. Neurology. 2008;71:1176–82.
27. Zhang JB, Liu LF, Li ZG, Sun HR, Ju XH. Associations between biomarkers of renal function with cerebral microbleeds in hypertensive patients. Am J Hypertens. 2015;28:739–45.
28. Wolf PA. Cerebrovascular risk. In: Izzo JL, Black HR, editors. Hypertension primer: the essentials of high blood pressure. New York: Lippincott, Williams & Wilkins; 2003. p. 239–42.
29. Wolf PA. Epidemiology of stroke. In: Mohr JP, Choi DW, Grotta JC, Weir B, Wolf PA, editors. Stroke: pathophysiology, diagnosis, and management. Philadelphia: Churchill Livingstone; 2004. p. 13–34.
30. Kato H, Izumiyama M, Izumiyama K, Takahashi A, Itoyama Y. Silent cerebral microbleeds on T2*-weighted MRI: correlation with stroke subtype, stroke recurrence, and leukoaraiosis. Stroke. 2002;33:1536–40.
31. Kinoshita T, Okudera T, Tamura H, Ogawa T, Hatazawa J. Assessment of lacunar hemorrhage associated with hypertensive stroke by echo-planar gradient-echo T2*-weighted MRI. Stroke. 2000;31:1646–50.
32. Kwa VI, Franke CL, Verbeeten Jr B, Stam J. Silent intracerebral microhemorrhages in patients with ischemic stroke. Amsterdam Vascular Medicine Group. Ann Neurol. 1998;44:372–7.
33. Fan YH, Mok VC, Lam WW, Hui AC, Wong KS. Cerebral microbleeds and white matter changes in patients hospitalized with lacunar infarcts. J Neurol. 2004;251:537–41.
34. Lee SH, Bae HJ, Yoon BW, Kim H, Kim DE, Roh JK. Low concentration of serum total cholesterol is associated with multifocal signal loss lesions on gradient-echo magnetic resonance imaging: analysis of risk factors for multifocal signal loss lesions. Stroke. 2002;33:2845–9.
35. Tsushima Y, Aoki J, Endo K. Brain microhemorrhages detected on T2*-weighted gradient-echo MR images. AJNR Am J Neuroradiol. 2003;24:88–96.
36. Lee SH, Park JM, Kwon SJ, et al. Left ventricular hypertrophy is associated with cerebral microbleeds in hypertensive patients. Neurology. 2004;63:16–21.
37. Roob G, Lechner A, Schmidt R, Flooh E, Hartung HP, Fazekas F. Frequency and location of microbleeds in patients with primary intracerebral hemorrhage. Stroke. 2000;31:2665–9.
38. Lee SH, Bae HJ, Kwon SJ, et al. Cerebral microbleeds are regionally associated with intracerebral hemorrhage. Neurology. 2004;62:72–6.
39. Jeong SW, Jung KH, Chu K, Bae HJ, Lee SH, Roh JK. Clinical and radiologic differences between primary intracerebral hemorrhage with and without microbleeds on gradient-echo magnetic resonance images. Arch Neurol. 2004;61:905–9.
40. Lee SH, Kim SM, Kim N, Yoon BW, Roh JK. Cortico-subcortical distribution of microbleeds is different between hypertension and cerebral amyloid angiopathy. J Neurol Sci. 2007;258:111–4.
41. Knudsen KA, Rosand J, Karluk D, Greenberg SM. Clinical diagnosis of cerebral amyloid angiopathy: validation of the Boston criteria. Neurology. 2001;56:537–9.
42. Martinez-Ramirez SRJ, Shoamanesh A, McKee AC, Van-Etten E, Pontes-Neto O, Macklin EA, Ayres AM, Auriel E, Himali JJ, Beiser AS, DeCarli C, Stein TD, Alvarez VE, Frosch MP, Rosand J, Greenberg SM, Gurol ME, Seshadri S, Viswanathan A. Diagnostic value of lobar microbleeds in individuals without intracerebral hemorrhage. Alzheimers Dement. 2015;11(12):1480–8.

43. Rosand J, Muzikansky A, Kumar A, et al. Spatial clustering of hemorrhages in probable cerebral amyloid angiopathy. Ann Neurol. 2005;58(3):459–62.
44. Ropper AH, Davis KR. Lobar cerebral hemorrhages: acute clinical syndromes in 26 cases. Ann Neurol. 1980;8:141–7.
45. Kase CS, Williams JP, Wyatt DA, Mohr JP. Lobar intracerebral hematomas: clinical and CT analysis of 22 cases. Neurology. 1982;32:1146–50.
46. Pfeifer LA, White LR, Ross GW, Petrovitch H, Launer LJ. Cerebral amyloid angiopathy and cognitive function: the HAAS autopsy study. Neurology. 2002;58:1629–34.
47. Vinters HV, Gilbert JJ. Cerebral amyloid angiopathy: incidence and complications in the aging brain. II. The distribution of amyloid vascular changes. Stroke. 1983;14:924–8.
48. Chabriat H, Bousser MG. CADASIL. Cerebral autosomal dominant arteriopathy with subcortical infarcts and leukoencephalopathy. Adv Neurol. 2003;92:147–50.
49. Singhal S, Bevan S, Barrick T, Rich P, Markus HS. The influence of genetic and cardiovascular risk factors on the CADASIL phenotype. Brain. 2004;127:2031–8.
50. Ruchoux MM, Maurage CA. CADASIL: cerebral autosomal dominant arteriopathy with subcortical infarcts and leukoencephalopathy. J Neuropathol Exp Neurol. 1997;56:947–64.
51. Lee JS, Kang CH, Park SQ, Choi HA, Sim KB. Clinical significance of cerebral microbleeds locations in CADASIL with R544C NOTCH3 mutation. PLoS One. 2015;10:e0118163.
52. Vernooij MW, Ikram MA, Wielopolski PA, Krestin GP, Breteler MM, van der Lugt A. Cerebral microbleeds: accelerated 3D T2*-weighted GRE MR imaging versus conventional 2D T2*-weighted GRE MR imaging for detection. Radiology. 2008;248:272–7.
53. Cheng AL, Batool S, McCreary CR, et al. Susceptibility-weighted imaging is more reliable than T2*-weighted gradient-recalled echo MRI for detecting microbleeds. Stroke. 2013;44(10):2782–6.
54. Goos JD, van der Flier WM, Knol DL, et al. Clinical relevance of improved microbleed detection by susceptibility-weighted magnetic resonance imaging. Stroke. 2011;42:1894–900.
55. Tsushima Y, Tanizaki Y, Aoki J, Endo K. MR detection of microhemorrhages in neurologically healthy adults. Neuroradiology. 2002;44:31–6.
56. Roob G, Schmidt R, Kapeller P, Lechner A, Hartung HP, Fazekas F. MRI evidence of past cerebral microbleeds in a healthy elderly population. Neurology. 1999;52:991–4.
57. Lee SH, Bae HJ, Ko SB, Kim H, Yoon BW, Roh JK. Comparative analysis of the spatial distribution and severity of cerebral microbleeds and old lacunes. J Neurol Neurosurg Psychiatry. 2004;75:423–7.
58. Horita Y, Imaizumi T, Niwa J, et al. Analysis of dot-like hemosiderin spots using brain dock system. No Shinkei Geka. 2003;31:263–7.
59. Jeerakathil T, Wolf PA, Beiser A, et al. Cerebral microbleeds: prevalence and associations with cardiovascular risk factors in the Framingham Study. Stroke. 2004;35:1831–5.
60. Romero JR, Preis SR, Beiser A, et al. Risk factors, stroke prevention treatments, and prevalence of cerebral microbleeds in the Framingham Heart Study. Stroke. 2014;45:1492–4.
61. Sveinbjornsdottir S, Sigurdsson S, Aspelund T, et al. Cerebral microbleeds in the population based AGES-Reykjavik study: prevalence and location. J Neurol Neurosurg Psychiatry. 2008;79:1002–6.
62. Poels MM, Ikram MA, van der Lugt A, et al. Incidence of cerebral microbleeds in the general population: the Rotterdam Scan Study. Stroke. 2011;42:656–61.
63. O'Donnell HC, Rosand J, Knudsen KA, et al. Apolipoprotein E genotype and the risk of recurrent lobar intracerebral hemorrhage. N Engl J Med. 2000;342:240–5.
64. Tatsumi S, Shinohara M, Yamamoto T. Direct comparison of histology of microbleeds with postmortem MR images: a case report. Cerebrovasc Dis. 2008;26:142–6.
65. Greenberg SM, O'Donnell HC, Schaefer PW, Kraft E. MRI detection of new hemorrhages: potential marker of progression in cerebral amyloid angiopathy. Neurology. 1999;53:1135–8.
66. Viswanathan A, Godin O, Jouvent E, et al. Impact of MRI markers in subcortical vascular dementia: a multi-modal analysis in CADASIL. Neurobiol Aging. 2010;31(9):1629–36.

67. Werring DJ, Frazer DW, Coward LJ, et al. Cognitive dysfunction in patients with cerebral microbleeds on T2*-weighted gradient-echo MRI. Brain. 2004;127:2265–75.
68. Henneman WJ, Sluimer JD, Cordonnier C, et al. MRI biomarkers of vascular damage and atrophy predicting mortality in a memory clinic population. Stroke. 2009;40:492–8.
69. Yakushiji Y, Noguchi T, Charidimou A, et al. Basal ganglia cerebral microbleeds and global cognitive function: the Kashima Scan Study. J Stroke Cerebrovasc Dis. 2015;24:431–9.
70. Kivipelto M, Helkala EL, Laakso MP, et al. Midlife vascular risk factors and Alzheimer's disease in later life: longitudinal, population based study. BMJ. 2001;322:1447–51.
71. Skoog I, Lernfelt B, Landahl S, et al. 15-year longitudinal study of blood pressure and dementia. Lancet. 1996;347:1141–5.
72. Mielke MM, Rosenberg PB, Tschanz J, et al. Vascular factors predict rate of progression in Alzheimer disease. Neurology. 2007;69:1850–8.
73. Tzourio C, Anderson C, Chapman N, et al. Effects of blood pressure lowering with perindopril and indapamide therapy on dementia and cognitive decline in patients with cerebrovascular disease. Arch Intern Med. 2003;163:1069–75.
74. Dufouil C, Chalmers J, Coskun O, et al. Effects of blood pressure lowering on cerebral white matter hyperintensities in patients with stroke: the PROGRESS (Perindopril Protection Against Recurrent Stroke Study) Magnetic Resonance Imaging Substudy. Circulation. 2005;112:1644–50.
75. Firbank MJ, Wiseman RM, Burton EJ, Saxby BK, O'Brien JT, Ford GA. Brain atrophy and white matter hyperintensity change in older adults and relationship to blood pressure. Brain atrophy, WMH change and blood pressure. J Neurol. 2007;254:713–21.
76. Saxby BK, Harrington F, Wesnes KA, McKeith IG, Ford GA. Candesartan and cognitive decline in older patients with hypertension: a substudy of the SCOPE trial. Neurology. 2008;70:1858–66.
77. Uiterwijk R, Huijts M, Staals J, et al. Subjective cognitive failures in patients with hypertension are related to cognitive performance and cerebral microbleeds. Hypertension. 2014;64:653–7.
78. van Norden AG, van Uden IW, de Laat KF, et al. Cerebral microbleeds are related to subjective cognitive failures: the RUN DMC study. Neurobiol Aging. 2013;34:2225–30.

Chapter 18
Neuroimaging of Hypertension and Related Cerebral Pathology

Alejandro Magadán

Continued refinement and improvement in neuroimaging allows for better evaluation of the effects of HTN on the brain. Nuclear magnetic resonance has seen (MRI) the most advancement and remains the gold standard for evaluating anatomy and pathology of the brain. MRI has become more widely available and new protocols allow for faster image acquisition times, which allow for the assessment of acute pathologies like stroke or intracranial hemorrhage (ICH). CT is widely available and has rapid acquisition times and is the most common imaging modalities used. Two other imaging modalities useful in the evaluation of HTN include 2-[^{18}F] fluoro-2-deoxy-D-glucose (FDG) PET (FDG-PET) and single photon emission computerized tomography (SPECT).

Effects of Hypertension

Effects of Hypertension on the Brain

The effects of hypertension on the brain affect the (1) cerebral vasculature, (2) cerebral parenchyma, and (3) brain metabolism and function either as a primary process or as result of a secondary effect. Cerebral hypertension pathology in a clinical setting can also be categorized as emergent in the case of ischemic stroke and intracranial hemorrhage or chronic as in the case of progression of white matter changes and cerebral atrophy.

A. Magadán, M.D. (✉)
Department of Neurology and Neurotherapeutics, University of Texas Southwestern Medical Center, 5323 Harry Hines Blvd., Dallas, TX 75201, USA
e-mail: Alejandro.Magadan@UTSouthwestern.edu

© Springer International Publishing Switzerland 2016
V. Aiyagari, P.B. Gorelick (eds.), *Hypertension and Stroke*, Clinical
Hypertension and Vascular Diseases, DOI 10.1007/978-3-319-29152-9_18

Effects of Hypertension on Cerebral Vasculature

There are acute and chronic effects of HTN on cerebral vasculature. Acute effects include vessel rupture, often in the territory of the penetrating lenticular striate arteries (putamen, thalamus, pons, cerebellum, and lobar white matter) presenting with concurrent high blood pressure. The effects of long-standing hypertension include the development of atherosclerotic plaque in larger arteries and hyalinosclerosis and lipohyalinosis weakening the small penetrating arterial walls and leading to the formation of microaneurysms, or the Charcot and Bouchard aneurysms, in small penetrating arteries [1–8]. Additionally, there is the development of centrally located cerebral microbleeds with long-standing uncontrolled blood pressure [9, 10]. Cerebral blood flow remains constant except with a shift in the curve to higher blood pressure with long-standing hypertension [11]. Regional blood hypoperfusion has been noted in the frontal, temporal, subcortical, and limbic regions in associated persons with hypertension [12, 13].

Effects of Hypertension on Cerebral Tissue

Ischemic stroke is an emergent secondary effect of hypertension on cerebral tissue and an important clinical and research target. Imaging remains key in the evaluation and treatment of stroke in the acute process for treatment candidacy and also further evaluation in order to discover a potential etiology for stroke and develop a treatment plan. Intracranial or parenchymal hemorrhage is primarily affected by hypertension with a correlation to malignant hypertension and ICH as well as by secondary effects through hypertensive arteriopathy of the cerebral vasculature and formation of microbleeds [9, 10] and predisposition for hemorrhage [14]. Over time, longstanding hypertension leads to the formation of white matter changes (leukoariosis), and both general and regional brain atrophy [15–23].

Effects of Hypertension on Cerebral Function and Metabolism

Long-standing hypertension at varying stages in life has led to increased incidence of cognitive impairment and spatial memory dysfunction [24–27], dementia of both Alzheimer's type, and vascular dementia [24, 28, 29] and has been associated with increased incidence of traditionally Alzheimer's dementia related pathology such as neurofibrillary tangles, neuritic plaques, and B Amyloid deposition [30–32]. Hypertension seems to accelerate cognitive impairment in genetically susceptible individuals with the APOE4 gene [33]. Blood pressure management of midlife systolic hypertension seemed to prevent late-life dementia [34] and non-pharmacologic preventive management of cerebrovascular risk factors and hypertension such as moderate exercise and Mediterranean diet also was associated with a decreased incidence of dementia and cognitive impairment [35–39] and a decrease in AB plaque using multimodal neuroimaging including Pittsburgh Compound B [40].

Computed Tomography

General Principles

Computed tomography (CT) images involve the use of X-ray tube housed in a gantry which in early CT scans, rotated 360° to capture an X-ray image. More modern CT scanners are spiral/helical CT scanners that allow for the gantry to rotate continuously as a patient moves along a Z-axis getting spiral/helical image data. The gantry is aligned in the X/Y axis and the table (patient) is aligned perpendicularly along the Z-axis. The technique relies on X-ray beams passing through tissue at a large number of angles. A detector array opposite to the X-ray source then collects the transmission projection data, which is then synthesized by a computer into a tomographic image. The transmission of the X-rays, or transmission projection data, through the body relies on the attenuation of X-rays (reduction in signal intensity) through different tissues, with bone, calcium and blood attenuating X-ray more than air or CSF. The slab of tissue image is divided into small volume elements, voxels, which have x, y, and z directions and is then converted into the gray scale units (Hounsfield units) based on the computed attenuation. CT scan continues to become faster and has less radiation exposure with increasing detector rows, or multi-slice CT scans.

Use in the Assessment of the Effects of Hypertension

The most common use of CT in hypertension is a rapid assessment for acute stroke, hemorrhage, and severe headaches primarily to determine the presence or absence of intracranial hemorrhage. Additional use of contrast allows for the assessment of intracranial vasculature, perfusion or potentially the presence of an expanding hematoma. The presence of contrast extravasation, "the spot sign," is associated with hematoma expansion [41]. Without contrast a heterogeneous signal within a hematoma may also represent an expanding hematoma [42]. Location of a hematoma elucidates an etiology of hypertension or malignant hypertension as a cause of an intracranial hemorrhage. The most common locations include the putamen, thalamus, pons, cerebellum, and the lobar white matter. A standardized score "ASPECTS" using a non-contrast CT scan has been shown to be able to predict outcome in ischemic stroke [43, 44]. Early ischemic signs, such as hyper-dense MCA sign, or attenuation of the basal ganglia insular cortex or cortical ribbon also appear on a non-contrast CT head [45, 46]. While ASPECTS score has show benefit, inter-rater agreement and detection of early signs of ischemic stroke on non-contrast CT remain poor [47, 48] and were often missed during rapid assessment for tPA administration [49].

CT Angiography

CT angiography (CTA) is useful for a minimally invasive and rapid assessment of extracranial carotid disease with a good degree of agreement compared to the "gold standard" digital subtraction angiography [50–52]. CTA also is used to evaluate plaque morphology such as degree of arterial stenosis, carotid wall thickness, and surface morphology [52]. CT angiogram is a fast method and has been used in the management of acute stroke and intracranial hemorrhage. In the rapid triage of acute stroke, CTA is able to evaluate vessel status and identify a cutoff or vessel occlusion. Recently, using novel stent-retriever devices in large anterior circulation strokes (distal carotid artery or proximal middle cerebral artery), the benefit of mechanical thrombectomy in addition to standard thrombolysis with tPA over IV-tPA alone has been shown [53] with a more robust improved clinical outcome combining CTA with a more methodical CT evaluation, the ASPECTS score [54]. CTA allows for the visualization of leptomeningeal collateral flow with better collateralization being associated with a better prognosis and absence of collateral vessels being associated with poor prognosis despite recanalization [55]. CTA use in intracranial hemorrhage allows for the detection of vascular malformations or aneurysms as potential etiology of the hemorrhage and contrast extravasation into the hematoma or "spot sign" predicts hematoma enlargement [41].

CT Perfusion

CT perfusion continued to improve with multi-detector technology allowing for faster scans and improving limited brain coverage. CTP tracks the "wash in" and "wash out" of iodinated contrast through a tissue capillary network. The main three parametric maps are cerebral blood volume (CBV), cerebral blood flow (CBF), and mean transit time (MTT). The MTT is the average time required by contrast (red blood cells) to cross the capillary network, cerebral blood volume is the volume of blood in milliliters per 100 g of brain tissue, and cerebral blood flow is the amount of blood flowing through each pixel in 1 min, measured as ml per 100 g brain tissue per minute. Tmax and time to peak (TTP) are two more parametric maps used to evaluate cerebral perfusion and are further described in the MR perfusion section. Quantitative measures of CBF, CBV, and MTT are generally more easily achieved with CT perfusion due the linear relationship between attenuation and iodinated contrast measured by Hounsfield units. Diffusion weighted imagining remains the most sensitive modality for determining infarct core in the acute phase in ischemic stroke, but a decrease in cerebral blood volume can be used with good correlation to final infarct volume [56–59]. CT perfusion has had little utility in the investigation of HTN in the absence of stroke but will likely mimic findings found with MR perfusion and arterial spin labeling.

General Advantages

The major advantages of CT over MRI are the more widespread availability, scan time speed, and lower cost. Major medical centers and most hospitals with an emergency department have a CT scanner. CT, CT angiogram, and CT perfusion can be completed within a few minutes. CT angiogram and CT perfusion studies are minimally invasive, requiring a venocatheter placement, usually in a large ante cubital vein, which will need to be of a sufficient bore width to accommodate the pressure and contrast injection. Newer multiphase CT angiography promises to reduce both scan time and iodinated contrast amount with improved vessel enhancement [60].

General Disadvantages

Overall, MRI is superior to CT for delineation of anatomy, lesions, and sensitivity in distinguishing hypertensive related pathologies. CT uses iodinated contrast with a significant risk for contrast-induced nephropathy, which carries a significant long-standing morbidity [61, 62]. CT perfusion provides only limited coverage of brain tissue around the circle of Willis versus whole brain coverage of MRI. Better multi-detector (multi-slice) CT can obtain more brain tissue coverage. CT perfusion values have significant variability over time, which is in part dependent upon the size as well as tissue heterogeneity of the imaged vascular territory [63]. MRI is the most sensitive and specific modality to image an acute ischemic stroke, though CBV may approximate the ischemic core, it requires additional contrast administration [64]. As such, the change in tissue perfusion must be greater than the observed variability in CTP sensitivity. This latter concern limits the usefulness of CTP in the assessment of HTN without significant TIA or stroke. Also, a significant issue in the quantification of this method is the lack of normative volume data for CTP at present [65]. CT also has a significant radiation exposure, with newer multiphase CT angiography having 5.73 mSv (millisieverts) of radiation [60]. A non-contrast CT of the head has an average dose of 2 mSv [66]. This has been associated with a varying degree of an increased incidence of cancer depending on the type of CT scans preformed [67].

Nuclear Magnetic Resonance Imaging

MR Imaging involves the interaction between a very powerful static magnetic field and the nuclear magnetic resonance properties of the proton (hydrogen nuclei), which are abundant within biological tissues. MRI is the most sensitive modality to image the effects of HTN on the brain. Due to the amount of hydrogen (in water) in tissue and blood, hydrogen is the most common atom used, but it can be used to measure any atom which has an odd number of protons and is abundant in the human body. Such atoms include carbon-13, sodium, fluorine, and phosphorus. Hydrogen is the most abundant atom in the body and most used in medical imaging, and sodium imaging has tremendous potential for evaluation of the effects of HTN on brain structure.

General Principles

Generally, six main factors contribute to MRI. These include the properties of nuclear spin, the properties of the radio frequency (RF) excitation, the properties of tissue relaxation, the strength of the static magnet field, the timing of RF pulses, and the sensitivity of signal detection. When placed into a magnetic field, the proton aligns parallel to the magnetic field (B0) generated by the MRI scanner and precess (wobbles) about an axis. As protons precess about an axis they are able to absorb radio frequency pulses causing an excited state leading to the protons leaving alignment along the magnetic field (B0) and spining at a different angle (spin angle). Typically, 90- and 180-degree radio frequency pulses are used, but any angle can be achieved. As the protons precess together at the same frequency, they realign to B0 (free induction decay) and will emit electromagnetic energy, which is the NMR signal. The total NMR signal is a combination of the sums of proton density reduced by T1, T2, and T2* relaxation. Relaxation occurs as longitudinal relaxation or longitudinal magnetization recovery, getting back into alignment with B0 and transverse relaxation or transverse magnetization decay, leaving the flip angle generated by the RF pulse. As such, each relaxation component offers distinct information about tissue character. T1 relaxation is characterized by a tissue specific time constant (Table 18.1). T1-weighted images are generally more spatially sensitive, making them useful in assessments of structure and volume. Long T1, such as a liquid (CSF) and a solid (hair), has a hypo-intense signal with short T1, such as viscous material (fat), has a hyperintense signal. Gadolinium causes T1 to shorten and appear hyperintense. T2-weighted images are more sensitive to pathology, especially when that pathology affects local water content, which appears as a hyperintense signal. T2 shortening as with gadolinium causes a more hypo-intense signal.

Table 18.1 T1 and T2 relaxation times by tissue type

Tissue	T1 (ms)	T2 (ms)
Fat	250	80
Liver	500	45
Kidney	650	60
White Matter	800	90
Grey Matter	900	100
CSF	2400	280
Water	3000	3000
Gadolinium	Reduces T1	Reduces T2

Note the longer relaxation times for T1 weighted images allows for better tissue contrast and better anatomic delineation

Use in the Effects of Hypertension

HTN is associated with not only large- and small-territory infarcts and rarefaction of white matter and more severe white matter lesions [15], but also cerebral tissue loss assessed by reduced cerebral volume [21, 68]. White matter hyperintensities are best noted on T2/FLAIR MRI imaging and are seen as hypodense lesions on CT scan. Age and HTN are directly correlated to the incidence of white matter hyperintensities, which approach nearly 100 % by age 85 and they are commonly observed in periventricular locations as well as subcortically [19, 20, 69–72]. White matter lesions are often attributed to "chronic microvascular ischemic changes," but depending on location and morphology, white matter lesions have different pathophysiology. Many of the small incidental white matter lesions are perivenous regions of demyelination [71, 73]. White matter lesions that are larger and more confluent tend to be associated with ischemic changes [73]. Apart from age, HTN is the cerebral vascular risk factor most associated with these more confluent white matter changes and progression of white matter changes [15, 17–19]. There is some evidence for an increased incidence in women [74]. A small study demonstrated a correlation to a reduced rate of white matter hyperintensity progression with blood pressure control [16] (Fig. 18.1).

A lifetime history of HTN has been associated with generalized and regional cerebral volume loss [16, 21, 75]. There is a correlation between cerebral atrophy and in particular, grey matter atrophy and white matter lesion burden [20, 23]. Blood pressure control has potential of reducing the risk of brain atrophy [16].

Cerebral microbleeds (CMBs) are small focal hemorrhages that are missed on CT scans and have been detected with T2* imaging (GRE or SWI) [76]. Centrally located CMBs are associated with long-standing hypertension and age and coexist with other hypertensive vasculopathies (lacunar infarcts and white matter lesions) [9, 10]. Detection of CMB is important as location distinguishes pathology with more lobar located CMBs being related to cerebral amyloid angiopathy [9, 77] and

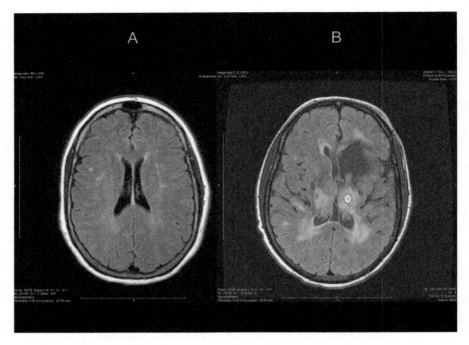

Fig. 18.1 Image A is a FLAIR sequence demonstrating small foci of T2 hyperintensity, consistent with non-specific white matter changes most likely regions of demyelination in a 59 years-old female with no vascular risk factors. Image B is a FLAIR sequence with more confluent white matter hyperintensities, prominent around the ventricles, a bright T2 hyperintensity in the left thalamus consistent with a late subacute hemorrhage and a region of encephalomalacia in the left frontal lobe that was a previous surgical sight for a ruptured MCA aneurysm in a 54 years-old female with long-standing uncontrolled hypertension

the presence of CMBs is associated with spontaneous intracranial hemorrhage risk and is thought to represent a potential risk of hemorrhage on antiplatelet agents or anticoagulants [78–80]. Thrombolysis in the presence of CMBs does not correlate to hemorrhagic transformation; studies were limited by the majority of the cases having less than 5 CMBs [81] and targeted intra-arterial thrombolysis instead of a systemic administration of thrombolysis [82] (Fig. 18.2).

Ischemic stroke can be visualized within a matter of minutes on diffusion-weighted imaging [83]. FLAIR may demonstrate a hyperintense vessel sign in association with vessel occlusion with more distal hyperintense vessels potentially representing collateral flow [84–86]. FLAIR also can be used as a tissue marker to time stroke onset with the lack of FLAIR hyperintensity associated with restricted diffusion thought to be stroke within 4.5 h time [87, 88]. Susceptibility weighted imaging also has a sensitive marker for vessel occlusion with a "blooming" or vessel susceptibility sign [89–91]. Both hyperintense vessels and T2* susceptibility signs are more sensitive than hyperdense a vessel sign on CT scan for identifying vessel occlusion. MRI has been validated for rapid assessment of stroke and administration of tPA within recommended time frame [92] and provides a wealth

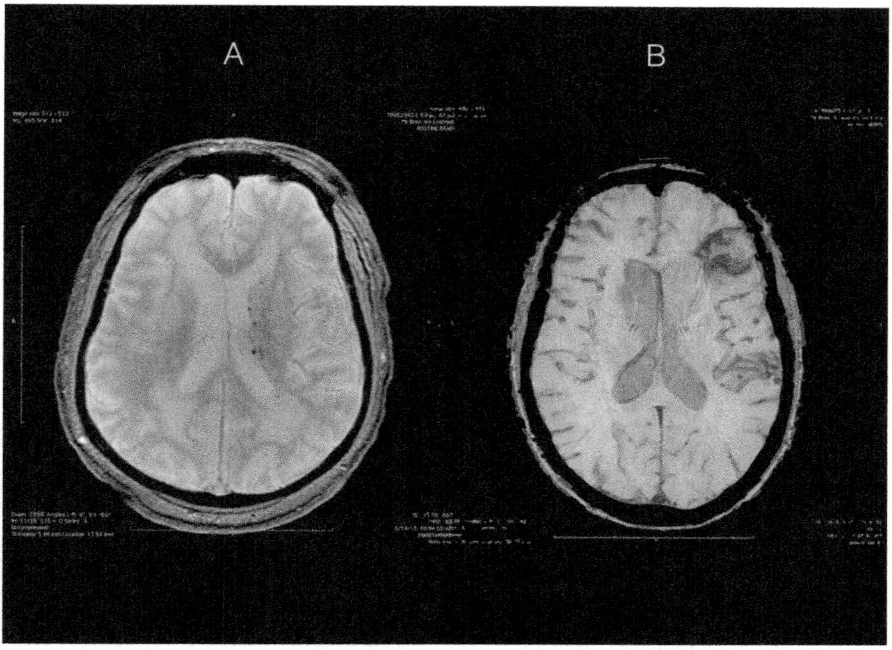

Fig. 18.2 Image A is a T2* sequence (GRE) demonstrating small microbleeds centrally in the left corona radiate in a 69 years-old male with HTN and other vascular risk factors with a hypertensive microbleed pattern. Image B is a T2* weighted sequence (SWI) demonstrating more lobar micro-bleeds, hypointensity of the sulci (superficial siderosis) and an old left frontal hemorrhage in an 81 years-old female with no vascular risk factors consistent with cerebral amyloid angiopathy and related bleeding events

of information about ischemic core, stroke age, and vessel patency, and it is poten-tially a valuable tool for patient selection into endovascular therapies and selection into clinical trials.

MRI use for the identification of vulnerable plaque morphology and composition is an active area of research. Typically, carotid stenosis of 60–70 % with symptoms is used as a guide for carotid endarterectomy or carotid stenting. MRI has high accuracy in the evaluation of carotid plaque [93] and MRI plaque morphology has been dem-onstrated to predict high stroke risk by identifying high risk or vulnerable characteris-tics such as lipid content, fibrous cap structure, calcium or intraplaque hematoma [94–96]. Most of the research has demonstrated feasibility and reproducibility of high resolution MRI plaque imaging [97–99]. Interpretation of high resolution MRI in the evaluation of carotid plaque has also demonstrated moderate to excellent inter-rater agreement in the evaluation of lipid core, intraplaque hemorrhage but only fair agree-ment for the evaluation of the fibrous cap [100]. MRI carotid plaque imaging is also combined with PET scan to associate increased inflammation with a lipid rich plaque core [101]. Ultra small super paramagnetic particles of iron (USPIOs) are small 30 μm diameter nanoparticles that are readily taken into macrophages that have accumulated in an area of active inflammation such as a rupture prone plaque causing a focal area of decreased signal intensity [102]. Importantly, MR imaging assessment of carotid plaque hemorrhage in asymptomatic carotid stenosis is suggested to be a cost-effective preventative method for stroke [103].

Magnetic Resonance Angiography

MR angiography is used to evaluate structural abnormalities caused by hypertension such as atherosclerotic plaques, arterial occlusion, and aneurysms. Both CT angiogram and MR angiogram have good inter-rater agreement and no significant diagnostic difference when evaluating intracranial aneurysms but are also limited in the evaluation of small aneurysms [104].

Recent advances in MRA technology include improving signal quality and assessment of more peripheral vasculature. Increased magnetic field strength allows for a better signal to noise ratio and higher spatiotemporal resolution and studies using 7 T MRA have demonstrated excellent proximal vessel architecture and comparative brain anatomy and with the addition of contrast, good to excellent visualization of the more distal arteries [105]. The application of phase-contrast techniques (phase-contrast MR angiography, 4D-MRA, PCMRA) has transitioned MRA from a purely diagnostic tool into a valuable technique for assessment of cerebrovascular anatomy and physiology. In addition to structural information, PCMRA allows the characterization of velocity of flow within any given vessel. PCA has been utilized as a means of minimally invasive monitoring of cerebral vascular malformations with a quality comparable to the gold standard—digital subtraction catheter angiograms [106, 107] and in particular of hypertensive related pathology, cerebral aneurysms [108]. In addition to measures of velocity and diameter, PCA also allows the relatively simple calculation of total cerebral blood flow (CBF). In MRA, total CBF is usually estimated as the sum of total flow in the three main arteries. PCA has been shown to demonstrate effects of age in the presence of cerebrovascular risk factors on CBF [109] as well as in patients with significant cerebrovascular disease [110, 111]. PCMRA has demonstrated a consistent and predictable difference in middle cerebral arterial mean flow velocities compared to the current clinical standard, Transcranial Doppler [112, 113], and has demonstrated a nonsignificant difference compared to carotid duplex with excellent inter-rater agreement [111]. PCMRA is able to combine physiologic and high-resolution anatomic data in feasible manner but needs further validation.

MR Perfusion-Weighted Imaging

MR-based perfusion-weighted imaging (PWI) or Dynamic Susceptibility Contrast (DSC) MRI is a semiquantitative measure of brain perfusion or microcirculation in the capillary network. Contrast passing through the cerebral vasculature alters the local magnetic fields causing a transient drop in signal intensity of the surrounding brain tissue due to the contrast agent's paramagnetic effect on the surrounding tissue. The variation is measured over the course of about 1 min. From this data, time-concentration curves are obtained by deconvolution of arterial input and calculations are made for different perfusion parameters, such as the cerebral blood flow (CBF), cerebral blood volume (CBV), mean transit time (MTT), time to peak (TTP), and Tmax. It is important to note that CBF=CBV/MTT. PWI map specifics include CBF representing blood supply to the brain and are most directly related to viability of the infarcted tissue, CBV correlates well with the final size of the ischemic infarct, MTT shows a wide range of perfusion deficit and will likely overestimate areas at risk (includes benign oligemia) and TTP is an indirect measurement of brain perfusion and will also overestimate tissue at risk. Tmax is the time it takes for the tissue residue function to reach its maximum intensity and is sensitive parameter to reflect changes of brain tissue into an infarction and changes in the perfusion state [114]. Tmax is the most widely accepted parameter to measure penumbra but it has yet to be validated with different studies using difference times to best predict final infarct [114]. MRP in the evaluation of HTN is used most often in the evaluation of acute stroke. The focus is on the evaluation of the perfusion-diffusion (PWI-DWI), which theoretically identifies the penumbra or tissue at risk. Presence of an ischemic penumbra on imaging does not affect appropriate use of IV thrombolysis, but in consideration of research and mechanical thrombectomy, the absence of a PWI-DWI mismatch predicts poor outcome regardless of intervention [115]. An automated computer map, RAPID, has demonstrated potential to identify a PWI-DWI mismatch pattern in patients who improved with successful recanalization [116, 117]. A small study demonstrated that short-term pharmacologically induced hypertension in a cohort of acute stroke patients demonstrated increased cerebral perfusion and was associated with improved NIHSS and poststroke cognitive testing [118]. Hypertensive vasculopathy has been demonstrated to induce persistent hypoperfusion in an animal model [119] as well as a strong association with leukoariosis and decreased cerebral perfusion of the abnormal white matter in human subjects [120, 121] (Fig. 18.3).

General Advantages

In assessing the effects of HTN on brain structure and function, the advantages of MRI, especially at high-fields, 3 t and above, are numerous. MRI is superior to CT in the assessment of brain anatomy, which is always more detailed and clinically useful than CT (Table 18.2). This applies for volumes of small structures where the potential tissue volume loss is small in otherwise healthy adults as well as for characterization of effects on cerebral white matter. Developments of quantitative phase-contrast techniques have huge potential in this application, although yet to be fully examined. MR perfusion is a rapid sequence and can be accomplished in about a minute and cover the entire brain compared to a short 5 cm margin of most CT perfusion studies. Post contrast-imaging acquisition can be competed afterward

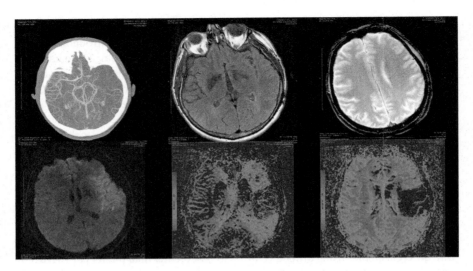

Fig. 18.3 A 62 years-old male with a left MCA stroke, image A is a CTA maximum intensity projection with a proximal middle cerebral artery cutoff, tPA was given, image B is a MRI with FLAIR hyperintense vessels, image C is a GRE with "blooming" of the penetrating vessels (increased cerebral blood volume), image D is a DWI with left frontal stroke and image E is a PWI-MTT map with a small amount of "mismatch" posterior to infarct (region of *light green*), image F demonstrates a PWI-CBV map with a dark core lesion correlating to the DWI lesion)

Table 18.2 Advantages and disadvantages of the major imaging modalities

Modality	Advantages	Disadvantages
Computed Tomography	• Fast	• Poor tissue contrast
	Can do angiography and perfusion scanning	• Radiation exposure
	• Widely available	• Uses iodinated contrast
MRI	• Excellent tissue contrast	• Time needed for scan
	• Can do angiography and perfusion scanning	• Interacts with medical devices Patient comfort limitation
	• Can evaluate fiber tract structure	• Contrast-induced systemic nephrogenic fibrosis in persons with renal failure
	• Representation of cortical function can be assessed	
	• Perfusion scan without need for contrast administration	
	• No radiation	
	• No iodinated contrast	
PET/SPECT	• Represent gold standard of cerebral metabolism and perfusion assessment	• Radiation exposure
	• Fast	• Limited availability
	• Repeatable	• Need special equipment to prepare contrast agents
		• Need CT or MRI to co-register for anatomic correlation

without adding significant time to imaging protocols. Advanced applications with MRI including diffusion tensor imaging (DTI), arterial spin labeling (ASL), and functional MRI (FMRI) also add to this significant list of advantages. Each of these will be discussed in detail in the following sections. Scan time has been argued as a general disadvantage for MRI but it has been demonstrated that MRI is feasible and able to meet current stroke guidelines for rapid administration of tPA with a 15-min protocol that includes DWI, FLAIR, GRE (SWI), time of flight MR angiogram, and a perfusion weighted study [92]. This allows for a more rapid and complete analysis of brain pathology and may have both research and clinical ramifications such as using FLAIR as an imaging tissue clock [87, 88]. MRI does not expose patient to radiation and gadolinium contrast is not nephrotoxic.

General Disadvantages

The main disadvantages with MRI relative to CT are cost and accessibility. MRI studies generally take significantly longer than CTs, about 15 min for a robust stroke study [92] and in general about 30–45 min. There are significant patient-related challenges in the use of MRI including foreign body ferromagnetic metals, some older aneurysm clips, medical stimulator, pace makers, and defibrillators. Many of these have been tested and approved for MRI, but in the case of a stimulator or pacemaker a qualified care provider is likely needed to assess these devices after a scan to ensure proper function and if needed reset the device. Another important contraindication is the limitation of gadolinium contrast in persons with end stage renal disease on hemodialysis as they may develop nephrogenic systemic fibrosis [122]. Most MRIs have stricter weight limits for patients than do CTs with the average allowable patient weight being under 300 lb. Finally, patient compliance in terms of motion and ability to lay still and claustrophobia are a common concern in many studies and affect not only the ability to conduct the study but also to interpret the images acquired.

Functional MRI

Functional magnetic resonance imaging (fMRI), a derivative of MR imaging, allows for the visualization of task-related brain activation [123]. During fMRI studies, a series of images (or volumes) are acquired as a participant performs a given task. The time-course of changes in local MR signal is then associated with the timing of the task being performed. To accomplish the temporal resolution required to investigate the time-course, spatial resolution is compromised. To overcome this significant limitation, the lower-resolution fMRI studies are generally statistically mapped onto a higher resolution anatomical scan. fMRI functions by utilizing the properties of blood flow and oxygen concentration changes that occur following neuronal firing as a marker for regional activity.

General Principles of FMRI

The link between neural activation and a local increase in CBF is the general basis of blood oxygen level dependent (BOLD) fMRI. When an area of the brain is activated by the demand to perform a task, the local neurons begin to fire and increase local metabolic activity in turn consuming oxyHb and increasing carbon dioxide and deoxyHb. Seconds after this drop in oxygenated hemoglobin, there is an increase in cerebral blood flow with an influx of fresh oxygenated hemoglobin. fMRI detects the change due to the difference in paramagnetic properties of oxyHb and deoxyHb, with deoxyHb being paramagnetic while oxyHb is not. On a T2* sequence, deoxyHb causes local dephasing of protons and reduces the return signal for tissues in the immediate vicinity which is the BOLD signal.

Uses

Functional MRI has not yet assumed a definitive role in the diagnostic evaluation of HTN and HTN-related disease. Animal model studies have demonstrated an increased BOLD response to moderate and severe hypertension as well as a decreased BOLD response to hypotension [124, 125]. BOLD imaging is being investigated at a potential marker for stroke related cerebral autoregulatory impairment. In studies with small sample sizes, a delay in BOLD signal response has been correlated to impairment of cerebral autoregulation [126, 127]. Here, the application of FMRI allows for the visualization of microvascular abnormalities, or hemodynamic impairment that may be associated with stroke risk. fMRI is now routinely used in poststroke research of brain function, plasticity, and prognostication of recovery. Generally, the primary measures used are the total volume of activation relative to controls both ipsilateral and contralateral to the infarct. These studies generally investigate the relative response either as a function of stroke or as a function of remapping of cortical controls following stroke [128, 129]. These studies not only offer information on cortical control of cognitive and motor functions but also on the local tissue perfusion during cognition. fMRI is in its infancy in regard to evaluation of HTN and its related diseases, but offers some direction into developing studies to evaluate poststroke motor recovery and HTN related cerebral autoregulatory impairment.

General Advantages

One of the major advantages of using fMRI is that it is a noninvasive technique requiring no use of intravenous contrast. Rather, fMRI relies upon the relative concentrations of oxyHb to deoxyHb in the blood as an endogenous contrast agent. This allows the clinician or researcher the availability to administer a number of scans on a single subject without sacrificing health or safety or having to control for change in contrast concentrations over time or over brain regions. The relevance of using fMRI to study HTN lies in its ability to visualize CBF as a function of neuronal activity. Unlike PET, studies using fMRI do not need to rely on an averaging across subjects because fMRI can accurately detect activation changes on the individual level. This is a crucial advantage as the effects of hypertension are highly variable and likely interact with a number of other factors (age, other cerebrovascular risk factors, significant medical history). Additionally, no ionizing radiation is needed as compared to PET. As MRI has become a mainstay clinical and research tool, availability of this technique has increased.

General Disadvantages

Despite FMRI's ability to provide spatially clear visualization of regional brain activation, it does have limitations imposed by the reliance on the cerebral microvascular system and the time-course of changes in blood flow. In a healthy adult, the time to a hemodynamic response from the initiation of cognitive or motor activity is 5–6 s. Also, since stressors, including claustrophobia, can transiently raise blood pressure and thus increase CBF, nonneural changes may have an influence on the BOLD signal, which, if they change over the course of the study, are difficult to account for in statistical models [125]. fMRI requires a high degree of patient compliance and is particularly sensitive to head movement and respiratory artifacts and requires significant amount of postprocessing.

Diffusion Tensor MR Imaging

Diffusion tensor magnetic resonance imaging (DTI) is a technique that allows quantitative assessment of mean diffusivity of water or metabolites and fractional anisotropy along organized white matter tracts. DTI allows for the visualization of microstructural organization, orientation, and the connectivity of the white matter fiber tracts in the brain based on the principal diffusion directions [130–133]. DTI allows for detection of microstructural changes of the brain related to different pathology such as traumatic brain injury, multiple sclerosis, CADASIL and of particular interest, hypertension related entities such as stroke and leukoariosis, before changes are noticed on traditional MRI sequences.

General Principles

DTI is a special form of diffusion-weighted imaging that allows the assessment and visualization of white matter and nerve fibers or the microstructure [133]. Conventional MRI pulse sequences do not allow for the examination of the integrity or directionality of white matter tracts. DTI takes advantage of the diffusivity of water and other metabolites and their diffusion parallel to white matter tracts with restriction noted perpendicular to the white matter tracts [130]. It is this shape of the restriction of diffusion that is assessed with DTI. In well-organized and intact white matter fiber tracts, the shape of water diffusion will occur preferentially along those tracts (anisotropy). When there is less organization or a lack of aligned and organized fiber structures, the shape of water diffusion will be more isotropic or in different directions [130, 132]. Commonly, the degree of alignment and anisotropy is calculated as the fractional anisotropy (FA). FA values range from 0 to 1, where 0 represents isotropic diffusion and 1 represents anisotropic diffusion [133]. Higher FA values are believed to represent such factors as degree of myelination and axonal density. The FA values are dependent upon the shape and primary direction of diffusion. These values can be combined in various methods to provide estimates of the axial and radial diffusivity in addition to more standard measures of water diffusion. DTI has been shown to distinguish between axonal and myelin injury by using axonal diffusivity as a marker of the integrity of axonal bodies and radial diffusivity as a measure of the degree of myelination [134–136].

Uses

Multiple studies have used DTI to determine microstructural changes in patients with small vessel disease/white matter changes or history of hypertension. A small study noted increased mean diffusivity (MD) and decreased FA in cohorts with clinical small vessel disease and leukoariosis and a nonclinical hypertensive cohort compared a normotensive cohort, but the study did not specify the region of interest as including leukoariosis or normal white matter [137]. Other studies have been able to identify microstructural changes in HTN patients prior to the appearance of white matter hyperintensities on FLAIR. Increased MD in normal white matter has been correlated to high diastolic blood pressure [138] and both decreased FA and increased MD are noted in normal appearing white matter prior to the development of FLAIR hyperintensities [139, 140]. Both cognitive impairment and gait difficulties have been correlated to increased MD in normal appearing white matter in hypertensive cohorts [141, 142]. DTI has found utility in monitoring research patients prior to visible imaging abnormalities or perhaps monitoring treatment effect and prognostication for cognitive impairment or worsening white matter changes.

General Advantages and Disadvantages

Diffusion tensor imaging shares many of the advantages and disadvantages of standard MR imaging. DTI is able to evaluate cerebral microstructure and correlate to other MRI sequences and be completed relatively quickly during a routine MRI protocol. The disadvantages of DTI are that it is not widespread in use and requires a significant amount of post processes and specific vendor software options.

Arterial Spin Labeling

Arterial spin labeling (ASL) is an alternative to the DSC method of MR perfusion scanning. Perfusion is quantified by measuring the magnetic state of inflowing blood in relation to the magnetic state of static tissue. ASL is, in particular, relevant to the study of the effects of HTN in the brain because differential vasodilatation effects potentially do not affect it.

General Principles and Technique

ASL allows for rapid quantitative measurements of perfusion in the brain taking about 2.5 min [143]. Arterial spin labeling takes advantage of the principles of endogenous tracers by taking advantage of arterial water as a feely diffusible tracer. First blood is magnetized proximal to the brain via a 180° radio frequency inversion pulse. The application of this pulse results in inversion of the net magnetization of the blood water; that is, the water molecules in the blood are now magnetically labeled and can be detected via MR imaging. After a period of time known as the "transit time," the magnetically labeled blood water travels to the region of interest and exchanges with the un-magnetized water present in the tissue altering total tissue magnetization. During this inflow of the inverted spin water molecules, total tissue magnetization is reduced, thereby reducing the MR signal and image intensity. At this point, a "tag image" is taken. The experiment is then repeated without labeling the arterial blood to create a control image. To produce an image showing blood perfusion, the tag image is subtracted from the control image. The resulting image reflects the total amount of arterial blood delivered to each voxel in the region of interest within the transit time.

Two major subgroups of ASL perfusion imaging exist, continuous ASL and pulsed ASL. In continuous ASL (CASL), a continuous radio frequency pulse is applied to the targeted region below the slice of interest, resulting in continuous inversion of the magnetization of arterial blood water. Because of this continuous inversion, a steady state develops in which regional magnetization in the brain is directly related to cerebral blood flow [144]. In pulsed ASL (PASL), a short 10 ms radio frequency pulse is used to label blood water spins over a very specific area which allows for minimization of the distance between the labeling region and the imaging slice [145]. Both have advantages and disadvantages.

Uses and Measures

ASL has been used in acute stroke research as a noninvasive way to evaluate perfusion. In patients who have renal disease and are at risk for developing nephrogenic systemic fibrosis, ASL provides a feasible and noninvasive method for assessing rCBF during imaging assessment of an acute stroke [143, 146–148]. Perfusion maps need varying amount of postprocessing and limitations include only moderate inter-rater agreement with visual assessment [148] and ASL tends to miss smaller perfusion deficits compared to DSC [143, 147]. ASL correlates well to NIHSS and outcome mRS during acute evaluation for stroke [146].

ASL has been used to measure the effects of cerebrovascular risk factors, such as HTN, on regional cerebral blood flow, in an attempt to correlate regional cerebral blood flow with specific risk factors. For example, HTN was found to be significantly associated with higher regional cerebral blood flow compared to other cerebrovascular risk factors such as body mass index (BMI), carotid artery stenosis, and diabetes mellitus [149].

General Advantages

Probably, the most noteworthy advantage of the ASL technique is that no exogenous contrast agent is needed. Acquisition times are fast and the technique has been used in time sensitive applications such as stroke. Additionally, multiple sequential ASL maps can be obtained and it can be used for functional applications as well as real-time cerebrovascular hemodynamic applications.

General Disadvantages

Some limitation of arterial spin labeling includes error in tagging blood as the time taken for the inverted-spin water molecules to travel from the region of inversion to the region of interest is nonzero. Additionally, visualization of small perfusion defects is often missed [147]. ASL is not widespread, and expertise in interpretation of images is limited to larger academic centers. Head motion artifacts are more significant because subtraction is necessary and it requires high concordance between subsequent images.

Positron Emission Tomography and Single Photon Emission Computerized Tomography

General Principles and Technique

PET imaging applications include functional neuroimaging, metabolic imaging, and evaluation of specific pathology that can bind to a given radiotracer. PET functional neuroimaging is based on an assumption that areas of high blood flow are also areas of high radioactivity. SPECT neuroimaging is similar to PET in that they both detect a radioactive tracer with gamma rays. Typically, SPECT radiotracers are ^{99m}Technetium, ^{123}Iodine, and ^{111m}Indium. PET imaging typically uses oxygen-15 labeled water (^{15}O) and fluorine 18-labeled deoxyglucose (^{18}F-FDG). The difference arises in that the tracer used in SPECT releases gamma rays that are directly detected. PET, on the other hand, uses a tracer that releases positrons that annihilate with electrons and subsequently form a pair of gamma photons that are emitted at a 180° direction from each other [150]. This allows for better localization of the source of the radiation. ^{15}O labeled water is typically used for measuring perfusion (CBV, CBF) and ^{15}O labeled oxygen is used for measuring oxygen extraction fraction (OEF). MTT and cerebral metabolic rate of oxygen (CMRO$_2$) are calculated from CBV, CBF, and OEF, respectively [150]. FDG-PET uses ^{18}F-FDG to monitor glucose metabolism.

Uses and Measures

PET scanning has been the modality of choice in the evaluation of the physiological and metabolic effects of HTN and related pathologies on the brain. PET parameters tested in hypertension as well as stroke and carotid disease are CBF, CBV, MTT, and OEF. Long-term HTN has been associated with a decrease in resting rCBF compared to healthy controls of similar age, noted in the prefrontal, anterior cingulate, and occipital areas [12] and task associated blunting of rCBF in the posterior parietal regions, thalamus, and middle cerebral artery watershed territory [151]. PET has been used to evaluate treatment effects of HTN in cognitive tasks. One study tested for improved regional blood flow of hypertensive patients on blood pressure treatment or control with memory tasks and acetazolamide challenge and found no improvement with rCBF [152]. The same group focused rCBF region of interest on the thalamus and found a blood flow response in treated hypertensive patients in the thalamus compared to control [153]. Mild hypertensive patients were found to have reduced rCBF in the prefrontal cortex and basal ganglia compared to normotensive patients, decreased CBF was found in moderate hypertensive patients compared to normal controls and in spontaneously hypertensive rats, there was a cortical and thalamic reduction in rCBF compared to normotensive rats [154]. PET has demonstrated the effect of hypertension on rCBF, the physiologic effect of cognition associated with long-standing HTN, and possibly improved rCBF with treatment of HTN [155].

Current clinical evaluation of treatment of carotid stenosis relies on a degree of stenosis, typically 60–70 % in a person with symptomatic disease. Research efforts have been directed in evaluating plaque morphology and composition in order to attempt to predict future stroke. PET identifies regions of inflammation with increased uptake of ^{18}F-FDG into the plaque but needs to co-registered with CTA [156–158], MRI [159], and carotid duplex [160] SPECT uses radiolabeled tracers to LDL or oxidized LDL (MDA2 epitopes on oxidized LDL), apo-B portion of LDL, macrophages expressive cell surface Fc receptors, and GPIIa/IIIb receptor antibodies for the identification of vulnerable plaque but has less resolution than

PET [161, 162]. Another use of PET is to correlate an increased oxygen ejection fraction (rOEF) as a region of tissue at risk that will progress to infarction with atherosclerotic carotid occlusion/stenosis, as OEF is an indicator of mismatch between metabolic demand and cerebral blood flow [150]. A study evaluating extracranial-intracranial bypass in persons with resent carotid occlusion was assessed using an OEF ratio suspected of being high risk for continued infarction; however, the procedure added no benefit compared to control [163].

General Advantages

^{15}O PET, FDG-PET, and SPECT all allow for quantification different quantitative parameters of brain hemodynamics, such as rCBFm rCBV, (rOEF) and metabolic rate (rCMRO2). PET gives physiological information, indirect information on neuronal and neurotransmitter activity. In addition, these modalities allow for evaluation of function both at rest and during neuropsychological testing. PET can be used to monitor pharmacologic efficacy as in a study that demonstrated decreased plaque inflammation with intensive statin use [164].

General Disadvantages

PET scan takes approximately 5–10 min [165]. The information regarding function allows for information co-registration with a CT scan or MRI which is needed in order to obtain structural correlation. In addition, it is quite expensive and reimbursement for clinical application may be limited to neuro-oncological evaluation. PET is subject to full width, half maximum (FWHM) and partial volume-averaging artifact phenomenon, due to detection of radiation in an area greater than the target tissue [123]. SPECT and FDG-PET are less expensive and more likely to be reimbursed [166]. PET has limited spatial resolution of about 5 mm; co-registration with CT or high resolution MRI can improve resolution. SPECT has a spatial resolution of about 10 mm, and like PET can be co-registered with CT to improve resolution [162]. The expense and radiation exposure of PET, FDG-PET, and SPECT make them all poor screening modalities, although their mechanism of detection makes them superior in screening vulnerable physiologic states for infarction, multiple modal MRI and CT can now provide much of the same physiological data. Additionally, many of the tracers in PET require a cyclotron nearby due to the short half-life of these tracers.

Summary and Conclusions

Recent advances in neuroimaging, together with the increasing availability of high-field MRI systems at most major medical centers, provide the foundation for the expectation that MRI-based measures will allow better quantification and qualification of the effects of HTN on the brain. MRI offers the most robust evaluation of anatomic and physiologic parameters. Arterial spin labeling has the added benefit of repeated perfusion studies without the need for contrast neither administration nor radiation exposure. MRI is clearly superior to CT for studies of brain structure and function and MRI also has been proven feasible for acute evaluation of HTN related pathologies, and CT remains relatively less expensive, fast, and more widely available. PET and SPECT represent the gold standard in evaluating and quantifying cerebral physiology and metabolism but require significant radiation exposure, have high cost, require MRI or CT co-registration for anatomical correlation and have limited availability.

References

1. Brott T, Thalinger K, Hertzberg V. Hypertension as a risk factor for spontaneous intracerebral hemorrhage. Stroke. 1986;17:1078–83.
2. Cole FM, Yates P. Intracerebral microaneurysms and small cerebrovascular lesions. Brain. 1967;90:759–68.
3. Fisher CM. Pathological observations in hypertensive cerebral hemorrhage. J Neuropathol Exp Neurol. 1971;30:536–50.
4. Fisher CM. Cerebral miliary aneurysms in hypertension. Am J Pathol. 1972;66:313–30.
5. Rosenblum WI. Miliary aneurysms and "fibrinoid" degeneration of cerebral blood vessels. Hum Pathol. 1977;8:133–9.
6. Rossrussell RW. Observations on intracerebral aneurysms. Brain. 1963;86:425–42.
7. Takebayashi S, Kaneko M. Electron microscopic studies of ruptured arteries in hypertensive intracerebral hemorrhage. Stroke. 1983;14:28–36.
8. Wakai S, Nagai M. Histological verification of microaneurysms as a cause of cerebral haemorrhage in surgical specimens. J Neurol Neurosurg Psychiatry. 1989;52:595–9.
9. Poels MM, Vernooij MW, Ikram MA, et al. Prevalence and risk factors of cerebral microbleeds: an update of the Rotterdam scan study. Stroke. 2010;41:S103–6.
10. Vernooij MW, van der Lugt A, Ikram MA, et al. Prevalence and risk factors of cerebral microbleeds: the Rotterdam Scan Study. Neurology. 2008;70:1208–14.
11. Paulson OB, Strandgaard S, Edvinsson L. Cerebral autoregulation. Cerebrovasc Brain Metab Rev. 1990;2:161–92.
12. Beason-Held LL, Moghekar A, Zonderman AB, Kraut MA, Resnick SM. Longitudinal changes in cerebral blood flow in the older hypertensive brain. Stroke. 2007;38:1766–73.
13. Dai W, Lopez OL, Carmichael OT, Becker JT, Kuller LH, Gach HM. Abnormal regional cerebral blood flow in cognitively normal elderly subjects with hypertension. Stroke. 2008;39:349–54.
14. Smith EE, Gurol ME, Eng JA, et al. White matter lesions, cognition, and recurrent hemorrhage in lobar intracerebral hemorrhage. Neurology. 2004;63:1606–12.
15. Chutinet A, Biffi A, Kanakis A, Fitzpatrick KM, Furie KL, Rost NS. Severity of leukoaraiosis in large vessel atherosclerotic disease. AJNR Am J Neuroradiol. 2012;33:1591–5.
16. Firbank MJ, Wiseman RM, Burton EJ, Saxby BK, O'Brien JT, Ford GA. Brain atrophy and white matter hyperintensity change in older adults and relationship to blood pressure. Brain atrophy, WMH change and blood pressure. J Neurol. 2007;254:713–21.
17. Schmidt R, Enzinger C, Ropele S, Schmidt H, Fazekas F, Austrian Stroke Prevention S. Progression of cerebral white matter lesions: 6-year results of the Austrian Stroke Prevention Study. Lancet. 2003;361:2046–8.
18. Schmidt R, Schmidt H, Kapeller P, et al. The natural course of MRI white matter hyperintensities. J Neurol Sci. 2002;203-204:253–7.

19. Schmidt R, Schmidt H, Kapeller P, Lechner A, Fazekas F. Evolution of white matter lesions. Cerebrovasc Dis. 2002;13 Suppl 2:16–20.

20. Wen W, Sachdev PS, Chen X, Anstey K. Gray matter reduction is correlated with white matter hyperintensity volume: a voxel-based morphometric study in a large epidemiological sample. Neuroimage. 2006;29:1031–9.

21. Wiseman RM, Saxby BK, Burton EJ, Barber R, Ford GA, O'Brien JT. Hippocampal atrophy, whole brain volume, and white matter lesions in older hypertensive subjects. Neurology. 2004;63:1892–7.

22. Gottesman RF, Coresh J, Catellier DJ, et al. Blood pressure and white-matter disease progression in a biethnic cohort: Atherosclerosis Risk in Communities (ARIC) study. Stroke. 2010;41:3–8.

23. Havlik RJ, Foley DJ, Sayer B, Masaki K, White L, Launer LJ. Variability in midlife systolic blood pressure is related to late-life brain white matter lesions: the Honolulu-Asia Aging study. Stroke. 2002;33:26–30.

24. Qiu C, Winblad B, Fratiglioni L. The age-dependent relation of blood pressure to cognitive function and dementia. Lancet Neurol. 2005;4:487–99.

25. Swan GE, Carmelli D, Larue A. Systolic blood pressure tracking over 25 to 30 years and cognitive performance in older adults. Stroke. 1998;29:2334–40.

26. Harrington F, Saxby BK, McKeith IG, Wesnes K, Ford GA. Cognitive performance in hypertensive and normotensive older subjects. Hypertension. 2000;36:1079–82.

27. Freitag MH, Peila R, Masaki K, et al. Midlife pulse pressure and incidence of dementia: the Honolulu-Asia Aging Study. Stroke. 2006;37:33–7.

28. Skoog I. Hypertension and cognition. Int Psychogeriatr. 2003;15 Suppl 1:139–46.

29. Skoog I, Gustafson D. Hypertension, hypertension-clustering factors and Alzheimer's disease. Neurol Res. 2003;25:675–80.

30. Petrovitch H, White LR, Izmirilian G, et al. Midlife blood pressure and neuritic plaques, neurofibrillary tangles, and brain weight at death: the HAAS. Honolulu-Asia aging Study. Neurobiol Aging. 2000;21:57–62.

31. Rodrigue KM, Rieck JR, Kennedy KM, Devous Sr MD, Diaz-Arrastia R, Park DC. Risk factors for beta-amyloid deposition in healthy aging: vascular and genetic effects. JAMA Neurol. 2013;70:600–6.

32. Sparks DL, Scheff SW, Liu H, Landers TM, Coyne CM, Hunsaker 3rd JC. Increased incidence of neurofibrillary tangles (NFT) in non-demented individuals with hypertension. J Neurol Sci. 1995;131:162–9.

33. Peila R, White LR, Petrovich H, et al. Joint effect of the APOE gene and midlife systolic blood pressure on late-life cognitive impairment: the Honolulu-Asia aging study. Stroke. 2001;32:2882–9.

34. Launer LJ, Hughes T, Yu B, et al. Lowering midlife levels of systolic blood pressure as a public health strategy to reduce late-life dementia: perspective from the Honolulu Heart Program/Honolulu Asia Aging Study. Hypertension. 2010;55:1352–9.

35. Feart C, Samieri C, Rondeau V, et al. Adherence to a Mediterranean diet, cognitive decline, and risk of dementia. JAMA. 2009;302:638–48.

36. Scarmeas N, Luchsinger JA, Schupf N, et al. Physical activity, diet, and risk of Alzheimer disease. JAMA. 2009;302:627–37.

37. Scarmeas N, Stern Y, Mayeux R, Manly JJ, Schupf N, Luchsinger JA. Mediterranean diet and mild cognitive impairment. Arch Neurol. 2009;66:216–25.

38. Yaffe K, Fiocco AJ, Lindquist K, et al. Predictors of maintaining cognitive function in older adults: the Health ABC study. Neurology. 2009;72:2029–35.

39. Larson EB, Wang L, Bowen JD, et al. Exercise is associated with reduced risk for incident dementia among persons 65 years of age and older. Ann Intern Med. 2006;144:73–81.

40. Matthews DC, Davies M, Murray J, et al. Physical activity, Mediterranean diet and Biomarkers-Assessed Risk of Alzheimer's: a Multi-Modality Brain Imaging Study. Adv J Mol Imag. 2014;4:43–57.

41. Wada R, Aviv RI, Fox AJ, et al. CT angiography "spot sign" predicts hematoma expansion in acute intracerebral hemorrhage. Stroke. 2007;38:1257–62.
42. Al-Nakshabandi NA. The swirl sign. Radiology. 2001;218:433.
43. Barber PA, Demchuk AM, Zhang J, Buchan AM. Validity and reliability of a quantitative computed tomography score in predicting outcome of hyperacute stroke before thrombolytic therapy. ASPECTS Study Group. Alberta Stroke Programme Early CT Score. Lancet. 2000;355:1670–4.
44. Pexman JH, Barber PA, Hill MD, et al. Use of the Alberta Stroke Program Early CT Score (ASPECTS) for assessing CT scans in patients with acute stroke. AJNR Am J Neuroradiol. 2001;22:1534–42.
45. Tomura N, Uemura K, Inugami A, Fujita H, Higano S, Shishido F. Early CT finding in cerebral infarction: obscuration of the lentiform nucleus. Radiology. 1988;168:463–7.
46. Truwit CL, Barkovich AJ, Gean-Marton A, Hibri N, Norman D. Loss of the insular ribbon: another early CT sign of acute middle cerebral artery infarction. Radiology. 1990;176:801–6.
47. Dippel DW, Du Ry van Beest HM, van Kooten F, Koudstaal PJ. The validity and reliability of signs of early infarction on CT in acute ischaemic stroke. Neuroradiology. 2000;42:629–33.
48. Wardlaw JM, Mielke O. Early signs of brain infarction at CT: observer reliability and outcome after thrombolytic treatment—systematic review. Radiology. 2005;235:444–53.
49. Hacke W, Kaste M, Fieschi C, et al. Intravenous thrombolysis with recombinant tissue plasminogen activator for acute hemispheric stroke. The European Cooperative Acute Stroke Study (ECASS). JAMA. 1995;274:1017–25.
50. Chen CJ, Lee TH, Hsu HL, et al. Multi-Slice CT angiography in diagnosing total versus near occlusions of the internal carotid artery: comparison with catheter angiography. Stroke. 2004;35:83–5.
51. Josephson SA, Bryant SO, Mak HK, Johnston SC, Dillon WP, Smith WS. Evaluation of carotid stenosis using CT angiography in the initial evaluation of stroke and TIA. Neurology. 2004;63:457–60.
52. Walker LJ, Ismail A, McMeekin W, Lambert D, Mendelow AD, Birchall D. Computed tomography angiography for the evaluation of carotid atherosclerotic plaque: correlation with histopathology of endarterectomy specimens. Stroke. 2002;33:977–81.
53. Berkhemer OA, Fransen PS, Beumer D, et al. A randomized trial of intraarterial treatment for acute ischemic stroke. N Engl J Med. 2015;372:11–20.
54. Goyal M, Demchuk AM, Menon BK, et al. Randomized assessment of rapid endovascular treatment of ischemic stroke. N Engl J Med. 2015;372:1019–30.
55. Nambiar V, Sohn SI, Almekhlafi MA, et al. CTA collateral status and response to recanalization in patients with acute ischemic stroke. AJNR Am J Neuroradiol. 2014;35:884–90.
56. Wintermark M, Flanders AE, Velthuis B, et al. Perfusion-CT assessment of infarct core and penumbra: receiver operating characteristic curve analysis in 130 patients suspected of acute hemispheric stroke. Stroke. 2006;37:979–85.
57. Wintermark M, Meuli R, Browaeys P, et al. Comparison of CT perfusion and angiography and MRI in selecting stroke patients for acute treatment. Neurology. 2007;68:694–7.
58. Wintermark M, Reichhart M, Cuisenaire O, et al. Comparison of admission perfusion computed tomography and qualitative diffusion- and perfusion-weighted magnetic resonance imaging in acute stroke patients. Stroke. 2002;33:2025–31.
59. Wintermark M, Rowley HA, Lev MH. Acute stroke triage to intravenous thrombolysis and other therapies with advanced CT or MR imaging: pro CT. Radiology. 2009;251:619–26.
60. Yang CY, Chen YF, Lee CW, et al. Multiphase CT angiography versus single-phase CT angiography: comparison of image quality and radiation dose. AJNR Am J Neuroradiol. 2008;29:1288–95.
61. Gleeson TG, Bulugahapitiya S. Contrast-induced nephropathy. AJR Am J Roentgenol. 2004;183:1673–89.

62. Mitchell AM, Jones AE, Tumlin JA, Kline JA. Incidence of contrast-induced nephropathy after contrast-enhanced computed tomography in the outpatient setting. Clin J Am Soc Nephrol. 2010;5:4–9.
63. Nabavi DG, Cenic A, Dool J, et al. Quantitative assessment of cerebral hemodynamics using CT: stability, accuracy, and precision studies in dogs. J Comput Assist Tomogr. 1999;23:506–15.
64. Gonzalez RG. Imaging-guided acute ischemic stroke therapy: From "time is brain" to "physiology is brain". AJNR Am J Neuroradiol. 2006;27:728–35.
65. Latchaw RE, Yonas H, Hunter GJ, et al. Guidelines and recommendations for perfusion imaging in cerebral ischemia: a scientific statement for healthcare professionals by the writing group on perfusion imaging, from the Council on Cardiovascular Radiology of the American Heart Association. Stroke. 2003;34:1084–104.
66. Mettler Jr FA, Huda W, Yoshizumi TT, Mahesh M. Effective doses in radiology and diagnostic nuclear medicine: a catalog. Radiology. 2008;248:254–63.
67. Smith-Bindman R, Lipson J, Marcus R, et al. Radiation dose associated with common computed tomography examinations and the associated lifetime attributable risk of cancer. Arch Intern Med. 2009;169:2078–86.
68. Strassburger TL, Lee HC, Daly EM, et al. Interactive effects of age and hypertension on volumes of brain structures. Stroke. 1997;28:1410–7.
69. Breteler MM, van Amerongen NM, van Swieten JC, et al. Cognitive correlates of ventricular enlargement and cerebral white matter lesions on magnetic resonance imaging. The Rotterdam Study. Stroke. 1994;25:1109–15.
70. Constans JM, Meyerhoff DJ, Norman D, Fein G, Weiner MW. 1H and 31P magnetic resonance spectroscopic imaging of white matter signal hyperintensity areas in elderly subjects. Neuroradiology. 1995;37:615–23.
71. Fazekas F, Kleinert R, Offenbacher H, et al. The morphologic correlate of incidental punctate white matter hyperintensities on MR images. AJNR Am J Neuroradiol. 1991;12:915–21.
72. Gunning-Dixon FM, Raz N. The cognitive correlates of white matter abnormalities in normal aging: a quantitative review. Neuropsychology. 2000;14:224–32.
73. Fazekas F, Kleinert R, Offenbacher H, et al. Pathologic correlates of incidental MRI white matter signal hyperintensities. Neurology. 1993;43:1683–9.
74. de Leeuw FE, de Groot JC, Achten E, et al. Prevalence of cerebral white matter lesions in elderly people: a population based magnetic resonance imaging study. The Rotterdam Scan Study. J Neurol Neurosurg Psychiatry. 2001;70:9–14.
75. den Heijer T, Launer LJ, Prins ND, et al. Association between blood pressure, white matter lesions, and atrophy of the medial temporal lobe. Neurology. 2005;64:263–7.
76. Offenbacher H, Fazekas F, Schmidt R, Koch M, Fazekas G, Kapeller P. MR of cerebral abnormalities concomitant with primary intracerebral hematomas. AJNR Am J Neuroradiol. 1996;17:573–8.
77. Vernooij MW, Ikram MA, Wielopolski PA, Krestin GP, Breteler MM, van der Lugt A. Cerebral microbleeds: accelerated 3D T2*-weighted GRE MR imaging versus conventional 2D T2*-weighted GRE MR imaging for detection. Radiology. 2008;248:272–7.
78. Lee SH, Ryu WS, Roh JK. Cerebral microbleeds are a risk factor for warfarin-related intracerebral hemorrhage. Neurology. 2009;72:171–6.
79. Soo YO, Yang SR, Lam WW, et al. Risk vs benefit of anti-thrombotic therapy in ischaemic stroke patients with cerebral microbleeds. J Neurol. 2008;255:1679–86.
80. Werring DJ, Gregoire SM, Cipolotti L. Cerebral microbleeds and vascular cognitive impairment. J Neurol Sci. 2010;299:131–5.
81. Fiehler J, Albers GW, Boulanger JM, et al. Bleeding risk analysis in stroke imaging before thromboLysis (BRASIL): pooled analysis of T2*-weighted magnetic resonance imaging data from 570 patients. Stroke. 2007;38:2738–44.
82. Kidwell CS, Saver JL, Villablanca JP, et al. Magnetic resonance imaging detection of microbleeds before thrombolysis: an emerging application. Stroke. 2002;33:95–8.

83. Schlaug G, Benfield A, Baird AE, et al. The ischemic penumbra: operationally defined by diffusion and perfusion MRI. Neurology. 1999;53:1528–37.
84. Kamran S, Bates V, Bakshi R, Wright P, Kinkel W, Miletich R. Significance of hyperintense vessels on FLAIR MRI in acute stroke. Neurology. 2000;55:265–9.
85. Lee KY, Latour LL, Luby M, Hsia AW, Merino JG, Warach S. Distal hyperintense vessels on FLAIR: an MRI marker for collateral circulation in acute stroke? Neurology. 2009;72:1134–9.
86. Schellinger PD, Chalela JA, Kang DW, Latour LL, Warach S. Diagnostic and prognostic value of early MR Imaging vessel signs in hyperacute stroke patients imaged <3 hours and treated with recombinant tissue plasminogen activator. AJNR Am J Neuroradiol. 2005;26:618–24.
87. Thomalla G, Cheng B, Ebinger M, et al. DWI-FLAIR mismatch for the identification of patients with acute ischaemic stroke within 4.5 h of symptom onset (PRE-FLAIR): a multi-centre observational study. Lancet Neurol. 2011;10:978–86.
88. Thomalla G, Rossbach P, Rosenkranz M, et al. Negative fluid-attenuated inversion recovery imaging identifies acute ischemic stroke at 3 hours or less. Ann Neurol. 2009;65:724–32.
89. Assouline E, Benziane K, Reizine D, et al. Intra-arterial thrombus visualized on T2* gradient echo imaging in acute ischemic stroke. Cerebrovasc Dis. 2005;20:6–11.
90. Chalela JA, Haymore JB, Ezzeddine MA, Davis LA, Warach S. The hypointense MCA sign. Neurology. 2002;58:1470.
91. Flacke S, Urbach H, Keller E, et al. Middle cerebral artery (MCA) susceptibility sign at susceptibility-based perfusion MR imaging: clinical importance and comparison with hyper-dense MCA sign at CT. Radiology. 2000;215:476–82.
92. Shah S, Luby M, Poole K, et al. Screening with MRI for Accurate and Rapid Stroke Treatment: SMART. Neurology. 2015;84(24):2438–44.
93. Yuan C, Beach KW, Smith Jr LH, Hatsukami TS. Measurement of atherosclerotic carotid plaque size in vivo using high resolution magnetic resonance imaging. Circulation. 1998;98:2666–71.
94. Fayad ZA, Fuster V. The human high-risk plaque and its detection by magnetic resonance imaging. Am J Cardiol. 2001;88:42E–5.
95. Yuan C, Zhang SX, Polissar NL, et al. Identification of fibrous cap rupture with magnetic resonance imaging is highly associated with recent transient ischemic attack or stroke. Circulation. 2002;105:181–5.
96. Takaya N, Yuan C, Chu B, et al. Association between carotid plaque characteristics and sub-sequent ischemic cerebrovascular events: a prospective assessment with MRI—initial results. Stroke. 2006;37:818–23.
97. Cai J, Hatsukami TS, Ferguson MS, et al. In vivo quantitative measurement of intact fibrous cap and lipid-rich necrotic core size in atherosclerotic carotid plaque: comparison of high-resolution, contrast-enhanced magnetic resonance imaging and histology. Circulation. 2005;112:3437–44.
98. Hatsukami TS, Ross R, Polissar NL, Yuan C. Visualization of fibrous cap thickness and rupture in human atherosclerotic carotid plaque in vivo with high-resolution magnetic resonance imaging. Circulation. 2000;102:959–64.
99. Saam T, Ferguson MS, Yarnykh VL, et al. Quantitative evaluation of carotid plaque composition by in vivo MRI. Arterioscler Thromb Vasc Biol. 2005;25:234–9.
100. Touze E, Toussaint JF, Coste J, et al. Reproducibility of high-resolution MRI for the identification and the quantification of carotid atherosclerotic plaque components: consequences for prognosis studies and therapeutic trials. Stroke. 2007;38:1812–9.
101. Silvera SS, Aidi HE, Rudd JH, et al. Multimodality imaging of atherosclerotic plaque activity and composition using FDG-PET/CT and MRI in carotid and femoral arteries. Atherosclerosis. 2009;207:139–43.
102. Kooi ME, Cappendijk VC, Cleutjens KB, et al. Accumulation of ultrasmall superparamagnetic particles of iron oxide in human atherosclerotic plaques can be detected by in vivo magnetic resonance imaging. Circulation. 2003;107:2453–8.

103. Gupta A, Mushlin AI, Kamel H, Navi BB, Pandya A. Cost-effectiveness of carotid plaque MR imaging as a stroke risk stratification tool in asymptomatic carotid artery stenosis. Radiology. 2015;277(3):763–72.
104. White PM, Teasdale EM, Wardlaw JM, Easton V. Intracranial aneurysms: CT angiography and MR angiography for detection prospective blinded comparison in a large patient cohort. Radiology. 2001;219:739–49.
105. Umutlu L, Theysohn N, Maderwald S, et al. 7 Tesla MPRAGE imaging of the intracranial arterial vasculature: nonenhanced versus contrast-enhanced. Acad Radiol. 2013;20:628–34.
106. Forkert ND, Fiehler J, Illies T, Moller DP, Handels H, Saring D. 4D blood flow visualization fusing 3D and 4D MRA image sequences. J Magn Reson Imaging. 2012;36:443–53.
107. Hadizadeh DR, Kukuk GM, Steck DT, et al. Noninvasive evaluation of cerebral arteriovenous malformations by 4D-MRA for preoperative planning and postoperative follow-up in 56 patients: comparison with DSA and intraoperative findings. AJNR Am J Neuroradiol. 2012;33:1095–101.
108. Parmar H, Ivancevic MK, Dudek N, et al. Neuroradiologic applications of dynamic MR angiography at 3 T. Magn Reson Imaging Clin N Am. 2009;17:63–75.
109. Buijs PC, Krabbe-Hartkamp MJ, Bakker CJ, et al. Effect of age on cerebral blood flow: measurement with ungated two-dimensional phase-contrast MR angiography in 250 adults. Radiology. 1998;209:667–74.
110. Amin-Hanjani S, Du X, Zhao M, Walsh K, Malisch TW, Charbel FT. Use of quantitative magnetic resonance angiography to stratify stroke risk in symptomatic vertebrobasilar disease. Stroke. 2005;36:1140–5.
111. Harloff A, Zech T, Wegent F, Strecker C, Weiller C, Markl M. Comparison of blood flow velocity quantification by 4D flow MR imaging with ultrasound at the carotid bifurcation. AJNR Am J Neuroradiol. 2013;34:1407–13.
112. Chang W, Landgraf B, Johnson KM, et al. Velocity measurements in the middle cerebral arteries of healthy volunteers using 3D radial phase-contrast HYPRFlow: comparison with transcranial Doppler sonography and 2D phase-contrast MR imaging. AJNR Am J Neuroradiol. 2011;32:54–9.
113. Enzmann DR, Ross MR, Marks MP, Pelc NJ. Blood flow in major cerebral arteries measured by phase-contrast cine MR. AJNR Am J Neuroradiol. 1994;15:123–9.
114. Kim BJ, Kang HG, Kim HJ, et al. Magnetic resonance imaging in acute ischemic stroke treatment. J Stroke. 2014;16:131–45.
115. Kidwell CS, Jahan R, Gornbein J, et al. A trial of imaging selection and endovascular treatment for ischemic stroke. N Engl J Med. 2013;368:914–23.
116. Lansberg MG, Lee J, Christensen S, et al. RAPID automated patient selection for reperfusion therapy: a pooled analysis of the Echoplanar Imaging Thrombolytic Evaluation Trial (EPITHET) and the Diffusion and Perfusion Imaging Evaluation for Understanding Stroke Evolution (DEFUSE) Study. Stroke. 2011;42:1608–14.
117. Lansberg MG, Straka M, Kemp S, et al. MRI profile and response to endovascular reperfusion after stroke (DEFUSE 2): a prospective cohort study. Lancet Neurol. 2012;11:860–7.
118. Hillis AE, Ulatowski JA, Barker PB, et al. A pilot randomized trial of induced blood pressure elevation: effects on function and focal perfusion in acute and subacute stroke. Cerebrovasc Dis. 2003;16:236–46.
119. Henning EC, Warach S, Spatz M. Hypertension-induced vascular remodeling contributes to reduced cerebral perfusion and the development of spontaneous stroke in aged SHRSP rats. J Cereb Blood Flow Metab. 2010;30:827–36.
120. Markus HS, Lythgoe DJ, Ostegaard L, O'Sullivan M, Williams SC. Reduced cerebral blood flow in white matter in ischaemic leukoaraiosis demonstrated using quantitative exogenous contrast based perfusion MRI. J Neurol Neurosurg Psychiatry. 2000;69:48–53.
121. O'Sullivan M, Lythgoe DJ, Pereira AC, et al. Patterns of cerebral blood flow reduction in patients with ischemic leukoaraiosis. Neurology. 2002;59:321–6.

122. Kuo PH, Kanal E, Abu-Alfa AK, Cowper SE. Gadolinium-based MR contrast agents and nephrogenic systemic fibrosis. Radiology. 2007;242:647–9.
123. Dickerson BC. Advances in functional magnetic resonance imaging: technology and clinical applications. Neurotherapeutics. 2007;4:360–70.
124. Qiao M, Rushforth D, Wang R, et al. Blood-oxygen-level-dependent magnetic resonance signal and cerebral oxygenation responses to brain activation are enhanced by concurrent transient hypertension in rats. J Cereb Blood Flow Metab. 2007;27:1280–9.
125. Wang R, Foniok T, Wamsteeker JI, et al. Transient blood pressure changes affect the functional magnetic resonance imaging detection of cerebral activation. Neuroimage. 2006;31:1–11.
126. Altamura C, Reinhard M, Vry MS, et al. The longitudinal changes of BOLD response and cerebral hemodynamics from acute to subacute stroke. A fMRI and TCD study. BMC Neurosci. 2009;10:151.
127. Amemiya S, Kunimatsu A, Saito N, Ohtomo K. Impaired hemodynamic response in the ischemic brain assessed with BOLD fMRI. Neuroimage. 2012;61:579–90.
128. Loubinoux I, Dechaumont-Palacin S, Castel-Lacanal E, et al. Prognostic value of FMRI in recovery of hand function in subcortical stroke patients. Cereb Cortex. 2007;17:2980–7.
129. Pineiro R, Pendlebury S, Johansen-Berg H, Matthews PM. Altered hemodynamic responses in patients after subcortical stroke measured by functional MRI. Stroke. 2002;33:103–9.
130. Basser PJ, Mattiello J, LeBihan D. MR diffusion tensor spectroscopy and imaging. Biophys J. 1994;66:259–67.
131. Basser PJ, Pajevic S, Pierpaoli C, Duda J, Aldroubi A. In vivo fiber tractography using DT-MRI data. Magn Reson Med. 2000;44:625–32.
132. Basser PJ, Pierpaoli C. Microstructural and physiological features of tissues elucidated by quantitative-diffusion-tensor MRI. J Magn Reson B. 1996;111:209–19.
133. Le Bihan D, Mangin JF, Poupon C, et al. Diffusion tensor imaging: concepts and applications. J Magn Reson Imaging. 2001;13:534–46.
134. Kraus MF, Susmaras T, Caughlin BP, Walker CJ, Sweeney JA, Little DM. White matter integrity and cognition in chronic traumatic brain injury: a diffusion tensor imaging study. Brain. 2007;130:2508–19.
135. Song SK, Sun SW, Ju WK, Lin SJ, Cross AH, Neufeld AH. Diffusion tensor imaging detects and differentiates axon and myelin degeneration in mouse optic nerve after retinal ischemia. Neuroimage. 2003;20:1714–22.
136. Song SK, Sun SW, Ramsbottom MJ, Chang C, Russell J, Cross AH. Dysmyelination revealed through MRI as increased radial (but unchanged axial) diffusion of water. Neuroimage. 2002;17:1429–36.
137. Nitkunan A, Charlton RA, McIntyre DJ, Barrick TR, Howe FA, Markus HS. Diffusion tensor imaging and MR spectroscopy in hypertension and presumed cerebral small vessel disease. Magn Reson Med. 2008;59:528–34.
138. Maclullich AM, Ferguson KJ, Reid LM, et al. Higher systolic blood pressure is associated with increased water diffusivity in normal-appearing white matter. Stroke. 2009;40:3869–71.
139. de Groot M, Verhaaren BF, de Boer R, et al. Changes in normal-appearing white matter precede development of white matter lesions. Stroke. 2013;44:1037–42.
140. Gons RA, de Laat KF, van Norden AG, et al. Hypertension and cerebral diffusion tensor imaging in small vessel disease. Stroke. 2010;41:2801–6.
141. de Laat KF, van Norden AG, Gons RA, et al. Diffusion tensor imaging and gait in elderly persons with cerebral small vessel disease. Stroke. 2011;42:373–9.
142. van Norden AG, de Laat KF, van Dijk EJ, et al. Diffusion tensor imaging and cognition in cerebral small vessel disease: the RUN DMC study. Biochim Biophys Acta. 1822;2012:401–7.
143. Bokkers RP, Hernandez DA, Merino JG, et al. Whole-brain arterial spin labeling perfusion MRI in patients with acute stroke. Stroke. 2012;43:1290–4.

144. Alsop DC, Detre JA. Multisection cerebral blood flow MR imaging with continuous arterial spin labeling. Radiology. 1998;208:410–6.

145. Calamante F, Thomas DL, Pell GS, Wiersma J, Turner R. Measuring cerebral blood flow using magnetic resonance imaging techniques. J Cereb Blood Flow Metab. 1999;19:701–35.

146. Chalela JA, Alsop DC, Gonzalez-Atavales JB, Maldjian JA, Kasner SE, Detre JA. Magnetic resonance perfusion imaging in acute ischemic stroke using continuous arterial spin labeling. Stroke. 2000;31:680–7.

147. Hernandez DA, Bokkers RP, Mirasol RV, et al. Pseudocontinuous arterial spin labeling quantifies relative cerebral blood flow in acute stroke. Stroke. 2012;43:753–8.

148. Mirasol RV, Bokkers RP, Hernandez DA, et al. Assessing reperfusion with whole-brain arterial spin labeling: a noninvasive alternative to gadolinium. Stroke. 2014;45:456–61.

149. van Laar PJ, van der Grond J, Hendrikse J. Brain perfusion territory imaging: methods and clinical applications of selective arterial spin-labeling MR imaging. Radiology. 2008;246:354–64.

150. Derdeyn CP. Positron emission tomography imaging of cerebral ischemia. Neuroimaging Clin N Am. 2005;15:341–50. x-xi.

151. Jennings JR, Muldoon MF, Ryan C, et al. Reduced cerebral blood flow response and compensation among patients with untreated hypertension. Neurology. 2005;64:1358–65.

152. Jennings JR, Muldoon MF, Price J, Christie IC, Meltzer CC. Cerebrovascular support for cognitive processing in hypertensive patients is altered by blood pressure treatment. Hypertension. 2008;52:65–71.

153. Jennings JR, Muldoon MF, Whyte EM, Scanlon J, Price J, Meltzer CC. Brain imaging findings predict blood pressure response to pharmacological treatment. Hypertension. 2008;52:1113–9.

154. Fujishima M, Ibayashi S, Fujii K, Mori S. Cerebral blood flow and brain function in hypertension. Hypertens Res. 1995;18:111–7.

155. Efimova IY, Efimova NY, Triss SV, Lishmanov YB. Brain perfusion and cognitive function changes in hypertensive patients. Hypertens Res. 2008;31:673–8.

156. Graebe M, Pedersen SF, Borgwardt L, Hojgaard L, Sillesen H, Kjaer A. Molecular pathology in vulnerable carotid plaques: correlation with [18]-fluorodeoxyglucose positron emission tomography (FDG-PET). Eur J Vasc Endovasc Surg. 2009;37:714–21.

157. Rudd JH, Warburton EA, Fryer TD, et al. Imaging atherosclerotic plaque inflammation with [18F]-fluorodeoxyglucose positron emission tomography. Circulation. 2002;105:2708–11.

158. Tawakol A, Migrino RQ, Bashian GG, et al. In vivo 18F-fluorodeoxyglucose positron emission tomography imaging provides a noninvasive measure of carotid plaque inflammation in patients. J Am Coll Cardiol. 2006;48:1818–24.

159. Davies JR, Rudd JH, Fryer TD, et al. Identification of culprit lesions after transient ischemic attack by combined 18F fluorodeoxyglucose positron-emission tomography and high-resolution magnetic resonance imaging. Stroke. 2005;36:2642–7.

160. Graebe M, Pedersen SF, Hojgaard L, Kjaer A, Sillesen H. 18FDG PET and ultrasound echolucency in carotid artery plaques. JACC Cardiovasc Imaging. 2010;3:289–95.

161. Davies JR, Rudd JH, Weissberg PL. Molecular and metabolic imaging of atherosclerosis. J Nucl Med. 2004;45:1898–907.

162. van der Vaart MG, Meerwaldt R, Slart RH, van Dam GM, Tio RA, Zeebregts CJ. Application of PET/SPECT imaging in vascular disease. Eur J Vasc Endovasc Surg. 2008;35:507–13.

163. Powers WJ, Clarke WR, Grubb Jr RL, et al. Extracranial-intracranial bypass surgery for stroke prevention in hemodynamic cerebral ischemia: the Carotid Occlusion Surgery Study randomized trial. JAMA. 2011;306:1983–92.

164. Tawakol A, Fayad ZA, Mogg R, et al. Intensification of statin therapy results in a rapid reduction in atherosclerotic inflammation: results of a multicenter fluorodeoxyglucose-positron emission tomography/computed tomography feasibility study. J Am Coll Cardiol. 2013;62:909–17.

165. Wintermark M, Sesay M, Barbier E, et al. Comparative overview of brain perfusion imaging techniques. Stroke. 2005;36:e83–99.

166. Miletich RS. Positron emission tomography for neurologists. Neurol Clin. 2009;27:61–88. viii.

Index

A

ABPM. *See* Ambulatory blood pressure monitoring (ABPM)
ACE-inhibiting properties, 218
ACR. *See* Albumin/creatinine (ACR)
Action to Control Cardiovascular Risk in Diabetes (ACCORD), 53, 139, 268
Acute ischemic stroke
    antihypertensive agents, 158–159
    blood pressure after stroke, 154–158
    cerebral hypoperfusion, 151
    cerebrovascular pathophysiology, 153
    neurological deterioration, 152
    SBP, 152
Adult Treatment Panel III (ATP III), 133
Advanced glycosylation end products (AGEs), 267
Albumin/creatinine (ACR), 11
Aldosterone receptor antagonists (ARAs), 253, 254
Alpha-adrenergic blockers, 254
Alzheimer disease (AD)
    AD-related brain atrophy, 268
    amyloid-β, 267
    APOE ε4 genotype, 267
    cardiovascular factor, 261
    neuritic plaque, 261
    neuropathology, 262
    pathophysiologic mechanisms, 262
    plasma homocysteine levels, 267
    risk factors, 261
    stroke pathogenic mechanisms, 261
Ambulatory blood pressure monitoring (ABPM), 5, 137
    advantages, 237, 238

    cost-effectiveness, 237
    data collection center, 237
    diurnal blood pressure variability, monitoring, 237
Ambulatory systolic–diastolic pressure gradient index (ASDPRI), 237
American and International Societies of Hypertension (ASH/ISH), 136
American College of Cardiology (ACC), 133
American Heart Association (AHA), 133
American Stroke Association, 198
Amyloid precursor protein (APP), 265, 271
Angiotensin-converting enzyme (ACE), 218
Angiotensin-converting enzyme inhibitor (ACEIs), 215
    CHD, 52
    diuretic, 50
    dose–BP reduction, response curve, 250–251
    metabolic routes, 219
    perindopril, 251
    ramipril, 250
    side effects, 250, 255
Angiotensin I (AT1), 218
Angiotensin II (AT2), 218
Angiotensinogen (AG), 219
Angiotensin receptor blocker (ARB), 227, 251
    diuretic, 50
    primary/secondary stroke prevention, 53
Angiotensin-receptor blocker candesartan for treatment of acute stroke (SCAST), 154, 186
Antihypertensive agents, 158
    blood pressure reduction, 184–185, 190
    clevidipine, 190

© Springer International Publishing Switzerland 2016
V. Aiyagari, P.B. Gorelick (eds.), *Hypertension and Stroke*, Clinical Hypertension and Vascular Diseases, DOI 10.1007/978-3-319-29152-9

352   Index

Small vessel disease (SVD) (*cont.*)
    lacunar infarctions, 285
    microvascular fibrosis, 285
Small vessel ischemic disease, 236, 237
Small vessel occlusion
    antihypertensive therapy, 116
    fibrinoid necrosis, 114
    hyaline arteriosclerosis, 114, 115
    immunohistochemistry and electron
        microscopy, 114
    lacunar infarction, 114
    lipohyalinosis, 115, 116
Small-vessel disease (SVD), 303
Spontaneously hypertensive rats (SHRs)
    baroreceptor function, 69
    ROS levels, 71
    RVLM, 71
SSSI classification, 113
STAT Registry. *See* Studying the Treatment
        of Acute hyperTension (STAT)
        Registry
Stress cardiomyopathy (SCM), 208, 211
Stroke, 19, 22, 23
    and blood pressure, 18, 19, 22
    cardiovascular disease, 262
    without dementia, 263
    epidemiological observational studies, 19
    hemorrhagic, 17, 24, 27, 28
    and hypertension, risk factors
        aging, 19, 22
        racial differences, 22, 23
    ischemic, 17, 23–24
    mechanisms, 63
    and mortality, 266
    pathogenic mechanisms, 261
    prevention
        antihypertensive drugs, 40, 217
        blood pressure, 217, 226
        BP-lowering, 51, 53
        cerebrovascular disease, 219
        indapamide, 228
        meta-analyses, 216
        perindopril, 228
        placebo-controlled trials, 45
        vascular events and mortality, 225
    recurrence, 28, 30
Study on Cognition and Prognosis in the
        Elderly (SCOPE), 226, 265, 294
Studying the Treatment of Acute hyperTension
        (STAT) Registry, 164
Subarachnoid hemorrhage (SAH), 120–122
    blood pressure and augmentation, 197
    brain injury, 202

cerebral aneurysm, rupture of, 28
    DCI, 203, 205
    genetic disorders, 198
    observational studies, 27–28
    risk factors, 28, 29
    sympathomimetic drugs, 198
    symptoms, 198
    "thunderclap" headache, 198
    traumatic brain injury, 197
Subfornical organ (SFO)
    circulating angiotensin binds, 69
    CNS receptors, 69
    endogenous renin–angiotensin system, 69
SVD. *See* Small vessel disease (SVD)
Sympathetic nervous system (SNS)
    baroreceptors, 66
    cardiovascular homeostasis, 64
    essential hypertension, 64
    neurohumoral reflexes, 65
    RVLM, 64
    splanchnic nerve activity, 64
Systemic hypoperfusion, 116
Systolic blood pressure (SBP), 132
    aging, 30–31
    epidemiological studies, 18, 31
    intracranial aneurysm rupture, 28
    observational studies, 18
    recanalization, 157
    risk factors, 28
    stroke, risk of, 19–21
    thrombolysis, 157
    transdermal glyceryl trinitrate, 156
Systolic Hypertension in Elderly Prevention
        (SHEP), 265
Systolic Hypertension in Europe (Syst-Eur),
        264, 294
Systolic Hypertension in the Elderly Program
        (SHEP), 216–217, 250, 295

T
Takotsubo cardiomyopathy, 210
Three-City Study, 269
Thrombolytic therapy
    ICH, 157
    NINDS, 157
Traditional lacunar infarction, 113
Transient ischemic attack (TIA), 245
Triple-H therapy
    dilutional hyponatremia, 204
    hemodilution, 202
    HTN, 211
    vasospasm, 203

CPSIA information can be obtained
at www.ICGtesting.com
Printed in the USA
LVOW02*1358161216

517609LV00001B/5/P

9 783319 291505